Annals of the American Society for Adolescent Psychiatry

ADOLESCENT PSYCHIATRY

DEVELOPMENTAL AND CLINICAL STUDIES

VOLUME 21

Edited by

LOIS T. FLAHERTY

HARVEY A. HOROWITZ

THE ANALYTIC PRESS

1997   Hillsdale, NJ   London

Published by The Analytic Press, Inc.
101 West Street, Hillsdale, NJ 07642

ISBN: 0-88163-195-7
ISSN: 0-226-24064-9

Printed in the United States of America
10 9 8 7 6 5 4 3 2 1

DEDICATION

This volume of *Adolescent Psychiatry* is dedicated to Richard C. Marohn and Herman D. Staples, both of whom were associated with the American Society for Adolescent Psychiatry throughout their professional careers and each of whom is important to the Society in a unique way.

When Richard Marohn died in November 1995, he was in the midst of editing what was to have been his second volume of *Adolescent Psychiatry* as Editor-in-Chief. He had already assembled and edited much of the material for this volume. As interim editors, we picked up where he left off, adding some new papers and organizing the papers into sections. Our goal was to continue the long tradition of *Adolescent Psychiatry* as a reference work for clinicians, incorporating research, clinical case presentations, and theoretical discussions in ways that reflect the growth and evolution of the field.

Aaron H. Esman, a long-time senior editor of *Adolescent Psychiatry*, will be the next Editor-in-Chief. We are grateful to have had the opportunity to contribute to the continuity of this distinguished series and look forward to Dr. Esman's leadership.

CONTENTS

IN MEMORIAM
RICHARD C. MAROHN, M.D. (1934–1995)

To say that Richard Marohn was a towering figure in adolescent psychiatry is to describe his influence as well as his physical characteristics. In many ways he epitomized the founding spirit of ASAP; the energy, enthusiasm, and dedication to a cause that had been, by and large, neglected by society and mainstream psychiatry— the psychiatric treatment of severely disturbed adolescents.

Richard Marohn was born in Milwaukee, Wisconsin, an only child raised by devoted parents. He was educated entirely in Jesuit schools through medical school and, although in his adult life not associated with any formal religious institution, brought from this background the rigorousness of thought and devotion to his profession, which for him was truly a calling. He undertook psychoanalytic training at the Chicago Institute of Psychoanalysis and eventually became a teaching analyst at this renowned institution. A student of Heinz Kohut, he was one of the leading exponents of selfpsychology, and the perspectives of this theoretical base inform much of his writing.

Dick Marohn was a pioneer in psychiatric services for youth. In the 1970s he developed and directed an adolescent inpatient service in the Illinois State Psychiatric Institute. Like most public sector programs, this unit served youngsters who had failed other forms of treatment and whose behaviors were violent and severely delinquent.

Dick brought the insights of selfpsychology to bear on work with severely disturbed adolescents. At the same time, as he peered into the abyss of the soul of the adolescent murderer, he offered the hope that even adolescents whose moral and emotional development had been warped could be reached by sensitive and empathic therapy. In 1969, with his colleagues Daniel Offer, Eric Ostrov, and others, Dick began a project, "The Psychological World of the Juvenile Delinquent," that looked beyond the surface and described the deeper levels that underlay the psychological topography of these youngsters. The outcome of this fertile collaboration was a series of papers and monographs that are landmark contributions to the understanding of adolescents with severe behavioral and emotional disturbances. Throughout his career, Dick continued to write about what would now be described as conduct-disordered youth. He looked beyond the façades of their often contemptuous, defiant exteriors to see the stunted emotional growth that lay underneath. A great many of his papers were published in *Adolescent Psychiatry*, including his last one, "Failures in Psychotherapy," which appears in this volume. This paper is about the tragic suicide of one of his adolescent patients and the successful adaptation of another many years after what seemed to be an unproductive course of psychotherapy. This essay typifies his relentless self-scrutiny and intellectual courage, as well as his willingness to share his mistakes and thereby teach others.

Dick brought to his endeavors with professional organizations a sense of fun and enjoyment, together with a dedication to the mission to be completed, that made working with him on projects a most rewarding experience. Dick's contributions to ASAP were numerous. He served as head of the New Directions Task Force that gave rise to the American Board of Adolescent Psychiatry, and he was one of the Directors for the Board; he was President of ASAP in 1983–84; he received the Schonfeld Award in 1990. In the year before his death, he had become chair of the Group for the Advancement of Psychiatry's Committee on Adolescence and Editor of *Adolescent Psychiatry*, and those of us who had the privilege of working with him looked forward to many years of his leadership in both these endeavors. Instead, his demise from herpes encephalitis in November 1995 left us to carry on with only the guidance of his spirit. I have felt this spirit as a very real presence during the past year as I have undertaken the task of completing the work he began on Volume 21 of *Adolescent Psychiatry* and assuming the chairmanship of the GAP Committee on Adolescence. We will miss you, Dick, but we will have you with us in your writings and your influence on ASAP, which will continue to enrich the field.

Lois T. Flaherty

IN MEMORIAM

HERMAN D. STAPLES, M.D. (1918–1994)

Herman D. Staples, M.D. was a Founding Member, fourth President (1971–72), and Convention Manager extraordinaire of the American Society for Adolescent Psychiatry.

Born, raised, and educated in Philadelphia, Herm and Mary, his wife of 52 years and our Executive Secretary for 25 years, were in the process of moving to Nashville, Tennessee, to be closer to Laura, their daughter, and her family. But, in one of life's great ironies, Herm collapsed and died of a coronary as he walked away from settlement on the sale of their home. They were to leave for Nashville the following day. As it turned out, Herm was not in the process of leaving, he was in the process of staying; this was a man of attachments and of roots, of enduring relationships and an energetic, generous loyalty.

The most enduring of relationships was with Mary. Herm liked to tell the story of how they met in sixth grade, during the summer when both were in school in order to skip a grade. "But," Herm used to kid, "I had my eye on her since third grade."

Friends from that summer of 1930 on, their relationship deepened and matured through the Great Depression and the beginning of World War II. They were married in 1942, while Herm was a medical student at Hahnemann Medical College. He received his medical degree in 1943, completed an internship at Mount Sinai Hospital, and by January 1944 he was Captain Herman Staples, Medical Corps, United States Army.

World War II continued, and the Army had little need for help in pediatrics, which was Herm's first choice of specially. So he requested training in psychiatry and was sent to Columbia to prepare to treat the psychiatric casualties of war. He joined the war in the Pacific, in places far from South Philly, places like Saipan, Okinawa, and finally

Korea, where, in 1945, Herm was the first American medical officer to establish a field hospital. Family mythology has it that while sitting in his tent in Korea, cold wind and rain blowing through unsecured tent flaps, Herman Staples decided that his future travel accommodations would be first class. And those of us who traveled to meetings organized by Herm and stayed in hotels selected by Herm are forever grateful.

Herm was discharged from the Army in 1946 and returned to Philadelphia, took his general psychiatry training in the Veterans Administration Training Program, and served a child psychiatry fellowship at the Philadelphia Child Guidance Clinic from 1947 to 1949. It was during these years that Herm and Mary welcomed their children, Laura in 1947 and Lee in 1950.

The decade of the 50s was stimulating and exciting for Herm. He began his career in the private practice of adult and child psychiatry, directed the Lancaster (PA) Child Guidance Clinic, and began his training in psychoanalysis. Mary tells the story of finding out from Herm about his plans to begin a training analysis. Late one night in bed, Herm said, "Tomorrow I'm going to be on the analyst's couch." Herm Staples could be a very private man of few words.

It was also during the 1950s that Herm and a small group of child psychiatrists began to meet regularly to discuss the ideas of the child psychiatrist and psychoanalyst Margaret Mahler. Two Saturdays a month, they traveled to New York to meet in Dr. Mahler's apartment and presented cases and received supervision from her. Herm developed a mentoring relationship with Margaret Mahler that he considered his most vital professional tie, as well as a deeply nurturing and healing relationship. Many of us will remember the great respect and affection he expressed when he introduced Dr. Mahler and presented her the Schonfeld Award in 1983. Mary recalls how startled and then moved she was in Portugal in 1980 at the first organized meeting of the World Association for infant Psychiatry. Herm, having organized the meeting, was having cardiac symptoms, and friends insisted that he take bed rest, to which he very reluctantly acceded. Mary returned to their room to check on Herm to find Dr. Mahler at his bedside taking his pulse and attending to him.

It was also at the 1980 meeting in Portugal that Herm and Mary became friends with Erik Erikson. Professor Erikson, suffering from glaucoma, was having difficulty seeing and getting around. He had lost his eyedrops, and did not recall the name of his prescription, leaving him further incapacitated. Enter Herm whose father had had glaucoma and together they determined that he and Erikson had used the same eyedrops. Herm obtained the drops for Erikson, and the meeting went on successfully. Later, Herm and Mary visited Erik and Joan Erikson at their home in Tiburon, California. In 1990, Herm and I were planning ASAP's annual meeting to be held in New Orleans and were talking about the Schonfeld Award. I suggested the names of Erik and Joan Erikson to our planning committee. There was concern that the Eriksons, then in their mid-80s, were no longer available for awards and meetings, but, when I spoke with Joan and mentioned Herm and Mary, she was enthusiastic and moved at being honored. People rarely forgot the kindnesses they received from the Staples.

Herm Staples was midwife at the birth of most of the major organizations in our field. He was a Founding Member of the American Academy of Child Psychiatry (1953), the Association for Child Psychoanalysis (1965), the American Society for Adolescent Psychiatry (1967), the World Association for Infant Psychiatry (1980), and the International Society for Adolescent Psychiatry (1985). In an article written in 1994 for *Adolescent Psychiatry*. Herm wrote, "The entire history of adolescent psychiatry lies in this century, with most of it concentrated in the years since World War II. It is sobering to think that I was an eyewitness to a good deal of it " (Staples, 1995). This statement reveals Hermes characteristic understatement and humility, for he was far more than an eyewitness. He helped create this history with his enormous energy, commitment, and decency. And what's more, his generosity, considerateness, and good humor helped make the whole journey a grand, good time for the rest of us.

Harvey A. Horowitz

REFERENCES

Staples, H. D. (1995), Reflections on the history of adolescent psychiatry. *Adolescent Psychiatry,* 20:39-40. Hillsdale, NJ: The Analytic Press.

PART I

DEVELOPMENT AND PSYCHOPATHOLOGY

1   A HIERARCHICAL MODEL OF ADOLESCENT DEVELOPMENT: IMPLICATIONS FOR PSYCHOTHERAPY

CHARLES M. JAFFE

Psychotherapy with adolescents has long been recognized as particularly challenging because young people come for help with specific problems in adaptation while they are in the midst of rapid developmental change. The rapid fluctuation and the range of behaviors typical of the period can make diagnosis and treatment perplexing (A. Freud, 1958). It may be difficult to understand adolescents because their modes of expression are often action oriented and engender strong responses in those around them. In addition, adolescents are often elusive with therapists, making the ordinary dialogue through which people learn about one another difficult (Katz, 1990).

Following Aichhorn's (1925) precedent, effective adolescent psychotherapists have flexibly employed a variety of interventions. For many of us, however, the psychoanalytically based developmental theory of adolescence and the practice of adolescent psychotherapy are not congruent. Adolescent therapists have always known that you do whatever works. But, it often seems a stretch to find a theoretical rationale for the wide range of interventions we all make. At the very least, the list of interventions includes giving advice, providing information about sex and educational and vocational opportunities; exploring the possibilities and planning of new ideas and actions; making self-disclosures about our own feelings and life decisions; offering a set of values, and helping the adolescent to develop a realistic acceptance of strengths and limitations. Often, helpful interventions include going to high school plays and graduations and joining patients on wilderness challenges. Occasionally, we might even interpret unconscious conflict.

Descriptions of psychotherapeutic technique with adolescents which use psychoanalytic models have emphasized synthesis over analysis (Gitelson, 1948) or the provision of ego support over the expression of regressive wishes and conflict (Masterson, 1958; Meeks, 1971). Although flexibility and availability are always recommended to adolescent therapists, an integrated rationale for the full range of interventions has been lacking. The result is that many of us feel constricted if we force our understanding into a framework that seems inadequate to describe and treat the problems we encounter, or we feel alienated as we work pragmatically and flexibly but with a sense of operating outside of, or in opposition to, standard practice.

Despite the challenge, every clinician is faced with the task of making sense of patients' problems in order to form a plan to help, to develop a therapeutic relationship that allows for adequate interventions, and to assess the progress of psychotherapy. In other words, we are always asking, What is wrong and what can I do about it? This task requires a theory to organize what is observed—a psychology of adolescence that can explain expected occurrences in the normal course of development, and that can then be used to understand deviations from the norm and serve as a rational guide to our therapeutic interventions.

I will first review some major psychoanalytic paradigms within which adolescence has previously been conceptualized and then discuss the revisions that have altered these theories. I will then present what I believe to be a broad and useful framework for understanding adolescents that has emerged out of clinical experience, revisions of psychoanalytic theory, and developmental research. Since my purpose here is to present perspectives on the adolescent's psychological organization, the many social, cultural (Rakoff, 1989; Galatzer-Levy and Cohler, 1993) and biological influences—including organic disorders affecting learning (Silver, 1993), mood (Golombek and Garfinkel, 1983; Cantwell, 1992), and thought (Volkmar, 1994)—are not addressed directly, but are considered from the perspective of their meaning to the psychologically developing individual. Finally, I illustrate how this model influences a theory of psychotherapy of adolescents and provides a rational guide to interventions.

Overview of Adolescence

We are all familiar with the normative spectrum of adolescent behaviors that generally delineate the passage through early, middle, and late adolescence. There are significant alterations in all aspects of life as the child explores new sexual and social behavior, new relationships with family and friends, and new intellectual skills. We generally accept that adolescent development reflects the confluence of physical and cognitive maturation and the expectations of the individual adolescent, the family, and society within an historical context (Blos, 1962; Erikson, 1968; Rakoff, 1989).

The progressive changes in adolescent behavior are understood to be the manifest expression of the developing child's efforts to master challenges and to manage anxiety. Successful mastery is accomplished through the reorganization of typical patterns of experiencing oneself, others, and the world. The "products" of this reorganization are familiar as the shibboleths of adolescent development: identity, character, mature super-ego and ego-ideal. Autonomy, individuation, and independence derive from these structural changes.

There is general agreement that the transformations of adolescence are influenced by prior development, that reorganization presents the opportunity for new growth through recapitulation of earlier experience in the light of new abilities, and that the transformations are molded by available avenues of expression. The progress toward mastery is monitored by reference to comfort with one's own body, the quality of relationships (with friends, family, and lovers), educational and later vocational vitality and direction, and the ability to plan flexibly and responsibly view one's life in the context of a generally optimistic and realistic attitude toward oneself and others. Because the achievement of self-maintenance and satisfying sexual, interpersonal, and vocational functioning is considered by adolescents and adults to be important to a productive and satisfying life, these are usually referred to as "the developmental tasks of adolescence."

Psychoanalytic Theories of Adolescence

Beyond this generic agreement, there really is no psychoanalytic theory of adolescence. Explanations for the psychological transformations in adolescence have always been based on some general theoretical orientation of mental organization, development, and psychopathology. Each orientation has its own assumptions about the basic motivation for the actions that organize psychological development and functioning (Greenberg and Mitchell, 1983). As a result, psychoanalytic theories of drive, ego, separation-individuation, social interaction, and the development of the self make different contributions to the definition, the process of psychological transformation, and the expected outcome of adolescence.

For example, theories that follow Freud's emphasis on the biphasic nature of sexual development, with instinctual discharge as the primary motivator for action, view adolescence primarily as the necessary revision of childhood sexuality in response to puberty (Blos, 1962, 1967, 1968, 1979). Independence, identity, intimacy, and realistic productivity reflect the successful reengagement of oedipal and preoedipal conflict so that the mature expression of sexual impulses is assured. Adolescence describes the process through which the child resolves restimulated preoedipal and oedipal conflicts and consolidates a stable character structure through the transformation of instinct, ego, superego, and ego ideal. The outcome of development depends on the child's ego strength, the strength of the instincts, and the adequacy of the child's defenses.

Other psychoanalytic theories emphasize the primary motive of object relations. Development and pathology are functions of the vicissitudes of their internal representations. In object relations theory, adolescence is the response to a normative thrust toward autonomy. The adolescent's task is to achieve autonomy with stable internal self- and object representations, intact reality testing, and secure ego boundaries. Disengagement from primary love objects recapitulates the separation-individuation phase of early childhood (Masterson, 1972). Psychopathology occurs in adolescence because the child is without the requisite internal structures to master the second individuation process.

Yet another theory, self psychology, views self-cohesion as the primary motive for action and development. Self psychology emphasizes the importance of empathic persons who are capable of fostering the selfobject experiences necessary to form and maintain a cohesive self (Kohut, 1971, 1977, 1984). In this view, adolescence is not a reaction to puberty; rather "the essential requirement for its occurrence seems to be the emergence of an inner necessity for new ideals, accompanied by opportunities encountered for such a transformation of the self" (Wolf, Gedo, and Terman, 1972, p. 269; Wolf, 1980, 1982; Kohut, 1972). The adolescent transformation involves a phase-appropriate deidealization of parental standards, resulting in disrupted self-cohesion that the adolescent regulates through selfobject experiences with peers, and culminating in restored self-cohesion through a transformation of the self. Satisfying sexual expression and, indeed, self-assertions in relationships and tasks of all kinds reflect stable selfobject experiences. Pathology occurs if empathic failures in childhood result in the persistence of an archaic idealizing and grandiose self that continues to seek satisfying selfobjects relations (Marohn, 1977).

In summary, each theory emphasizes some aspect of adolescence, and together they provide a sense of the rich adolescent process. Problems arise, however, when one looks more carefully at the individual theories or attempts to integrate them.

Influences of Revisions in Psychoanalytic Theory On Approaches to Adolescence

In the past few years extensive attention has been devoted to clarifying the psychoanalytic theory of motivation and development and to providing a useful theory of therapy. Psychoanalytic theory has been influenced reciprocally by investigations of motivation, theory formation, new discoveries in clinical process and technique, and observational research. These have been usefully applied to understanding and treating adolescents.

For example, Freud's method of theory formation has been vigorously criticized and his basic assumptions about thought and motivation examined and revised (Peterfreund, 1971; Basch, 1973; G. Klein, 1976; Schafer, 1976). Freud's assumption that motivation is based on sexual and aggressive instincts that drive a closed system mental apparatus with the aim of tension discharge has been convincingly replaced by the more useful concept of motivation as the search for order mediated by affective communication (Basch, 1976). Motivation and development are more usefully understood to proceed from the fact that the brain integrates information rather than from a need to insure instinctual discharge and to avoid danger. Consistent with this view, child observation studies have demonstrated that infants enter the world as information-processing and organizing individuals very responsive to the environment (Lichtenberg, 1983, 1989; Stern, 1985) and with a propensity for organizing behavior and internal representations in concert with other people (Sameroff and Emde, 1989).

In addition to the motivational theory of instinct, Freud's assumption that infants' thinking includes symbols in much the same way that

7

adults use words has been replaced by our knowledge that infants do not think like adults, but go through a progression of cognitive changes involving the increasingly complex use and manipulation of symbols (Piaget and Inhelder, 1969). Freud thought that the fantasies he had recovered through dreams and parapraxes represented the earliest form of thought—the primary process. In fact, he recovered complex symbolic transformations of experience. These revisions of the basic assumptions about human thought and motivation significantly affect any theory of development, defenses, and psychopathology.

The theory of adolescence has also been influenced by discoveries from the clinical process. Observations of transference, countertransference and necessary alterations in technique have broadened our understanding of factors that affect therapeutic change (Eissler, 1953; Racker, 1968; Tansey and Burke, 1989). For many patients, transference issues seemed directed to the patient–therapist relationship and could not be profitably managed solely by interpretation of defense, resistance, or conflict. For these patients, progress in treatment seemed more connected to the stabilizing effects of the relationship than to insight into repressed wishes. From a theoretical standpoint, this emphasis on the patient–therapist relationship in therapeutic change encouraged clinicians to look for an explanation for these phenomena in that period of life involving the emergence of a self-sufficient individual from the nutritious or deficient soil of the dyadic relationship in infancy. Clinicians were encouraged to view these phenomena as renewed developmental striving and not simply as resistance (Kohut, 1984).

The resulting shift in focus to the subjective experience of the individual striving for wholeness through relationships rather than defending against impulses (Goldberg, 1978) has been especially salutary for understanding adolescents' need for guidance, for genuine affective responses, and for help in forming a realistic assessment of themselves and others. It gives a theoretical underpinning for the range of interventions necessary for work with adolescent patients.

A Revised Conceptualization of the Adolescent Process

These cumulative revisions have produced an encompassing, rational model of development, pathology, and intervention that is usefully applied to the psychotherapy of adolescents. The model I review here represents an amalgamation. Although the model joins elements born of clinical experience and developmental research, I believe that the grounding of the clinical models in sound developmental principles permits their combination.[1] These common principles include several factors. First, development throughout life relates to the ordering of internal and external stimulation mediated through affective communication. Second, development proceeds in a dialectic between child and caretakers that may be described in terms of feedforward and feedback cycles that include assimilation, accommodation, identification of invariants, and associational learning. Third, the epigenetic principle encompasses development. Specifically, increasingly complex organizations of internal models of oneself, the world, and patterns of interaction occur throughout development, each affecting the next. These increasingly complex organizations comprise constellations of affect, cognition, and behavioral integration, subjectively experienced in domains of self. Although organizations seem to appear in some predictable sequence determined by biobehavioral shifts during infancy and early childhood, once in place they co-exist and are transformed throughout life. And, fourth, psychopathology is related to problems integrating affectively meaningful information and the consequences of that behavior on subsequent adaptations.

Integration of Information: Motivation and the Cycle of Competence

The basis for the developmental theory is that motivation is based on the brain's function of organizing information in the service of adaptation, a process that Basch (1988) refers to as the self system: "a collective term encompassing the hierarchy of neurologically encoded, goal-directed feedback cycles whose activity constitutes character and governs behavior" (p. 106). Inborn constellations of behavior become motives because they generate and organize affect that guides behavior, that is, in the process of "minding" (Basch, 1976; Lichtenberg, 1989).

---

[1]Such assertions inevitably raise questions. In making the arguments in this essay, I am endorsing the view that psychoanalytic views of development, pathology, and interventions need to be considered within the context of related fields. Earlier I have considered some of the issues involved with integrating data derived from empirical research and clinical methods for the purpose of theory formation (Jaffe and Barglow, 1989; Jaffe, 1994) and conducting treatment (Jaffe and Ryan, 1993).

In this view, the organizing principle of development may be understood as the achievement of competent functioning, or what C. Daly King (1945) called "function in accordance with design" (p. 493). In the most generic sense, development proceeds through the affectively mediated integration of increasingly complex information, allowed by cognitive maturation, in the context of a more or less supportive environment, which results in increasingly complex behavioral organizations subjectively experienced.

From birth there is an error-correcting feedback cycle between caretakers and infants whereby the infant learns (Basch, 1988; Zeanah et al., 1989). Information from internal and environmental sources is received, amplified, and communicated through an inborn system of affects, such as startle, interest, anger, pleasure, distress, disgust, and fear (Tomkins, 1962). This affective tone of communication determines the meaning of the experience and thus influences later motivation for actions (Basch, 1976; Stern, 1985).

These very early interactions, which combine learning in a particular affective tone, become the patterns of expectation with which new information is met and that determine how new information will be understood and what response will occur. Whenever the child encounters something new, it attempts to make a match with something already known in order to feel a continuous sense of integration and be able to muster an effective response (Stern, 1985; Zeanah, 1989). If there is a match, the infant experiences a sense of competence (Basch, 1988). When there is a mismatch, the infant will continue to try responses until a match can be made but will eventually employ available strategies to preserve a subjective sense of competence through selective attention (Basch, 1983a; Jaffe, 1988). If all goes well, the infant is able to elicit predictable responses that can be integrated subjectively as self-experiences (Stern, 1985; Sameroff and Emde, 1989).

This general cycle of interaction, for which Basch has coined the term the "cycle of competence," may be envisioned as a helical unfolding of a reciprocal process over time of meaning, decision, behavior, feedback, and assessment of competence (experienced eventually as self-esteem).

The cycle of competence occurs in the context of a number of factors. A full review and integration is beyond the present scope, although we can get a flavor for the richness of human experience by looking at each of these components: 1) functional-motivational systems, 2) other people, 3) cognitive maturation, 4) self-organization, and 5) domains of self.

Functional-Motivational Systems

First, overall competent functioning may be assessed within a number of functional-motivational systems (Lichtenberg, 1989). Motivational systems begin as biological propensities and are experienced over time as subjective aims within the child's evolving inner world because they organize experience. Drawing on accumulated research and clinical observations, Lichtenberg suggests that development may be assessed within five motivational systems: that based on the regulation of physiological requirements; attachment-affiliation; aversion; exploration; and sensual/sexual stimulation. Throughout life these systems are operant, taking shape commensurate with cognitive ability, personal meanings, and age appropriate concerns. They combine in kaleidoscopic fashion, resulting in shifts in emphasis at various times. Although this classification is certainly open to revision, it captures the critical idea that no single motivational system can account for overall adaptation. Various behaviors—such as regulation of eating, sleeping, and elimination; communication, emotional sharing, guidance seeking and giving; efficacy pleasures in engaging novel opportunities; and sensual stimulation seeking—all deserve to be assessed on their own merits as well as by each being viewed as it either facilitates or inhibits the others as they are transformed over a lifetime.

Other People

The caretakers who provide phase-appropriate stimulation and responses in each motivational system provide an influential context for development. The earliest periods of development involving basic regulation, reciprocal exchange, initiative, focalization, self-assertion, and recognition and continuity (as reviewed by Sroufe, 1989) and culminate in memories of patterns of experience are all intimately related to caretaker responsiveness. Throughout these stages and those over the subsequent four or five years, the child's ability to experience competence remains dependent on the responses of caretakers. To maintain integration while remaining open to new information, the child utilizes the affectively attuned responses of supportive and encouraging caretakers. The child's internal experience of those relationships that help to maintain the integrity of self-functioning are termed kinship, mirroring and idealizing selfobject experiences (Basch, 1988).

I should note that this is a somewhat different definition of selfobjects than Kohut's. Kohut's view was that sustaining self-cohesion through selfobject ties is a primary motive for development. In my current usage selfobject experiences—internal experiences of supportive and guiding relationships—enhance overall integration. Certainly people need and seek such relationships with varying intensity throughout life, but that does not elevate them to the status of a supraordinate organizing principle of mental life.[2] I will return to this point later, as it plays an important role in my discussion of empathy in psychotherapy.

A variety of circumstances may be associated with problems in establishing the affective attunement necessary for a child to recruit adequate selfobject experiences. In an erratic environment or one lacking adequate stimulation, the infant cannot develop the clear patterns of expectation and response that lead to competence and self-stability. There may also be problems when the infant is unable to process ordinary communications as a result of some neurologic deficit (Palombo, 1979; Rothstein et al., 1988; Silver, 1992) or from differences in temperament between the infant and its parents (Chess and Thomas, 1987).

Perhaps more common is a problem that arises when aspects of the infant–caretaker interaction are so idiosyncratic that they are not usable in a more general context. In such circumstances, a moment that offers the potential for greater integration becomes instead a destabilizing threat to the relationship with the caretaker and reinforces a continued need to remain within the context of the original situation in order to maintain competence and self-esteem. In a moment of self-assertion, the child is forced to ignore what is felt naturally and substitute a

---

[2]Considerations of adolescent phenomena by some Self Psychologists do place self cohesion through selfobject ties as the primary organizer of development (Lage and Nathan, 1991; Palombo, 1988, 1990). While I agree with the phenomenology presented by these authors, and with the importance of selfobject experiences in development and in the therapeutic process, I do not subscribe to the implication that one can construct a general psychology of normal development from concepts derived within the clinical situation.

different person's response. The child, rather than having new information and explorations meet with affirmation, finds it impossible to integrate new experiences either because the skills for managing the new experience have not been taught or because to engage the new experience would threaten a needed mode of organizing one's self (Gedo, 1988). In the future, when similar circumstances arise, they are experienced as disruptive because they are humiliating or threaten the loss of integration once again.

Cognitive Maturation

In the normal course of events, we are in the process of continuous selective attention to information depending on its personal relevance (Basch, 1983a; Jaffe, 1988). We sleep through the sound of fire engines unless we also smell smoke. This normal process is used in the service of defense when overall integration is threatened. At such a moment, a person may use a variety of means to exclude affectively meaningful, motivating information because it stimulates anxiety. In short, cognitive ability serves the purpose of both normal (i.e., typical for a period of development) and pathological (i.e., fixed and repetitive at the price of continued development) defense. The earliest mode of protection is withdrawal. Later, in the period of preoperational thought the child may maintain integration by ignoring the affective significance of incompatible information or aims through disavowal. With the advent of concrete operations in cognitive functioning, the child now has a more realistic understanding of caretakers and protects itself by excluding affectively significant information from conscious awareness (Basch, 1977). In other words, the child can use repression to reconcile conflicting interests and preserve self-competence. The particular defense employed to protect the child's functioning thus relates to child's cognitive abilities and the stability of self-cohesion during the period when problematic experiences were encountered.

Self-Organization

Over time, affect and cognitive maturation within each motivational system in a particular environmental matrix results in a typical epigenetic hierarchy of overall behavioral integrations that Gedo (1979, 1988) terms the self-organization. Gedo classifies the hierarchy of self-organization as tension regulation, coordination of aims, tolerance for reality over illusion, and appropriate avenues of expressing desire. Self-organization is based on the premise that in the earliest months of life biobehavioral aims become organized into a "primary identity," or internal patterns of behavior and expectation that are evident throughout life and are repeated to preserve self-integration. This is the compulsion to repeat. Aspects of self-organization may or may not be subjectively or symbolically represented.

This classification is useful for understanding states of behavioral function and dysfunction. Terms that we ordinarily associate with different motivational theories may be understood as useful descriptions of behaviors that signify various self-organizations. For example, when the period of problems relates to the earliest development of tension regulation and a self fluctuating in the ability to maintain a coherent set of goals, the issues of splitting, projective identification, separation, and abandonment may apply. If the problems occur later, when the child is better able to maintain overall integration and competence but is still in need of caretaker support to maintain integrated functioning, then narcissistic vulnerability and relationships marked by disavowal, grandiosity, or idealizations may dominate the clinical picture. Still later, usually when the child has progressed to being able to use more complex manipulations of symbols and when issues of sexuality and competition have emerged in a more reliably intact self, reaction formations, displacements, and repression of unacceptable wishes may dominate the clinical picture.

An important aspect of Gedo's theory is the fluidity of self-organization. Much as in Lichtenberg's motivational systems, in Gedo's view all states of self-organization exist at all times (though the prominence of one or another shifts). It is the limitations resulting from foreclosure of any of these adaptive achievements that results in psychopathology. In other words, although thoughts and wishes are not pathogenic, patterns of organization may be.

For example, we can all recall times when we attempted a task that was important and that made us anxious. In such situations it is not unusual to have a moment of disorientation when considering how to approach the task, or some anticipation of shame at the idea of failure. To compensate for these feelings, we might find ourselves either denigrating the task or being critical of the person who put us in the position of having to perform in the first place. Quickly these thoughts and feelings pass, and our perspective returns, usually as soon as we focus on the task at hand. This process is, in itself, totally mundane. To organize a life around one aspect of this sequence would, however, be pathological. As Gedo (1988) states, "The subject matter of human thought is never pathological—only the manner in which it is processed may be maladaptive" (p, 8).

Before proceeding, and for purposes of clarification, I should note here that self-organization is defined in terms of behavioral organizations and is not subjectively experienced. It is distinct from "senses of self" (Stern, 1985), which can be understood as the subjective experience of one's state of integration, one's "self" (Basch, 1988), which connotes a subjectively whole person who triggers error-correcting behaviors when integration is disrupted; and "self-esteem," which connotes a person's overall verbalizable assessment of his or her performance in integration and adaptation.

Domains of Self-relatedness

From a different vantage point, we can say that a child's holistic experience of affect, cognition, the interactional matrix, synthesized in a behavioral or self-organization, may be classified in an epigenetic unfolding of senses of self. In essence, although abilities, thought, and patterns of action change throughout life, we experience ourselves subjectively as a continuous whole from start to finish. Stern (1985) suggests a hierarchy of subjective experiences, which he classifies as the emergent, core, subjective, verbal, and narrative self. The emergent self concerns the infant's experience of the process of the emerging organization of the basic rhythms of life. The emerging self involves amodal (cross-modal) perception (translation of stimulation between sensory modalities), physiognomic perception (translation of stimulation into a category of affect), and "vitality affects" (qualities of feeling in dynamic terms). The core self involves a sense of one's self as stable while other things change. Embodied in the core self are self-agency (a sense of authorship and control over self-generated action, expecting consequences of action), self-coherence (a physical whole with boundaries), self-affectivity (experiencing related patterns of affect), and self-history (a sense of continuity). The subjective self and domain of intersubjective relatedness involve the recognition that one's own experiences are shareable. Affect attunement plays a crucial role in the preverbal sharing of joint attention, intention, and affective states. The verbal self involves self-reflection, the capacity for symbolic action, and the acquisition of language. An important aspect of the development of language is that, while it opens new avenues for relatedness, it also makes aspects of experience less shareable; there is a division between life as lived and life as it is verbally represented. The narrative self discusses one's internal world with others, possibly leading to revisions or confirmation of one's private world. As with self-organization, each sense of self emerges in sequence but, once established, continues as a domain of self-relatedness throughout life.

Adolescence

This integrative approach may be extended into adolescence. Within a model that views development as the progressive integration of increasingly complex information allowed by cognitive maturation within the context of an empathic environment, adolescence is a period of necessary change to accommodate greater complexity. Between the second and third decades of life the young person is challenged to integrate a number of occurrences within the self system in which motivational systems, self-organization, and domains of self all come into play.

The process of adolescence may be considered in terms of the shifting equilibrium of the self system, that is, in terms of the developing child's ability to remain open to new affect-laden information. The young person's need and desire to meet the tasks of adolescence results in a period of self-disorganization that necessitates the use of stabilizing experiences. The adolescent's ability to maintain overall integration and competence and to use selfobjects during the time of transition determines how this period of transformation is negotiated. Teachers, friends, rock stars, literary figures, and a variety of other persons and activities may serve a mirroring or idealizing function, eroticized or not, in the service of maintaining and revising self-functioning.

The emphasis on adolescence as a major reorganization of the self system in the service of maintaining competence helps organize the various definitions of adolescence as a biological, psychological, cognitive, and social phenomenon within a subjective perspective rather than one of external observation. Thus, adolescence is defined not by any of the component phenomena of the period but, rather, by the meaning of the changes to the young person (Gedo, 1979). Such a conceptualization of adolescence, which separates the physical from the psychological transformations during the second decade of life is consistent with the clinical finding that some postpubertal people remain psychologically frozen in latency (Gedo, 1979) and with the historical perspective that adolescence as we know it is a recent historical phenomenon (Rakoff, 1989).

To elaborate, a number of motivational systems maintain continuity with early development but are significantly and actively altered during adolescence. These include psychological regulation (e.g., diet, exercise, sleep), exploration (e.g., creative play and work), attachment-affiliation (e.g., friendships and integration in the social world), and sexual and sensual stimulation involving affectively charged behaviors (e.g., sex, drugs, and rock 'n roll). The need to develop new skills in adolescence with respect to physiologic regulation, attachments and affiliations with family, groups, and value systems; explorations in school and vocation; and sexuality requires expanding the range of the cohesive self. Problems remaining from childhood in these areas may be advantageously revised during the adolescent process because self-organization and domains of self are formed in childhood, providing the adolescent with abilities not available in early life but within which continuing issues may be reworded (Lichtenberg, 1982, 1989).

Tension regulation, organizing oneself according to a coherent plan, placing reality over illusion, and exploring appropriate avenues to channel desires are particularly related to master of the tasks of adolescence. Problems in any area of behavioral organization, results in maladaptive behavior. The same may be said of the adolescent's domains of self. With life's increasing complexity, new demands are made on perceptions and affects; new contingencies are presented for effective actions; a more complex intersubjective experience occurs; and there is a need to further weave one's personal narrative within a larger lifespan viewpoint. If the necessary revisions in any of these areas is blocked because new challenges threaten to disrupt a cohesive self, problems in adaptation may ensue.

The adolescent's task of developing a stable sexual identity and satisfying sexual relationships illustrates the confluence of these issues. Competence in sexual behavior requires the integration of multiple motivational systems, especially exploration and attachment-affiliation in addition to the sexual/sensual. In order to develop a relationship and then perform sexually within it, one must first tolerate the stimulus intensity and associate it with pleasure. Emergent self-processes of amodal and physiognomic perception, as well as vitality affects, all play a role. Next, one must be able to organize coherent action toward a goal of satisfaction and have the expectation of being effective and affirmed. Involved are core self-experiences of a sense of authorship and volition in one's actions and feelings and an expectation ofpredictable contingent responses to them. Also involved are experiences of shared affects, intentions, and attention relevant to the domain of the subjective self. Finally, an adolescent has to find an appropriate partner for the sexual experience and appreciate sex without illusion. That is, sex may satisfy physiologic urgencies and bring about a temporary feeling of warmth and security, but it is not a whole life. In particular, it will not in itself assure the positive self-esteem that reflects overall competent functioning by substituting for all motivational systems and self domains. Perhaps the most complex culmination of the sexual experience is the self-reflection that integrates the meaning of sexual behavior in the context one's overall self-concept and verbal communication with partners about one's own private world, issues related to the domains of the verbal and narrative self.

Implications for a Theory of Psychotherapy

GENERAL IMPLICATIONS

Having reviewed this revised model of adolescence, I now want to address some issues related to psychotherapy. I believe that we can approach treating adolescents through understanding them within this broad-based framework of normal development. In addition, the model provides rational guidance for employing a variety of creative and flexible interventions used by adolescent psychotherapists. I am not suggesting new interventions, but rather an organizing theory for their use.

Let me set the stage with two short vignettes.[3]

First, Toni. Toni was a 14-year-old ninth grader. At the insistence of her mother she came to see me to talk about "feeling like killing herself." Toni had performed reasonably well in school until seventh grade, but since then her grades were failing. During the same period she gained and then lost a lot of weight, started cutting classes,

---

[3]The clinical vignettes are composites.

smoked pot, and became promiscuous, which resulted in a pregnancy and an abortion. Her mother said she had become viciously oppositional and saw any input as a violation of her rights. When I talked with Toni, she became enraged and took everything I said as deeply assaultive and a show of misunderstanding and a lack of confidence. Her attitude was, "If my mother left me alone everything would be fine." She considered herself to be more open minded and understanding, and generally a better person, than her mother. Toni's mother said that she had tried everything to change Toni, from absolute laissez-faire to frequent confrontation and limit setting, all to no avail.

Toni's parents were divorced. Her father was an alcoholic who left home when Toni was five. She still saw him and even lived with him for periods of time. Mother was deeply attached to Toni but often felt that her own life was such a struggle that she did not have the energy to deal with her child.

I saw Toni for a short time to see if she would respond to my attempts to engage her in treatment. I also wanted to see if mother could be helped to respond usefully to Toni. My efforts were to no avail. Toni continued her oppositional and sexual behavior in dangerous and self-destructive ways and often lied to evade confrontation. I recommended hospitalization for her. The process took some time, however, because, despite mother's frequent emergency calls about Toni's behavior and complaints that she was not responding fast enough, mother opposed more rigorous interventions by minimizing the severity of the problems with Toni and within the family.

The second story is about Dan, an 18-year-old freshman in college who called me during his Christmas vacation. He said he wasn't sure if he could go back to school and was feeling panicky about it. He had started out all right but then couldn't concentrate and failed a course. He wasn't interested in his friends or sports and felt angry and tearful most of the time. He always had been able to handle things on his own and was scared by his inability to get ahold of himself. The immediate reason for calling was that he had begun to have thoughts of killing himself.

Dan's background was strikingly similar to Toni's. His parents divorced in his early childhood, and his father, too, was an alcoholic with whom Dan lived at times. Like Toni's, Dan's mother felt deeply attached to her child but often was herself overwhelmed.

As Dan told his story, it emerged that last summer he discovered that his father had cancer. His father was very secretive about it and would not discuss it with Dan. They began to have fights—what would start as an intellectual debate would escalate into a big fight. Dan felt that his father did not appreciate his intellect and refused to see his point of view. He felt morally and intellectually superior to his father.

What emerged was that Dan felt he was losing his father just when he needed his dad to help him feel confident about leaving his parents and going out into the world. Specifically, Dan wanted his father to share his experience of growing up by telling Dan of his own experiences starting out on his own. He also felt enraged that his father was treating him as if he could not empathize with his father's experience of his illness; yet he felt guilty and ashamed of his selfishness and explosive behavior.

Over about five visits, my acknowledgment that Dan had a legitimate developmental need and that his rage was in response to his feeling afraid and cheated, not because he was selfish (as he had accused himself of being), relieved his suicidal ideation, calmed his explosive behavior, and enabled him to talk more productively with his father and to return to school with the plan to seek continued help in sorting out his feelings about his needs and his father's.

Two youngsters, similar backgrounds, very different courses of treatment. How can we be guided rationally toward intervention?

Psychotherapy seeks to help remove obstacles to competent functioning through empathic immersion in the patient's subjective experience. The goal of psychotherapeutic intervention with adolescents is to enable them to experience competence by helping them to regulate, organize, integrate, and articulate an increasingly complex life. The fulcrum for change is the establishment of a relationship wherein the patient can use the therapist to enable self-stability by recruiting appropriate selfobject experiences during the therapeutic process. The avenue for relationship formation is empathy.

Resistance in psychotherapy and regression in adaptation are viewed as manifestations of the patient's inability to use selfobjects productively because experiences in the therapy revive previously problematic efforts at overall integration. A number of symptoms and phenomena of the adolescent period may be reexamined in the light of the idea that failures to adapt to new affect-laden information represent the inability to match the information with preexisting expectations and thus result in increased anxiety and confusion. In other words, they may be understood as the manifestations of attempts to preserve a failing self-organization (Gedo, 1979). The particular symptom reflects the degree to which the self is disorganized and the self-concept is concretized or experienced as a physical sensation. General symptoms, such as lethargy, emptiness, and periods of hopelessness, may be the manifestations of fluctuating self-organization. Obsessional concerns represent a heightened self-aware-ness. The adolescent may obsess about alternatives (doubting) but still have a self-concept as one who remains able to select between various alternatives. Or the very ability to be a problem solver may come into question with a preoccupation with the mechanics of mental functions. Hypochondriasis represents a self-experience at the level of actual body functioning with loss of the symbolizing capacity and a return to operating in a sensorimotor mode.

The clinical emphasis here is on the level of self-organization and domain of self-relatedness as expressed within motivational systems. Some adolescents may manifest the earliest sensorimotor patterns in addictions, or they may become hypochondriacal or obsessional. Other adolescents, with more resilient self-cohesion, may experience revived incestuous wishes primarily and may act in the service of keeping these from consciousness. Consistent with Daniel Offer's (Offer and Offer, 1975) continuous growth group, some adolescents may even be able to continue to make use of their own parents during the transformation. Failure to find any avenue for self-maintenance may result in major depression or suicide (Basch, 1975).

IMPLICATIONS FOR RECONSTRUCTIONS OF PAST EXPERIENCE

In psychotherapy we attempt to understand our patient's motives. Although most often psychotherapy with adolescents does not involve the sustained analysis of transference that leads to a shared conviction about the antecedents of current dysfunction (Peterfreund, 1983), we nevertheless make assumptions about motivation and believe that current maladaptation has developmental roots. Viewing a patient's past is often like looking at the bottom of a pool through rippling, muddy water—some things may show through to the surface, but intervening distortions make accurate identification of what is there and where it is located highly speculative. What emphasis does this model place on the value of reconstruction of past experiences in the service of therapeutic change? What connection can we make between current and past dysfunction in various areas?

Clinically, it appears that the particular methods for preservation of competence and self-esteem that first appeared in a particular developmental phase may be subsequently employed to manage disruptions relevant to any problem with self-integrity, not simply problems relevant to that developmental phase. Disavowal, although arising in the preoperational phase, may be employed to manage disruptions in any previous or subsequent phase of development (Jaffe, 1988). For example, in practice we see patients in whom disavowal covers repression, and repression covers disavowal (Basch, 1983a). This differs from the view that particular constellations of defenses or enactments are associated with points of fixation.

Lichtenberg (1989) makes a similar point in discussing the interwoven relationship of motivational systems. A full review is beyond our scope here, but a few examples should suffice. First, "each group of patterns constituting one motivational system has an effect on motives derived from other motivational systems" (p. 8). The effect may be facilitating (eating affects physiologic regulation, enhances attachment motives, and stimulates the senses) or inhibiting (in playing with a spoon, eating competes with exploring and may disrupt smooth interaction with a caretaker). Also, although all motivational systems are present at each stage in life, they are not in themselves determinants of the overall mode of organization in any phase. In infancy all motivational systems are in play, but it appears that the dominant issue is "change in state and its relationship to regulation by caregivers" (p. 10). In adolescence, however, the overall mode of organization is characterized by each motivational system taking center stage in turn (p. 10). In addition, at any moment, one motivational system may predominate and appear to explain the whole system. This is similar to the situation where proponents of drive, attachment and object relations, or self psychology assert that their system encompasses the others. Lichtenberg argues that it is a property of motivational systems that they each relate to a core function, but that, within that core, subsidiary functions relating to the other systems are served. Each system, then, has a holistic appearance. We have all had the clinical experience of listening to a patient and suddenly being certain that all his or her pathology is understandable within the context of oedipal conflict, or the vicissitudes of early object relations, or some character distortions secondary to chronic panic disorder or neurologic deficit. Of course, this may be a countertransference commitment to some theoretical stance, but it may also be one system presenting in relief.

Similar issues arise in self-experiences. Stern (1985) argues that whether we view the origin of pathology in abandonment, empathic failures, or pathologic defenses is more a function of which domain of self-experience we address—in this example core relatedness, intersubjective relatedness, or verbal relatedness—than of any direct tie to the past (pp. 264–266). Furthermore, although he considers each phase of self-formation as a "sensitive period" that casts a shadow over further development, he cautions against using a domain of self-relatedness as a route to reconstruction, because all senses of self are seen as actively evolving throughout life, making the idea of "fixation" less useful.

The same principle applies to self-organization. In any treatment, any patient, no matter how well integrated under optimal circumstances, shifts between modes of integration (Gedo and Goldberg, 1973; Gedo, 1988). What distinguishes one patient from others is the most persistent mode of organization, not defense or history.

What does this mean for the clinician struggling to integrate current and past motives? In terms of defenses as well as clinical diagnoses, the conventional view that current symptoms reflect specific derailments in development (the fixation-regression hypothesis, however described) no longer seems trustworthy. Certainly the shared view of behavioral and subjective hierarchies suggests considerable caution for reconstruction of pathogenic events or periods (Zeanah et al., 1989). These various shifting permutations of hierarchical organizations of systems, defenses, and behavioral integrations help us see the way a person reshapes original meaning in the current context and the way current context can reshape meaning (and thus behavior). This shifting tapestry of integrations seems to give some support to the argument by some that we cannot make reconstructions in treatment, but can only construct some coherent and useful model of a personal past (Spence, 1982). Attachment research, however, makes a convincing argument that broad-based patterns of interaction do seem to have continuity over time (Sroufe, 1989), so the issue may not be whether or not current events are related to past events, but rather that the transformations are so rich as to make the original derailments hard to identify. Stern (1985) captures this when he distinguishes the "actual point of origin" from "narrative point of origin" of pathology (p. 257).

IMPLICATIONS FOR THE ROLE OF EMPATHY
AND THE RANGE OF INTERVENTIONS

The model that I have reviewed points us toward intervening with patients with flexible technique. In psychotherapy patients form many images of their therapists, as threatening objects of suspicion, devalued parents, admired teachers, allies against society, erotic sexual partners. These transferences may be the manifestation of repressed or disavowed affects in any motivational system and may express issues relevant to any self domain. Additionally, they may be shame-avoidant efforts to engage the therapist for help in functioning.

A flexible stance is well suited to adolescents when fluctuations between modes of behavior and self-concept are frequent, and the therapist is required to maintain empathic contact with patients by understanding and intervening in accord with these the sometimes momentary shifts. Our interventions are guided by our assessment of our patient's current presentation of self domain and self-organization within motivational systems, as we understand them, through empathy.

The shift in emphasis from conflict to overall competent functioning in developmental theory and a theory of psychotherapy has placed empathic understanding of adolescents' experiences in a central role (Goldberg, 1978). Both attachment theory (Main and Goldwyn, 1984; Bowlby, 1988) and self psychology (Kohut, 1984; Wolf, 1988) point to the instrumental role of caretaker empathy in normal development. Many practitioners have taken up the banner of empathy, focusing as it does on the intersubjective field, as equally important in the etiology of psychopathology and as a technique of cure (Atwood and Stolorow, 1984). Some practitioners of self psychology place great value on the effect of empathic immersion and feel that it results in a curative bond of empathy (Atwood and Stolorow, 1984; Wolf, 1988; Terman, 1989). I feel that this overstates the therapeutic effectiveness of empathy and places an unnecessary burden on the therapist. In effect, it overemphasizes the therapist's verbal recognition and acceptance of the patient's conscious point of view and the interpretation of childhood trauma in a way that supports this view. In the worst circumstances, it supports a patient's self-pity and indulgent sense of entitlement (Gedo, 1988). In summary, Kohut's contribution was to broaden the arena for Freud's method by adding the selfobject transferences to the interpretive realm. The current model further enlarges the therapeutic field to allow for a range of flexible interventions based on empathic understanding.

How can we view the role of empathy in adolescent psychotherapy? Empathy is probably best understood in a broad interpersonal and a narrow therapeutic sense. In the broad view, empathic understanding is the process through which one comes to appreciate the affective as well as cognitive experiences of another (Basch, 1983b). Through the therapist's synthesis of his or her affective resonance with the patient's communications, interpretation of the resonance in the light of the therapist's own experiences, and the evaluation of the personal meaning of the communication within the larger context of the therapist's general knowledge of development and of the patient, the patient's experiential state may be ascertained. This is a neutral process that implies only understanding, not sympathy or kindness or help.

In therapy, then, the empathic mode of understanding is the generic way that the therapist comes to understand the patient. When used in the service of helping, this very process of dialogue creates the therapeutic environment wherein an interpersonal matrix of acceptance, support, and affirmation are supplied. Furthermore, the understanding that results from this process may be applied in a wide repertoire of interventions. In other words, in this view empathy is a mode of understanding that leads to possibilities for curative interventions but is not necessarily curative in itself.

When is empathy a therapeutic intervention? It probably would lead to too much confusion to label empathy an intervention per se. Therapists often mistakenly think that "saying something empathic" is a useful intervention. Nevertheless, sometimes the fact of its existence is salutary. Adolescence itself is a time of maturation of the empathic appreciation of others' emotions. Basch (1983b) describes a developmental sequence of affect (an autonomically mediated communication system), feeling (the word labelling affect), emotion (the combination of feelings), and empathy that reaches maturation in adolescence. Mature empathy involves the ability to decenter, or to objectively view one's own emotions in order to appreciate another's. It is enhanced by the advent of formal operations (Piaget and Inhelder, 1969). Not only is empathic understanding the route to appreciating the adolescent patient's subjective world, but it is also something the adolescent is learning and for which the therapist's behavior and the very process of therapy serves as a model.

When empathic understanding leads us to believe that the patient is struggling to maintain competence through a selfobject transference reflecting a need for self-affirmation, communicating our empathic understanding to the patient may support sufficient sharing of affect, attention, and intention to enable the patient to consolidate the ability to recruit the necessary self-affirming experiences. In other words, communicating our understanding of the patient's needs for our attunement as he or she struggles for competence is curative for disruptions in the domain of the intersubjective self, once resistances to the awareness of these needs have been overcome.

This was the case with Dan. My empathic attunement to his need for self-affirmation was beneficial. It was sufficient to enable him on his own to tolerate his strong emotions and to approach his life realistically. He was no longer directionless. No direct attention to other domains of self was necessary. In fact, Dan could see that his father could actually be fairly open and talkative if he approached him in a more self-reliant, less imploring style that demonstrated respect for his father's need to protect his own sense of self-determination.

At other times, our empathic dialogue may lead us to believe that the patient is operating in other modes of organization or domains of self where intersubjectivity is not so much the issue. In these circumstances, communicating an empathic understanding of the patient's experience usually makes little difference.

For instance, if our empathic listening to a patient's reports of actions, associations, and perhaps dreams reveals that the patient is inhibited about exploring lusty, playful sex with his girlfriend because of displaced hostile wishes toward his father, then empathy for the patient's frustrated needs for self-affirmation through sex is not sufficient. Interpretation of the symbolic transformation is necessary to promote the return of the patient's ability to discriminate between his hostile and sexual aims in addition to the empathic immersion that recognizes selfobject needs.

Alternatively, if the patient's behavior is organized around issues of tension regulation or coordination of aims, the patient may require a variety of direct interventions. At such times the "talking cure," even the "understanding cure," is not enough. This was the case with Toni. No amount of interpretation or affect attunement, however accurate, enabled her to reestablish competent functioning. Over much time and with much struggle she attained needed inpatient treatment, then day treatment that revolved around the provision of a predictable environment where she could learn to identify her affects and relate them to her own body signals in the service of managing her eating disorder and substance abuse, reestablish effective actions that she could use in a way that would not drive people away or lead her to become overinvested, and eventually to develop the mutually consensual feeling that she was worth all the effort. The primary mode of intervention was in the lived "life-space" (Redl, 1959) rather than the realm of verbal interactions. Self-reflection was the icing on the cake.

For adolescents operating in the domain of the emergent or core self, empathy is the vehicle through which needs (or first the defenses against them) can be discerned and then met. In essence, this is akin to the idea that empathic understanding of an infant's need for milk does not nourish babies—milk nourishes babies. The therapist's and the hospital staff's empathic understanding enabled them to use "optimal responsiveness" (Bacal, 1985), a flexible approach wherein they ascertained Toni's psychological state and responded in synchrony with her evolving organization and domains of experience.

In Toni's case and with many less dysfunctional adolescents, much of the treatment seems to involve interventions such as confrontation, clarification, validation, direction, encouragement or a variety of nonverbal interventions through activities. Examples include helping patients to order their lives, to read social signals with greater accuracy, or to enable learning or mood-disordered patients to get appropriate remedial instruction or stabilizing medication. These interventions have been traditionally labeled "noninterpretive," an unfortunate term because it suggests that these interventions play some sort of supporting role on the way to a mutative interpretation. Sometimes these interventions do seem to enhance the appearance of an interpretable transference (Hollinger, 1989), but for many adolescents these interventions play a leading role in therapy. These so-called noninterpretive interventions seem to address directly self-disorganization, or issues not involved with self-reflection but relevant to the emergent and core self. In summary, empathic understanding and optimal responsiveness promote stabilizing experiences with the therapist that enable the adolescent to maintain self-esteem while learning new skills that are necessary for competent functioning. This view supports the idea that psychotherapy is a technology of instruction (Gedo, 1988). Specifically, psychotherapy provides the context wherein the patient can learn.

Gedo and Goldberg (1973) have offered a useful classification of interventions that fits nicely with our model. When the patient is operating in the organizational mode of the emergent or core self, without the capacity for verbal expression or self-reflection, pacification is the term used for the provision of a soothing and consistent environment.

Practically, this may include hospitalization or medications. Unification involves presenting oneself as a real and affectively responsive person to help reestablish an organized and coordinated plan of activity when self-coherence or self-agency is disrupted, or, in other words, when the patient is functioning in the mode of the core self. This may include confronting patients about the impact of their behavior on others or actively helping to structure their lives. It may also include educating patients about affective, cognitive, and social awareness. Optimal disillusionment may be used when a patient is functioning with fairly stable self-cohesion but needs help with functioning realistically without self-sustaining illusions. This is really the realm of empathy in the narrow sense, as affect attunement to help with self-cohesion. Finally, interpretation is used if the patient is operating in the realm of the verbal or narrative self and explication of symbolic transformations is indicated.

Conclusion

A number of theoretical orientations have been applied to understanding adolescent development and to developing a theory of psychotherapy. I have tried to present an integrative model that I believe may be applied to understanding adolescence and to a theory of psychotherapy that affords a variety of interventions flexibly employed. Of course, any developmental theory is only as useful as the amount of information it organizes and as it points to rational interventions. Like the adolescent struggling with the reality of the probabilistic nature of life, we must be prepared to struggle with the fact that we are still describing adolescence and developing a theory that will adequately capture the complex tapestry of human development, of which the adolescent experience is only a part.

REFERENCES

Aichhorn, A. (1925), *Wayward Youth*. New York: Viking Press.
Atwood, G. & Stolorow, R. (1984), *Structures of Subjectivity*. Hillsdale, NJ: The Analytic Press.
Bacal, H. (1983), Optimal responsiveness and the therapeutic process. In: *Progress Self in Psychology, Vol.1*, ed. A. Goldberg. New York: Guilford Press, pp. 202–227.
Basch, M. F. (1973). Psychoanalysis and theory formation. *Annual of Psychoanalysis*, 1:9–52. New York: International Universities Press.

_____ (1975), Towards a theory that encompasses depression: A revision of existing causal hypothesis in psychoanalysis. In: *Depression and Human Existence*, ed. J. Anthony & T. Benedek. Boston: Little Brown, pp. 483–534.

_____ (1976), The concept of affect: A re-examination. *J. Amer. Psychoanal. Assn.*, 24:759–777.

_____ (1977), Developmental psychology and explanatory theory in psychoanalysis. *Annual of Psychoanalysis*, 5:229–263. New York: International Universities Press.

_____ (1983a), The perception of reality and the disavowal of meaning. *Annual of Psychoanalysis*, 11:125–153. New York: International Universities Press.

_____ (1983b), Empathic understanding: A review of the concept and some theoretical considerations. *J. Amer. Psychoanal. Assn.*, 31(1): 101–126.

_____ (1983c), Interpretation: Toward a developmental model. In: *Progress in Self Psychology Vol 1*, ed. A. Goldberg 1:33–42. New York: Guilford Press, pp. 33–42.

_____ (1988), *Understanding Psychotherapy*. New York: Basic Books.

Blos, P. (1962), *On Adolescence*. Glencoe, IL: Free Press of Glencoe.

_____ (1967), The second individuation process of adolescence. *The Psychoanalytic Study of the Child*, 22:162–186. New York: International Universities Press.

_____ (1968), Character formation in adolescence. *The Psychoanalytic Study of the Child*, 23:245–263. New York: International Universities Press.

_____ (1979), Modifications in the classical psychoanalytic model of adolescence. *Adolescent Psychiatry*, 7:6–25. Chicago: University of Chicago Press.

Bowlby, J. (1988), Developmental psychiatry comes of age. *J. Amer. Psychiat. Assn.*, 145(1):1–10.

Cantwell, D., ed. (1992), *Mood Disorders. Child and Adolescent Psychiatric Clinics of North America*, Vol 1(1). Chicago: University of Chicago Press.

Chess, S. & Thomas, A. (1987), *Origins and Evolution of Behavior Disorders*. Cambridge, MA: Harvard University Press.

Eissler, K. (1953), The effect of the structure of the ego on psychoanalytic technique. *J. Amer. Psychoanal. Assn.*, 1:104–143.

Erikson, E. (1968), *Identity*. New York: Norton.

Freud, A. (1958), Adolescence. *The Psychoanalytic Study of the Child*, 13:255–278. New York: International Universities Press.

Galatzer-Levy, R. & Cohler, B. (1993), *The Essential Other.*. New York: Basic Books.

Gedo, J. (1979), *Beyond Interpretation*. Hillsdale, NJ: The Analytic Press.

———— (1988), *The Mind in Disorder*. Hillsdale, NJ: Analytic Press.

———— & Goldberg, A. (1973), *Models of the Mind*. Chicago: University of Chicago Press.

Gitelson, M. (1948), Character synthesis: The psychotherapeutic problem of adolescence. *Amer. J. Orthopsychiat.*, 18:422–431.

Goldberg, A. (1978), A Shift in emphasis: Adolescent psychotherapy and the psychology of the self, *J. Youth Adoles.*, 7:119–134.

Golombek, H. & Garfinkel, B. (1983), *The Adolescent and Mood Disturbance*. New York: International Universities Press.

Greenberg, J. & Mitchell, S. (1983), *Object Relations in Psychoanalytic Theory*. Cambridge, MA: Harvard University Press.

Hollinger, P. (1989), A developmental perspective on psychotherapy and psychoanalysis. *J. Amer. Psychiat. Assoc.*, 146:1404–1412.

Jaffe, C. (1988), Disavowal: A review of applications in current literature. *Annual of Psychoanalysis*, 16:93–110. New York: International Universities Press.

———— (1994), Psychoanalysis and cognitive science: The multiple code theory. Discussion of a paper by Wilma Bucci. *Annual of Psychoanalysis*, 22:261–270. Hillsdale, NJ: The Analytic Press.

———— & Barglow, P. (1989), Adolescent psychopathology and attachment research: Mutual contributions. *Adolescent Psychiatry*, 16:350–371. Chicago: University of Chicago Press.

———— & Ryan, K. (1993), The adolescent psychotherapist: Research producer and research consumer. In: *The Handbook of Clinical Research and Practice with Adolescents*, ed. P. Tolan & B. Cohler. New York: Wiley, pp. 411–426.

King, C. D. (1945), The meaning of normal. *Yale J. Biol. Med.*, 17:493–501.

Katz, P. (1990), Engaging the difficult adolescent patient. *Adolescent Psychiatry*, 17:69–81. Hillsdale, NJ: The Analytic Press.

Klein, G. S. (1976), *Psychoanalytic Theory*. New York: International Universities Press.

Kohut, H. (1971), *The Analysis of the Self*. New York: International Universities Press.

_____ (1972), Thoughts on narcissism and narcissistic rage. *The Psychoanalytic Study of the Child*, 27:360–400. New Haven, CT: Yale University Press.

_____ (1977), *The Restoration of the Self.* New York: International Universities Press.

_____ (1984), *How Does Analysis Cure?*, ed. A. Goldberg & P. Stepansky. Chicago: University of Chicago Press.

Lage, G. & Nathan, H. (1991), *Psychotherapy, Adolescents, and Self-Psychology*. Madison, CT: International Universities Press.

Lichtenberg, J. (1982), Continuities and transformations between infancy and adolescence. *Adolescent Psychiatry*, 10:182–198. Chicago: University of Chicago Press.

_____ (1983), *Psychoanalysis and Infant Research*. Hillsdale, NJ: The Analytic Press.

_____ (1989), *Psychoanalysis and Motivation*. Hillsdale, NJ: The Analytic Press.

Main, M. & Goldwyn, R. (1984), Predicting a mother's rejection of her infant from representations of her own childhood experiences. *Internat. J. Child Abuse Neglect*, 7:203–217.

Marohn, R. (1977), The "Juvenile Imposter": Some thoughts on narcissism and the delinquent. *Adolescent Psychiatry*, 5:186–212. Chicago: University of Chicago Press.

Masterson, J. (1958), Psychotherapy of the adolescent: A comparison with psychotherapy of the adult. *J. Nervous Ment. Dis.*, 127:511–517.

_____ (1967), *The Psychiatric Dilemma of Adolescence*. Boston: Little, Brown.

_____ (1972), *Treatment of the Borderline Adolescent*. New York: Wiley-Interscience.

Meeks, J. (1971), *The Fragile Alliance*. Baltimore, MD: Williams & Wilkins.

Miller, D. (1983), *The Age Between*. New York: Aronson.

Offer, D. & Offer, J. (1975), *From Teenage to Young Manhood.*. New York: Basic Books.

Palombo, J. (1979), Perceptual deficits and self-esteem in adolescence. *Clin. Soc. Work*, 7:34–61.

_____ (1988), Adolescent development: A view from self psychology. *Child Adoles. Soc. Work*, 5:171–186.

_____ (1990), The cohesive self, the nuclear self, and development in late adolescence. *Adolescent Psychiatry*, 17:338–359. Chicago: University of Chicago Press.

Peterfreund, E. (1971), *Information, Systems, and Psychoanalysis. Psychological Issues*, Monogr. 25/26. New York: International Universities Press.

———— (1983), *The Process of Psychoanalytic Psychotherapy*. Hillsdale, NJ: The Analytic Press.

Piaget, J. & Inhelder, B. (1969), *The Psychology of the Child*. New York: Basic Books.

Racker, H. (1968), *Transference and Countertransference*. New York: International Universities Press.

Rakoff, V. (1989), The emergence of the adolescent as a special patient. *Adolescent Psychiatry*, 16:372–386. Chicago: University of Chicago Press.

Redl, F. (1959), Strategy and techniques of the life space interview. *Amer. J. Orthopsychiat.*, 29:1–18.

Rothstein, A., Benjamin, L., Crosby, M. & Eisenstadt, K. (1988), *Learning Disorders*. Madison, CT: International Universities Press.

Sameroff, A. & Emde, R., ed. (1989), *Relationship Disturbances in Early Childhood*. New York: Basic Books.

Schafer, R. (1976), *A New Language for Psychoanalysis*. New Haven, CT: Yale University Press.

Silver, L. (1992), *Attention-Deficit Hyperactivity Disorder*. Washington: American Psychiatric Press.

————, ed. (1993), Learning disabilities. *Child and Adolescent Psychiatric Clinics of North America*, 2(2). Chicago: University of Chicago Press.

Spence, D. (1982), *Narrative Truth and Historical Truth*. New York: Norton.

Sroufe. A. (1989), Relationships, self, and individual adaptation. In: *Relationship Disturbances in Early Childhood*, ed. A. Sameroff & R. Emde. New York: Basic Books, pp. 70–94.

Stern, D. (1985), *The Interpersonal World of the Infant*. New York: Basic Books.

Tansey, M. & Burke, W. (1989), *Understanding Countertransference*. Hillsdale, NJ: The Analytic Press.

Terman, D. (1989), Therapeutic change: Perspectives of self psychology. *Psychoanal. Inq.*, 9:88–100.

Tomkins, S. (1962), *Affect, Imagery, Consciousness*, Vols. I & II. New York: Springer.

Volkmar, F., ed. (1994), *Psychoses and Pervasive Developmental Disorders. Child and Adolescent Psychiatric Clinics of North America*, 3(1). Chicago: University of Chicago Press.

Wolf, E. (1980), Tomorrow's self: Heinz Kohut's contributions to adolescent psychiatry. *Adolescent Psychiatry*, 8:41–50. Chicago: University of Chicago Press.

——— (1982), Adolescence: Psychology of the self and self-objects. *Adolescent Psychiatry*, 10:171–181.

——— (1988), *Treating the Self*. New York: Guilford Press.

Wolf, E., Gedo, J. & Terman, D. (1972), On the adolescent process as a transformation of the self. *J. Youth Adoles.*, 1(3):257–272.

Zeanah, C., Anders, T., Seifer, R. & Stern, D. (1989), Implications of research on infant development for psychodynamic theory and practice. *J. Amer. Acad. Child Adoles. Psychiat.*, 28(5):657–668.

2 THE AWARENESS OF THE PAST IN ADOLESCENCE

CLAUDE VILLENEUVE

The search for identity, the most crucial developmental task of adolescence, reaches completion towards the end of the adolescent period (Erikson, 1968). The adolescent's view of self and identifications whose interplay is closely connected in adolescence are, by then, reshaped. The continuity in the relationships and the formation of a coherent identity are determined by the development of a historical sense of the past and the integration of the past into the present (Blos, 1977).

The process of reappraising and integrating the past is not, however, without difficulties and contradictions. Adolescents redefine themselves through both the selective repudiation and the assimilation of childhood identifications. They withdraw their cathexis from their parents and their imagoes, on the one hand; on the other hand, they build their identity on a new appraisal of their past relationships. As they try to master the past, they disidentify and deidealize archaic parental imagoes (Deutsch, 1967). In their quest for identity, late adolescents may also develop a narrative of their own development, which has the characteristics of a "personal myth" (Kris, 1956). They can construct the past as though it had designed them, or, better, they had designed the past (Erikson, 1958; Fisher, 1992). That reassessment serves as defensive purpose.

The adolescent's awareness of the past is usually poor and obscured by earlier conflicts, leaving unchecked the influence of unconscious forces on the integrative process. As analysts, we realize that key portions of the parents' experience, in particular, remain unknown, which affects the reappraisal of the parental imagoes. The adolescent analysand often has a superficial image of his parents' personality. Rare are the analysands, adults or adolescents, who look for deeper exploration of their origins. The psychic reality of the parents is "reduced to stereotyped images of which only the color seems to have changed" (de Mijolla, 1987, p. 401).

Secrets or withholding of information also make the adolescent ill informed about the past. The revealing of the child's or of his or her parents' experience may be shrouded in uncertainty and mystery, leading the child to fill the gaps with fantasies. The phenomenon is well illustrated by adopted children and offspring of Holocaust survivors (Jucovy, 1985). Lacking information about their genealogical background, adopted children tend to develop elaborate fantasies about their origins (Colarusso, 1987). To cope better with their identity lacunae, some adoptees are encouraged to search for their past and to get some background information (Weider, 1978). That knowledge promotes a greater sense of identity and is particularly positive for adoptees when the biological parents' difficulties are considered in the context of their life situation. Some offsprings of Holocaust survivors also tend to develop elaborate fantasies, including pathological family romance, as a way to deal with their parents' preoccupations and silences in regard to their horrendous experiences in camps (Auerhahn and Prelinger, 1985). Barely guessed family secrets or mysteries also may instill imaginary constructions in which children substitute a character from their family history for part of ego or superego. These unconscious identification fantasies (de Mijolla, 1987) compel adolescents to live out something from somebody else in the prehistory of their family, which may interfere with the identity process and the integration of some past experiences.

Because defensive processes and unconscious representations play an important role in identity formation, can a better awareness of their unconscious history and of the fantasy and representation potential thus conveyed help adolescents to rehabilitate their imagoes and strengthen their identity? That question will be addressed here through the analysis of two adolescents presenting some identity problems.

Awareness of the Past through Reconstruction in Adolescence

Stating the importance of the past to psychoanalysts is like preaching to the converted. The use of the past in analysis has, however, decreased over the years in favor of focusing on current issues. Deemphasizing reconstruction, in particular, is seen by Kernberg (1993) as part of a psychoanalytic fashion. Along with less emphasis on the past, as well as on the recovery of memories and on external reality, there is an increased focus on the analysis of unconscious meanings of the transference. As will be described, the difficulties inherent in the analysis of adolescents may also impede the exploration of the past. Reconstruction remains important in the analysis of adolescents (Friend, 1970) and is crucial in the treatment of some identity-problem adolescents.

In adult analysis, the process of development of the transference gives good evidence of what happened with the parents. Reconstructive work allows access to the patient's past. The focus is not, however, on the search for historical truth but on the formation of a narration (Spence, 1989). The scope of reconstruction has widened with the ego psychologists to cover past external realities and their later overlays (Lowenstein, 1951). Information that the child was unable to appreciate, in particular, the motivation of the other participants in his or her earlier experience becomes subject to scrutiny (Wetzler, 1985). Reconstruction is thus used to fill the gaps and to get a second look at the family and at the motives of people (Novey, 1968).

The particularities of the analysis of adolescents may not permit an adequate reconstruction of the past. The transference neurosis and the working through are less complete. The necessary regression may be too threatening, which can make part of the past escape any deep questioning (Klumpner, 1975). The decathexis of the old objects and the fear of revival of painful experiences also do not foster the exploration of the past. Focusing on the immediate situation characterizes therapy with adolescents (Sugar, 1992). The adolescent's past experiences and the unconscious family history cannot, however, be ignored. The reawakening in the transference of fantasies about archaic objects and of the peculiarities of early parenting have to be analyzed.

Adolescents may deny the importance of knowing their origins, but in analysis some of their ego attitudes reveal the opposite. Many adolescent analysands complain about not knowing enough about their parents. During anamnestic interviews, adolescents are very attentive when their parents talk about the family history and their own parents. When that exploration goes beyond the stereotypical qualifications of parents idealizing or criticizing their own parents to reach significant material, adolescents are often quite moved.

Some modifications may be used for the exploration of the adolescent's past experiences and related fantasies. As part of being more active when dealing with adolescents, the analyst may, at times, leave the free associations of the adolescent and evoke the material from the past without interpreting the hidden fantasy. Such specific reconstruction is facilitated with adolescents insofar as some direct or indirect information about the family background may be available to the analyst before starting analysis. The continuing relative proximity of the adolescent to his or her family may also be helpful. A few adolescents will even seek out significant persons from early life, which is relatively common in analysis of adults (Novey, 1966).

The use of the past is often important in dealing with adolescents' inability to discuss their feelings toward the analyst and to cope with the negative transference in particular. A better understanding of the reality of the parents and of the work of defense that has transformed their images into what now transpires in the transference could follow. Previously not invested id derivatives, countercathected as they appear in the transference, may then be used to reidentify with the parents.

Awareness of the Past and Some Identity Problems

An ill-informed and defensively reappraised past may have an indelible influence on the adolescent's identifications and identity and could lead to some identity problems. Secrets and withholding of information about the adolescent's background are often present.

IDENTITY CRISIS

Facing new psychosocial tasks, adolescents may manifest anxieties and preoccupations concerning their identity and the internal cohesiveness of their own person. The crisis is usually preceded by the sudden rejection of the parental imagoes as well as of their ideal self-representations and of other narcissistically based object representations. Faulty preoedipal or oedipal identifications are involved. A conflictual identification with the parent of the same sex may lead to narcissistic uncertainty and to a weak identity. The formation of the ego ideal may be prevented, leaving unchecked a primitive superego.

Paul, who started analysis at age 17, had important hypochondriacal preoccupations and somatizations. He was fearful of meeting girls and concerned with sexual potency, which were related to castration fear and an incestuous fixation on his mother. As a consequence of the early differentiation of a strict superego, he showed a tendency for asceticism built against sexual and aggressive impulses. This inclination was, then, giving him some feeling of coherence. The reawakened oedipal and preoedipal urges led to tremendous anxieties related to fantasies that were under repression during latency. Facing the oedipal danger and decisions concerning his future career, he had loosened ties to his mother. Decathecting the object brought mourning and loss with narcissistic withdrawal and inability to transfer to new objects. Paul showed a return to body language with somatization of affects and drives. As will be described later, the analysis revealed dreadful fantasies related to his unconscious family history and unveiled his anxious search for his own identity. He had difficulty identifying with his father, which meant relinquishing an anaclitic attachment to his mother. He felt weak as a male, with passivity and little sexual striving. He had regressed to a state of primitive dependence, preventing the oedipal situation. Paul had been prone to intellectual activities as a defense against instinctual demands. These activities had remained ego autonomous as they were not symbols of identity conflicts.

IDENTITY DIFFUSION

Along with the decathexis of the parental imagoes, misrepresentations of the past and faulty identifications may lead to identity diffusion or identity confusion. Identity-diffuse adolescents are fixed in the present, wishing to forget the past and unable to imagine a future (Josselson, 1987). They cannot make a commitment to a chosen role, and feel uncertain about goals and values. These adolescents do not have a historical sense of the past. They can be confused about their sexual identity, with fear of identification or competition with the same-sex parent and conflicts with the other parental figure. The need to reject the parents may, then, be masked. Depressive symptoms can appear, signifying battle against identifications to parental imagoes and rejection of the sexual self.

Jane was referred at 17 for depressed feelings and school refusal for many months. She spent most of her time in her room watching television, doing nothing, and communicating little. She perceived her father as stoic, self-centered, and critical of everybody in the family and her mother as submissive, depressed, and ineffectual. Her analysis showed a strong amnesia for her childhood and poor awareness of her parents' background. In her search for identity, Jane had engaged in premature sexuality, which had been traumatic for her. A problematic identification to her oedipal parents was present. The resurgence of the oedipal conflict made her feel that, on one hand, identifying with her mother meant taking her place, destroying her, but also being ineffective and inferior. On the other hand, identifying with her father was linked to being aggressive, sadistic, and assuming a virility while acknowledging castration. Jane was unconsciously identifying with her mother by her passivity and with her father through a strict superego. Her rigid conscience prevented her autonomy and the development of her own ideals. Jane felt uncertain about goals and values and did not know how she wished to grow as a person. She was judging herself as no good but she could not define who she was. She had found a compromise to her identity problems by denying her identity, being nothing and doing nothing.

Illustrations Through the Analytic Work

Some material that partly summarizes reconstructive work in Paul's and Jane's analyses may illustrate how a better awareness of the past helps consolidate the adolescent's identity.

Paul vividly experienced in the transference his past relationship with his intrusive mother and his peripheral father. He had difficulty, though, tolerating these early experiences whose genesis was surrounded by dreadful unconscious fantasies. He had built a personal myth of a rosy childhood, raised as a defense against traumatic memories and as a narcissistic barrier, preventing awareness of his parents' weaknesses. During the sessions, he often drifted into intellectualizing monologues and somatic ruminations. To tackle the resistance to exploration and reach significant material, the analyst was led to evoke the past. Through his phase-specific need to identify with the analyst and the analyst's function, Paul was then induced to use his considerable intellectual capacities to investigate his mood states and reconstruct their origins. He became active in reappraising his past and received some information from his maternal uncle and later from his father. He had been told little, was misinformed about his family background, and had filled the gaps with fantasies.

A narrative of a very sad childhood and of a morbid family background was built. Many family secrets emerged. Both his mother and his maternal grandmother had experienced depression. Paul's grandmother had lived a secluded and austere life under the tyranny of a sadistic husband. She had sent their daughter, in late adolescence, to a Catholic convent to become a nun and redeem the family. Paul's mother became depressed and was forced to leave the convent, feeling lost and a failure in her mission on earth. Soon after, her own mother died and her father broke contact with her. She quickly married a submissive, uneducated man and kept her past experiences secret. She remained depressed and withdrawn except for involvement in religious activities, which served as an umbrella under which everything was hidden. She showed a delayed expression of her conflicts in brooding preoccupations and developed an unempathic symbiosis with her son, her only child, while Paul's father was kept away. She could not cease being overwhelmed by her past experience. Imagery of his mother's past became an unconscious pillar of Paul's identity. A pact of silence was set between the two that led the son to develop nightmarish stories about his mother. This transpired in analysis through his difficulty verbalizing. The mother's fears of sin and eschatological fantasies had been transformed into calamities by Paul as a young child. He felt invaded by demons that could magically make his mother dead and force him to follow her into Satan's world.

The past that Paul had strongly denied suddenly resurfaced during adolescence, following the breakdown of his defenses. Paul felt pain and terrors. Primitive affects that seemed to come from nowhere were threatening his identity. These affects had to be bound to their origins and integrated. Reconstructing helped Paul fill the breach about his early parenting and correct the distortions related to the vicissitudes of his mother's silence. The narrative gave coherence to the biographical material. Paul had been a well-behaved lonely child who could hardly play. As a defense against a threatening and desperate internal world, he molded himself to his mother's wishes and dreams and never gratified himself. Becoming aware of his history, he finally tore off the shroud in which he was wrapped with his mother. He had foreclosed his identity, committing himself to a matriarchal ideological goal. His mission of redemption that was used to fulfill his mother's ambition and his own narcissism was scrutinized. Its link to the maternal grandmother through unconscious identification became evident. A character from his family history had been substituted for part of his superego and ego ideal to compensate for previous family losses.

A better knowledge of his mother's motivation helped Paul work through in the transference his tremendous rage at the maternal object.

Repressive forces were lifted and other emotionally charged material, including his sexual mythology, resurfaced. Sexual fantasies hinted at before in a casual manner by the analyst had remained unexplored. The use of the past facilitated the resurgence of fantasies of violence related to Paul's early sexual arousal. These fantasies were analyzed in relation to his early parenting and feelings toward the archaic mother.

The analyst as a male figure of identification invested in the transference brought reassurance to Paul's identity and protected him against the bad object. He rediscovered his devalued father. He revived through the transference some good moments he had had with him. These experiences had been distorted by the son as an oedipal child and had not been acknowledged by his mother. Paul realized he had identified with his "idealized dyadic father" (Blos, 1985) as a soft and caring man. Through the resurrection of the past, the paternal image became more important to him. The confrontation between the father who had been fantasized and the newly discovered one, led to some restructuring of Paul's identity.

Paul's regained continuity helped him prevent further collapse and allowed the emergence in the transference of his real self. His deep conviction that both he and his family were unfit and doomed to fail was shaken up. A shift from a moralistic view of right and wrong to more personal values became evident. He showed more acceptance of his identity as revealed in his dreams. Benevolent male figures, with whom he identified, replaced witches and sad stories. His genitality became more integrated as his harsh superego gave way to a more appropriate ego ideal. Paul's scholastic interests shifted toward literature, a field in which be excelled. The decrease of his narcissistic withdrawal was accompanied by a recathexis of new objects. Paul responded to social demands with a more integrated sense of self, developed from a new understanding of the genetic roots of his problem.

Reconstructing the past should not, however, detract from the basic work, the working through of the infantile conflict that occurs in the analysis of the transference. Awareness of past experiences, on the contrary, helps validate old memories and facilitate the elucidation of the transference. Acting out and premature termination, recurring phenomena in the treatment of adolescents, may thus be prevented. The psychic representation of the past and the realities from which distortions come are both used. In line with the adolescent's developmental phase, some early structures are dissolved. The reexperiencing of emotions provides new memory structures and a frame of reference that are much needed, especially for the adolescent presenting with identity problems. A reappraisal of the parents' past and of their motivations helps adolescents rework their imagoes and reidentify with better estimated images of the parents. When seen in their background context, the parents may also stimulate more empathy and be more easily forgiven. The process of rehabilitating the parental imagoes which is activated and hastened by analysis is usually at work later when the individual becomes a parent.

In Jane's analysis, some significant material was kept repressed for a long time: She could not remember much and was very vague about her past. The strength of the material repressed, however, let derivatives enter consciousness. Her defensive maneuvers and distortions in the transference showed the conflictual area of earlier years. The infantile conflicts were revived, but Jane withdrew to avoid her infantile attachments to the archaic maternal imago and the surge of aggressive impulses. Her mood swings and shifting psychopathology, which frequently occur in adolescent analysands, did not leave much time for the analyst to adjust. Jane's sadomasochistic traits appeared in the transference as her rebelling against any move of the therapist by her mutism and being late. Jane's revolt against the analyst threatened the continuation of the treatment. The well-defended aggressive urges that had transpired in the transference could not be analyzed as Jane strongly opposed the exploration of her background.

The past was subtly brought in through the discussion of the current and past family living experiences and through Jane's childhood interests. Her unconscious history was thus slowly infiltrated and circumscribed as much as she could bear it. Interpretation of the repressed ego and superego finally led to the recovery of other memories and to the sources of her aggressive feelings. As a child, Jane was seen as normal even though she was reserved and rather solitary. Her parents had high expectations of her and she thought they were gods. She had rationalized their attitudes, repressed angry feelings toward them, and blamed herself instead. Her resentment, manifested in the transference toward the parental figures could not, however, be worked through. She refused to explore her parents' motivations. She swore she would never forgive her mother. Jane acknowledged her mother did not do harm to her intentionally but wondered why she should have to know her mother while her mother did not reciprocate. Reconstructing past experience with her parents meant to Jane getting closer to them, identifying with them and giving up splitting the good therapist and the bad parents. As she relived some forgotten early experiences that appeared in dreams and in the transference in a more empathic context, she slowly became interested in her parents' background.

Jane knew little about her stoic father who never talked about his past. She learned he'd had a difficult childhood, feeling rejected by his stepfather and having been sent to a boarding school until his late teens. Even though she had sometimes heard her mother complaining about her own childhood, she had not made links between her mother's past and hers. From early on, Jane's mother had taken care of her own sick mother and of her younger sisters while her father kept criticizing her.

Interweaving the adolescent's psychic truth and external reality, the analyst helped Jane reconstruct the past atmosphere at home. Jane's mother had reexperienced pain and depression raising her own children, more so with a daughter, which reminded her of taking care of her own sisters. She was closer and emotionally more available to her son. That new information was then returned to the context of Jane's own conflicts as a child. Her resentment against the maternal figure that held her development back decreased and was finally worked through in the transference.

With regard to some of her identity issues, Jane went through a moratorium period. She had given up childhood resolutions, but she was in a state of uncertainty, facing psychic reorganization and having to make choices with regard to young adulthood. She had not yet committed herself to values and occupational goals, but she became actively involved in exploring various alternatives. Her counteridentification toward the maternal imago lessened, and Jane stopped building her identity against her mother. She realized she resembled her mother and found herself thinking more often about her. Jane's self-blaming finally abated as the negative aspects of her idealized mother were decathected. Her female identity was also consolidated, following a reappraisal of her father's imago. Through the analyst as a more benevolent figure, the paternal imago was felt as more sensitive and accepting. Her receptivity to femininity and to her sexual self became apparent in her clothing and manners. Jane's symptoms proved to be neurotic in nature.

Changes in her dynamic equilibrium and identity also became evident through her associations and dreams. In a dream that symbolizes change, Jane is in the middle of a lake, alone in a canoe. She is unable to move, busy looking at another boat in which there are men and women she knows. Jane vaguely feels there is a lot of tension in the group. She cannot recognize these people because it is too foggy. Jane feels very anxious, and the two boats are drifting. The fog dissipates. Jane is alone on the lake, relaxed and paddling toward the shore. The dream confirms the analytic work. Many latent thoughts related to the transference, to the reconstruction, and to the past are evoked. This is an identity dream. Jane's origins through traces of the past chaos are alluded to. She finally has found some goals and has defined who she is.

Jane's confusion and bewilderment abated. She left analysis and within a year, moved away from her parents. She had been in treatment for two and a half years. Some analytic work was left undone, but Jane had developed a stable view of self and some freedom of choice. She could then assume her identity without breaking off with her origins.

For late adolescents with some identity problems, the analytic treatment and its emphasis on the past allows the young people to experience themselves in novel ways and offers identity-formation possibilities. Their identity would have likely remained problematic, otherwise. Their analysis demonstrates the relevance for late adolescents of knowing their origins, which has an impact on their identity process. As we have seen, the ambivalent characteristics of earlier object relations may interfere with the adolescents' identification with parental objects in their roles as adults and with new objects (Ritvo, 1971). The liquidation of childhood residual conflicts, which is promoted by a greater awareness of the past, serves to modify earlier identifications and to strengthen the new identity. The new internal representations of the parents become more attuned to what the real parents are, leading to changes in the ego ideal that, in turn, influence identity. New meanings given to the adolescents' family prehistory also help them to find new directions for the future, enabling them to choose more freely values and career.

Conclusion

Analysis in late adolescence allows a closer view of the process of reappraising the parents in the light of infantile idealization and the adolescent's deidealization. As Deutsch (1967) pointed out, in our societies where durable values and adequate ego ideals in the form of appropriate heroes for the adolescent are scarce, the devaluation of the parents may lead to identificatory groups opposed to the parents' ideals and toward pop culture idols and even street gangs. For many youngsters, that route is the only alternative available to fill the identity void they experience.

The study of identity formation has not been sufficiently related to adolescents' and their families' unconscious history. The reappraisal and integration of the past are under the sway of unconscious and defensive forces related to earlier conflicts that obscure the evaluation of early parenting and of the parent's background. A better informed reappraisal could help late adolescents locate their own self-perception in a meaningful context and reidentify with some adequate components of the parental imagoes. Continuity in relationships, which is essential for the preservation of identity, is thus ensured. Knowing their origins better, adolescents experience their identity as more integrated, and drastic maneuvers away from the parental figures may be prevented. The rejection of parental values is not a necessary condition for the successful completion of adolescence. Rather, the consolidation of a personal identity, promoted by an adequate awareness of one's past, is the most important criterion.

REFERENCES

Auerhahn, N. C. & Prelinger, E. (1983), Repetition in the concentration camps survivor and her child. *Internat. Rev. Psycho-Anal.,* 10:31–46.

Blos, P. (1965), *Son and Father.* New York: Free Press.

———— (1977), When and how does adolescence end: Structural criteria for adolescent closure. *Adolescent Psychiatry,* 5:5–17. New York: Aronson.

Colarusso, C. A. (1987), Mother, is that you? *The Psychoanalytic Study of the Child,* 42:223–237. New Haven, CT: Yale University Press.

de MiJolla, A. (1987), Unconscious identification fantasies and family prehistory. *Internat. J. Psycho-Anal.,* 68:397–403.

Deutsch, H. (1967), *Selected Problems of Adolescence*. New York: International Universities Press.

Erikson, E. H. (1958), *Young Man Luther*. New York: Norton.

———— (1968), *Identity: Youth and Crisis*. New York: Norton.

Fisher, C. P. (1992), Beyond identity: Invention, absorption, and transcendence. *Adolescent Psychiatry*, 18:448–460. Chicago: University of Chicago Press.

Friend, M. P. (1970), Youth unrest: Reflections of a psychoanalyst. *J. Amer. Acad. Child Psychiat.*, 17:224–232.

Josselson, P. (1987), Identity diffusion: A long-term follow-up. *Adolescent Psychiatry*, 14:230–258. Chicago: University of Chicago Press.

Jucovy, M. E. (1985), Telling the Holocaust story: A link between the generations. *Psychoanal. Inq.*, 5:131–149.

Kernberg, O. F. (1993), The current status of psychoanalysis. *J. Amer. Psychoanal. Assn.*, 41:45–62.

Klumpner, G. H. (1975), On the psychoanalysis of adolescents. *Adolescent Psychiatry*, 4:393–400. New York: Aronson.

Kris, E. (1956), The personal myth: A problem in psychoanalytic technique. *J. Amer. Psychoanal. Assn.*, 4:653–681.

Lowenstein, P. (1951), The problem of interpretation. Psychoanal. Quart., 20:1–14.

Novey, S. (1956), Why some patients conduct actual investigations of their biographies. *J. Amer. Psychoanal. Assn.*, 14:376–387.

———— (1968), *The Second Look: The Reconstruction of Personal History in Psychiatry and Psychoanalysis*. Baltimore, MD: John Hopkins University Press.

Ritvo, S. (1971), Late adolescence. Developmental and clinical considerations. *The Psychoanalytic Study of the Child*, 26:241–263. New Haven, CT: Yale University Press.

Spence, D. (1982), *Narrative Truth and Historical Truth*. New York: Norton.

Sugar, M. (1992), Late adolescent development and treatment. *Adolescent Psychiatry*, 18:131–155. Chicago: University of Chicago Press.

Weider, H. (1978), On when and whether to disclose about adoption. *J. Amer. Psychoanal. Assn.*, 26:793–811.

Wetzler, S. (1985), The historical truth of psychoanalytic reconstructions. *Internat. Rev. Psycho-Anal.*, 12:187–197.

3   ADOLESCENCE, AUTHORITY, AND CHANGE

PHILIP KATZ

Some 2300 years ago, Aristotle commented on the adolescents of ancient Greece:

> The young are . . . prone to desire and ready to carry any desire they may have formed into action. Of bodily desires it is the sexual to which they are the most disposed to give way, and in regard to sexual desire they exercise no self-restraint. They are changeful too, and fickle in their desires, which are as transitory as they are vehement. . . . They are passionate, irascible, and apt to be carried away by their impulses. . . . They have high aspirations; for they have never yet been humiliated by the experience of life. . . . If the young commit a fault, it is always on the side of excess and exaggeration. . . . They regard themselves as omniscient and are positive in their assertions; this is, in fact, the reason of their carrying everything too far [pp. 18–19].

Our studies of European culture indicate that in ancient Greece and ancient Rome there were adolescents who questioned and challenged the status quo. They were primarily from the aristocracy and the middle class. With the coming of the dark ages in the 400s and the concomitant shortening of life expectancy, adolescence, and indeed most of childhood disappeared. Infancy lasted until somewhere between four and six, and the child was then plunged directly into the adult work world, to either survive it or die. The life expectancy was less than 30 years and there was no time to be wasted. Even with the children of the aristocracy, responsibilities and hard work were thrust at them in childhood. It was at the beginning of the Renaissance, in the late 14th century, that adolescents began to reappear, initially in the families of the Italian aristocracy who with more time and better health were able to give their teenagers a few years in which to be adolescent: to think, to question, and to try to develop some sort of individual identity. Adolescence, as a developmental phase, gradually spread through the aristocracy of western Europe, and began to reach down into the middle classes in the late 1500s and the 1600s. Adolescence as a stage of development finally appeared in the lower and lower middle socioeconomic classes at the beginning of this century, due to the introduction of longer periods of compulsory schooling and child labor laws that limited the hours of work for early adolescents.

Indeed, adolescence not only has become widespread throughout the western world, but also has been greatly prolonged. While adolescence begins with a biological phenomenon, the onset of puberty, it gradually ends with a sociological phenomenon, the assumption of an adult economic role, that of the breadwinner, or homemaker, or mixtures thereof. A lengthened educational process, child labor laws which postpone full entry into the work force, and a delayed age of marriage, have pushed the ending of the stage of adolescence into the late teens or early 20s. The unexplained biological shift in the average age of the onset of puberty, which now comes some three years earlier than it did a century ago, has also prolonged adolescence. These ten years or so of adolescence provide many opportunities for clashes between adolescents and adult authority, especially in the area of adolescent sexual behavior.

In the early 1700s, the French government of what is now Quebec fined all 14 year old males if they were not married. Life expectancy was 30 years and they had to get on with having families—but in reality, many of the boys were married before they were pubertal and even interested in heterosexual relationships. It was easy to impose a standard of no premarital intercourse back then. Facing an eight to ten year period between puberty and marriage, most of today's adolescents challenge the traditional standards of sexual behavior. During that six- to ten-year period between the onset of adolescence and the restricting effects of work, marriage, and family, the adolescent has plenty of time to question and challenge everything: Who said so? Why do they say that? Who are these so-called authorities? What gives them the right to power?

It is interesting to note that the progress of western civilization parallels the existence of the stage of adolescence. In Greek and Roman times there was a great explosion of creativity, of scientific knowledge, and of philosophy. Progress in these fields slowed with the dark ages, but began to reappear with the Renaissance, and has accelerated with the steady spread of the adolescent stage of development amongst the western peoples. The adolescent search for his or her identity, with the eternal questions of Who am I? What do I believe? Why am I this way? What is true and what is not? Why is this so? have led to many of the great philosophical and scientific works of our time. Many of the great writers and great scientists, Einstein and others, have said that a lot of their major works were first formulated in the adolescent period when they were asking the question Why?. It is that unceasing challenge to the pronouncements of the authorities, to the rules of the authorities, that has led to many of the breakthroughs in science and politics. The Group for the Advancement of Psychiatry (GAP) issued a report on "Power and Authority in Adolescence" (1978) in which they stated, "It must be remembered that many of today's heroes were yesterday's malcontents" (p. 165). I remember attending an international congress where one of the papers was on the Danish underground in World War II. Initially the Danish adults had accepted the Nazi occupation, but the refusal of the Danish adolescents to accept it led to the formation of the Danish underground, which was responsible for helping many allied airmen, and played a significant role during the war.

The GAP report concluded, "The adolescents' struggles with authority . . . may serve as the basis for change in laws, codes, and social practices. The conflict creates moments of challenge and fluidity within social codes and practices. These can stimulate constructive societal growth or, alternatively, they can provoke regressive societal constriction and rigidification" (p. 70). Examples of the latter would be Tiananmen Square or Kent State, where adult authority brutally attacked adolescents in the midst of peaceful protest.

On an individual level, each adolescent must work out his or her own responses to authority and power. The GAP report said,

> A basic feature in the emotional maturation of every human being consists of his or her continued encounters with relationships of power and authority, encounters that involve interactions of both conflict and collaboration. . . . Every human must resolve the problems of these encounters in order to establish an adult capacity to relate to others and to the social environment. There is a range of possible solutions, from adaptive to maladaptive to disastrous, and these have been undergoing significant changes due to the rapid evolution of social structures and functions [p. 61].

Power is the ability to coerce, it is demonstrable and can be measured. Authority has no physical meaning, it resides in the belief systems of people, it depends on interpersonal agreements that enable the authority to have control, because he or she or an institution is perceived to be the best choice to do so. That perception has to be constantly validated. When the capacity of authorities to dispense justice, to act morally, or to cope with change is questioned, their authority is eroded; frequently the response of authorities, whether parents or political leaders, is to escalate the exercise of coercive power in the assertion of control [p. 62].

An example: One of my patients, who was approaching his 16th birthday, filled out his application for a driver's license and then gave it to his parents for their required signature. They saw that he had filled in the portion donating his body, in case of death, to the local medical school. Mother said, "I don't want that."

He said, "But it's only worm food."

She said, "We don't do those things."

He said, "Why not? I can't take it with me in a carry-on."

Father said angrily, "It's not our way!"

He said, "I don't see what's so great about being ten toes up in an underground condo."

Father said, "Erase it, or we won't sign the application."

Whether one speaks of scholarly authority, religious authority, political authority, or parental authority, the situation is inherently a dynamic one. There will be fluctuations, with moments of greater stability that may alternate with periods of unease and insecurity. The essence of authority, however, is that it must forever be worked at to be maintained, both by those who bear it and those who accept it.

Erich Fromm (1947) differentiated between rational authority and irrational authority. Rational authority has its source in competence. The person whose authority is respected functions competently in the task with which he is entrusted by those who conferred it upon him. He need not intimidate them nor arouse their admiration by magic qualities. Rational authority not only permits but requires constant scrutiny and criticism by those subjected to it; it is always temporary, its acceptance depending on its performance. The source of irrational authority, by contrast, is always power over people. This power can be physical or mental, it can be realistic or only relative in terms of the anxiety and helplessness of the person submitting to this authority.

Power on the one side, fear on the other, are always the buttresses on which irrational authority is built.

There have been many discussions about the use and abuse of power. The use of power is helpful when an authority, someone with knowledge, shares it with others, thus lessening the difference between them. The abuse of power occurs when an authoritarian figure, someone with a lot of power, uses it to lessen the power of those below, thus widening the gap between them.

It is most interesting that in many of the traditionalist Amerindian tribes, the parents do not exercise authority over their children. They do not tell them to go to school, to go to bed, or what to do, and they are not considered to be the major sources of wisdom, that is the province of the grandparents and the elders of the tribe.

These concepts of power and authority come into clinical focus when we look at the adolescent and his or her encounters with authority. Adolescent rebellion is a common catchphrase, and a headline grabber, used to describe anything from challenging the parents' neurotic decisions to violent clashes with established authority. For a long time, adolescent psychiatry accepted Anna Freud's formulation that an adolescent who did not overtly rebel was too constricted and inhibited, and heading for trouble. Daniel Offer (1987) laid that theory to rest with an extensive study that showed that many healthy adolescents wended their way through their adolescence in peace and quiet. James Masterson (1967) found that many tumultuous adolescents develop into borderline adults.

The child's first involvement with authority is with the parents. The vagaries of the parental exercise of authority will be sharply reflected in the adolescent's dealings with other adults. As the early adolescent proceeds into the deidealizing of the parents, the parents' stability, integrity, knowledge, and tolerance for the deidealization will enable the young adolescent to maintain a working relationship with parents' and other's authority (Lage, 1991). It is very difficult for the adolescent to respect authority when his or her life experience has been with dysfunctional parents—abusive, alcoholic, promiscuous, antisocial, criminal.

In recent years, because of the rapid changes in the world of the adult, parents have increasingly come to doubt the givens—religious, moral, legal, and governmental codes and mores—upon which they have based their authority. The result has been an insidious and public erosion of adult authority.

For thousands of years, one could read the future by looking back at the past. If one's father and grandfather had been a farmer, then in all likelihood one would become a farmer. Girls could safely assume that they would grow into the roles of mothers and housewives, because that was the role that women had always played. Fathers and mothers, grandfathers and grandmothers, shared their experiences and wisdom with their children and grandchildren to prepare them for the future. Their authority over the adolescent was based on their knowledge and the adolescent's respect for that knowledge. A rapidly changing world has disenfranchised these parents and grandparents. To most of them, the changes are so rapid that they feel lost, as they see the jobs they always knew disappearing, political lines that they always knew fading, their knowledge base being challenged and eroded by new discoveries, and new technologies appearing that outdate and destroy their world. We are told that the amount of knowledge in the world today doubles every two years. Kenneth Boulding said that "the world of today . . . is as different from the world in which I was born as that world was from Julius Caesar's. I was born in the middle of human history. Almost as much has happened since I was born as happened before" (cited in Toffler, 1970, p.13). Today, he would have to say that he was born near the dawn of human history.

About the same time, Margaret Mead (1970) suggested that parents were like immigrants in a strange land, a land that differed from the land where they grew up, not in location, but in time. She suggested that the only real natives of this new land were the youth of the day, and that the older generation were visitors from elsewhere. Kenneth Kenniston (1965) stated that many adolescents feel that the world of their parents is so far estranged from their world, the present world, that it does not even merit consideration, and they feel pity for their parents. From mid-childhood on, our future adolescents have been aware of the confusion of their parents, of their division on many important issues, of their frustration with society. Consequently, the authority of the adult culture is compromised in the eyes of many adolescents, and with it the authority derived by parents from their position as family representatives of that culture (Conger, 1971). This means that the authority of the parents no longer comes from their status as representatives of a unified adult society, it must come from their own individual strengths and resources.

Lack of confidence in the effectiveness and basis of their authority has led many parents to assume postures without conviction and to make assertions that lack substance. Instead of operating from a base of functionally earned authority, adults have often relied upon coercive power or upon evoking guilt in the adolescents. . . . Power struggles follow soon and under conditions unfavourable for both the adolescent's development and the well-being of adults [GAP Report. 1978, p. 168].

The parent of today, because of the rapid changes in society, is not in a good position to teach the adolescent about the world. He or she is, however, in the position of being able to teach the adolescent how to cope with the world and its changes: how to analyze a situation, how to obtain information, how to weigh the pros and cons of each choice, and how to change in case his or her choice proves wrong. These skills will help the young person proceed with the tasks of adolescence, which despite all the changes in the world remain the same: the development of independence, the establishment of a sexual identity, the choice of a vocational identity, and the development of a system of values.

John Janeway Conger (1971) wrote:

The fact that in today's rapidly changing world these tasks may be more complex, and that both parent and child have fewer consistent blueprints to guide them in their accomplishment, does not fundamentally alter the situation. Sexual and social roles of men and women may change, as indeed they are changing today; the responsibilities and privileges associated with independence may change; the difficulties of projecting the vocational needs of the future may increase; and the kind of personal and social identity that will be viable in both today's and tomorrow's world may alter. But each remains a critical and indispensable task of adolescent development [p. 1122].

One of the major changes in our society, and one that has greatly complicated the tasks of adolescence is the removal from the world of the adolescent of adults with whom they could relate, adults who could help them in their struggles around issues of authority. The average American family moves once every five years, often from one city to another. Many adolescents rarely see, and hardly know their grandparents, aunts and uncles, because they live in other cities. The only adults they know in their families are those in the nuclear family, and that, because of separation and divorce may be only a single parent family. If the parents or parent has major problems, such as alcoholism, depression, and criminality, the children are exposed to it full bore, without any intervening protection from the extended family, who could have presented a different image of authority.

This family mobility moves adolescents away from the neighbours, and from the possibility of having adult neighbours as friends, and it also moves them away from their close friends, and their friend's parents. The result is that adolescents often find that the only adults available for them that they can bounce their ideas off of are their parents. Many cannot use their parents for this purpose because of the state of their struggles for independence at that time, so there is no influence from loving authority on their newly conceived concepts of society. Several of my patients have told me about similar situations to that of my patient, Jeff, who told me how amazed he was that his girlfriend liked to talk to his parents, discussing her ideas and problems with them, while he could not stand to talk to his parents. But he enjoyed talking with her parents, whom she could not stand.

It used to be that an adolescent boy could see his father at work, and sense his father's role in society, his capabilities, and knowledge. As parents rarely work in or near the home now, today's adolescent rarely has that authority-endowing opportunity. This change also interferes with the adolescent's development of a vocational identity.

There used to be a time when one went to school and had only one teacher, someone who had taught your siblings, and knew that your dad was alcoholic, and could be understanding when there were family problems. Today, adolescents have a different teacher every hour, and the teachers often do not ever know the names of all their many students. This changed structure has removed a significant adult authority with whom the adolescent could relate.

Also amongst the adults who have been removed from the adolescent's world has been the policeman who walked the beat every day, and knew a lot of the kids on the beat. Today, he drives around, out of conversational reach inside his automobile fortress.

The clergy also have disappeared from the adolescent world. In the eyes of today's adolescents, the clergy are not as relevant as they were earlier in this century, they are seldom seen to be within the family circle, and are generally considered to be out of touch.

Adolescents have also lost opportunities for contact with adults because of the changed ways in which adults socialize. In times past, families visited families, and children and adolescents got to know

56

their parents' friends, almost as another extended family. Not only do adults party by themselves nowadays, but the children tend to socialize within their own age group, so that they do not get exposed to the thinking, and the needs of other age groups.

To return to my earlier stated premise that authority in its best sense involves the sharing of knowledge between the persons in authority and those subject to authority, it is axiomatic that there must be opportunities for the sharing to occur in order for it to happen. Sharing between people takes place through talking, observing, and doing things together. With adolescents and adults, discussions, working alongside each other, or just observing each other, provide opportunities for such sharing of knowledge. It can be seen from the examples above that forces in society preclude these opportunities for many adolescents. Many of the adults who could best take part in such discussions have been removed from the world of the adolescent. Some years ago a White House Conference on Children took an even broader view of that topic when they wrote that children and adolescents are currently

> deprived not only of parents but of people in general. A host of factors conspire to isolate the young from the rest of society. The fragmentation of the extended family, the separation of residential and business areas, the disappearance of neighbourhoods, zoning ordinances, occupational mobility, child labor laws, the abolishment of the apprentice system, consolidated schools, television, separate patterns of social life for different age groups, the working mother, the delegation of child care to specialists—all these manifestations of progress operate to decrease opportunity and incentive for meaningful contact between children and persons older, or younger, than themselves [p. 1111].

They go on to say,

> The young cannot pull themselves up by their own bootstraps. It is primarily through observing, playing, and working with others older and younger than himself that a child discovers both what he can do and who he can become—that he develops both his ability and his identity. It is primarily through exposure and interaction with adults and children of different ages that a child (or adolescent) acquires new interests and skills and learns the meaning of tolerance, cooperation, and compassion. Hence to relegate children to a world of their own is to deprive them of their humanity . . . Yet, this is what is happening in America today [cited in Conger, 1971].

There are many indicators of trouble between North American society and its youth. The increasingly high rate of juvenile crime speaks to the refusal of so many of our youth to accept society's laws. The high number of adolescent runaways, many of whom become involved in crime and prostitution speaks to the battle between youth and their families. The increasing rate of high school dropouts, and the mounting numbers of violent incidents in the schools speak to the inability of society and its schools to establish their authority in the eyes of our youth. And I would suggest that we would have much more intergenerational upheaval, if not for the suppressive effects of these severe economic times, which have our youth fearfully trying to position themselves to cope with a terrifying, unpredictable future.

Over the past three decades, there have been some changes in the social world of the adolescent that have had profound effects on his or her view of society. There has been a steady increase in the amount of violence and killing, mostly due to the spread of street drugs. The advent of the drug scene, with its steadily increasing involvement of organized crime, street and biker gangs, seems to be accepted by the police forces, who ignore the gangs, and steal the confiscated drugs. The turning of a blind eye to this situation by adult society, this abdication of responsibility, has brought into question the respectability of adult authorities. The obvious inequity of the justice system, where children from the lower socioeconomic class are treated much more harshly than those from the upper middle and upper socioeconomic classes, is common knowledge amongst the adolescents. If one cannot afford a good lawyer the mechanical function of the justice system becomes monolithic and impersonal. Anna Freud (1965) referred to one aspect of this when she wrote that "'to be equal before the law' implies that all claims for benefits, privileges, and preferential treatment on personal grounds have to be abandoned. It remains a difficult step, and one not achieved by everybody, to accept that the community enforces its laws, and punishes transgression, without reference to the [individual's] intellectual and characterological status which either fits him or incapacitates him for compliance with the law."

"By the book" adherence to "equality before the law" is perceived by many adolescents to be cold, inhumane, and unfair, particularly since the rich get preferential treatment. If you steal a videotape you go to jail, but if you scam several million dollars off a Savings and Loan institution, nothing happens. If the courts and the police are not deserving of respect, is it any wonder that so many adolescents do not accept society's laws?

This unempathic, insensitive, often callous approach of the legal system is repeated in the educational system where it has far more impact. Society's desire to provide mass education economically, has created a factory for the production of alienated youth, if I may use an outdated but accurate term. Anna Freud (1965) wrote, "School rules take less or no notice of individual differences . . . within the age group all individuals are expected to conform to a common norm, whatever sacrifice this may mean to their personalities" (p. 182).

Kenneth Kenniston (1975), in describing the progression from adolescence to what he calls the stage of "youth," says that the adolescent struggles to define who he is, the youth begins to sense who he is, and recognizes the possibility of conflict between his emerging selfhood and his social order. Kenniston states that the struggle for individuation is with the family in adolescence, and with society during youth; and that the failure of individuation, that is, to cope with social reality, is alienation, whether from self or from society.

Edgar Friedenberg (1965) wrote extensively about alienation, attributing much of the responsibility for it to the schools, which he felt fostered a bland, vacuous, affable, "all-American" youth with no depth, and little capacity for commitment. He used the scenario of a youngster in a class, discussing the current topic, which happens to have been of particular interest to him, and in which he has therefore developed a significant expertise. He is interrupted by the teacher who says, "That's an interesting point. Now let's hear what other pupils think of it." The message is clear that his personal interest and expertise is not important, that what counts is what everybody has to say about it, and that it is the working relationship within the group that is important. Friedenberg (1959) wrote, "Students are likely to find that they can only win esteem by how they look and behave, not for what they are. The effect of this is a severe form of alienation; they lose faith in their right to an independent judgment of their own worth" (p. 108). They are alienated from themselves.

In talking about the alienating effects of the school, Friedenberg (1965) wrote, "The students want to discover who they are; the school wants to help them 'make something out of themselves.' They want to know where they are; the school wants to help them get somewhere. They want to learn how to live with themselves; the school wants to teach them how to get along with others. They want to learn how to tell what is right for them; the school wants to teach them to give the responses that will earn them rewards in the classroom and in social situations" (p. 212). How they look and behave, not for what they are.

Other writers have commented that when a student comes into the school, the system does not want to hear that his father beat up on his mother the night before, or that his dog was killed, they want him to do his math, and do it now. This mechanistic approach to education has been tabbed as one of the major causes of alienation from the self, with the youngster being forced to suppress his emotions, and being put out of touch with who he is, and what his capabilities are. He only knows how to get along in society. If a youngster is in difficulty, the focus is not on the understanding of why he is in that situation, but on the necessity of his not being in such a situation.

How they look and behave, not for what they are.

What message does society, through its surrogate, the educational system, give its adolescents, when it hails the educational success of a youngster who is mean, vicious, selfish, and ungiving? It says, in effect, "We don't care what kind of a louse you are, put down on paper what we want to see, and we will graduate you, magna cum laude"

How they look and behave, not for what they are.

I am reminded of the comment that a Cree medicine man made to me after I asked him about the meaning of the circle in the Indian religion. He talked about the circle being a natural form in nature, how the spheres of the earth, sun, and moon, and their orbits, are based on circles; that the winds and the waters move in circles, and therefore the natives live in circular houses and sit in circles when they talk. He then commented to me that he could not understand the white man, who puts his children in rows in school where they can only relate to the back of the neck of the child in front of them.

And then there was a 15-year-old patient of mine who came in raging. He got a "D" on an essay on "Nonconformity" because he did not put down what had been discussed in class.

During the Gulf War, a group of adult organizers of an antiwar protest in Toronto were jolted by the number of teens who phoned up to ask how they should dress for the event, and what the signs should say.

If the schools, with parental approval, are teaching the kids that it is appearance that counts, and are suppressing their sense of self, if we alienate them from themselves, we then produce a generation of adolescents who do not care about anyone else, who do not feel for those in distress or trouble, and who only think of themselves.

Recently, a prominent Canadian pollster, Michael Adams of Environics Research Group (1992), surveyed today's teenagers in several cities and reported, "Most of today's teenagers are in the remarkable and almost unprecedented situation of having no sense of themselves as being members of an exceptional generation. Every generation since perhaps the conformist Edwardians has had its own myth, has known for sure it had something new to offer . . . not these kids. These kids don't think in terms of 'we.' For them the imperative is the first person singular. . . . They simply do not understand why they would want to change things. . . . Adolescence today is not the home of dreams or even ideas. It is the boot camp for adulthood. Today, the prime occupation of most teenagers is to find their niche in society and nestle into it like a hand in a fur-lined glove."

The educational system, along with the work world, have long been fingered as major contributors to the alienation of our youth from society. Youngsters are told, over and over again, that in order to get a job in the adult world they will need an education. They are told that with today's changing job market, and the development of labor-saving machinery, that they are doomed to years in the unemployment lines if they do not get their high school diploma. Yet, the reality is that even with a high school diploma, they know that the chances of getting jobs are greatly diminished from what they used to be. Furthermore, many of the high schools are set up so that only a fraction are able to graduate. Many students have access to only a handful of technical-vocational high schools. By contrast, there is a whole armada of academic high schools where only about half the pupils will ever go straight through to graduation. Many of the pupils will require extra years in order to stumble through to graduation. The message that many of the youngsters get is that this is not their world, that they cannot make it in this world, that their skills, talents and abilities are not valued by the authorities, and therefore they will not be able to get all the good things in life that they see advertised on television. Their response is a rejection of the adult world and its authority and its laws. This is one of the major causes of juvenile crime. One AmerIndian youngster with whom I had worked for several years told me, while terminating treatment, after he had become settled in a quite good working situation, that the main thing he had gotten from me was the realization that he could make it in this world, that he did not have to resort to crime to avoid poverty.

We need to take an honest look at the attitude to authority that results amongst members of the lower socioeconomic class, when siblings are constantly sick or dying from the effects of poverty, whether it be inadequate housing or poor nutrition, or in the U.S. an absence of medical care. One has to ask, how can these adolescents have respect for the authority of the adult world, when that adult world turns a blind eye to their pain?

I would like to take a moment to look at another educational system—the television. A Minister of Education in France stated that their studies indicated that before the advent of television, 80% of what an adolescent knew came from what he learned in school; now 80% of what he knows comes from watching television. Television teaches its lessons directly and indirectly. Direct teaching is in the form of documentaries, school lessons, and the various educational programs such as those on PBS. They are usually well prepared, informative, and presented in an interesting way. Inevitably, students will contrast the quality of the teaching in school with the teaching on television. The anger that results is not at the school for lacking fancy production facilities, but at those teachers who lack the commitment to make the studies interesting, at those authorities who rob them of their right to a good education. As psychiatrists, we know that being boring is a hostile act.

Indirect teaching is by way of the implications of the programming. A number of studies have reported that the average high school graduate has watched some 15,000 hours of television, much of it in prime time while he was wide awake. During that time, the graduate had watched some 31,000 murders, and an unbelievable number of beatings. If this is what his family serves up to him in his own living room as entertainment, what underlying message does the child and adolescent draw about the value of life, and the sanctity of the human body? How often do the shows that they watch portray the authority figures as bumbling fools, and how seldom are they portrayed as being competent and respectable?

Finally, a brief look at society as a whole. Robert Lindner (1956) wrote that initially society was formed by a group of individuals banding together for their protection from enemies, for the provision of necessities, and for fellowship.

In return, Lindner says, the individual gave his strength against the enemy, the product of his labour, and the comfort of his presence. . . . Society then could be regarded largely as the product of separate units, as a consensus established and maintained by its component parts. This is no longer true. No more is society the servant of man, no more does it reflect and implement his personal requirements, no more does it find its source in the consent of its parts, and no more can it be held that society is man. For it has come about over the centuries that the organism originally created by the participation of its individual units has assumed a life of its own. It has also acquired a disposition unfriendly to humans. In short, society has become a stranger to man, and a hostile stranger at that [p. 150].

A few years ago a Marxist philosopher said that if Karl Marx were alive today, he would not be focusing on the oppression of the masses by the capitalists, but on the oppression of the masses by the bureaucracy. I am sure that everyone has their favorite story about bureaucratic oppression. As physicians, we are aware of how easily hospitals lose their focus on the well-being of patients for the sake of easing the work of the hospital staff. A high school student speaking about his school said that it would run perfectly if only there were no students in it. In every institution there is a tension, a natural tug-of-war, between the need to provide service to a specific population, and the desire of the institutional staff to have life as easy as possible. Unfortunately, the staff often wins the battle, and an obstructive monolith is created.

We need our adolescents to challenge those institutions that fail to serve humanity, to challenge those institutions that alienate them, and to challenge all of us adults to prove the wisdom, knowledge, and understanding that qualifies us as authorities.

At an American Orthopsychiatric Association meeting that I attended in about 1969, Fritz Redl, famous for his work with delinquents, was chairing a panel discussion on the anti-Viet Nam war protesters. About 25 of the protesters suddenly marched in, placards and all, protesting our discussing them. Redl invited them to join us. Their leader demanded to know why we were discussing them. Redl said, very sincerely, that sadly, on the campus where he worked, there were no stirrings of protest, and he hoped by studying the protesters that he might then be able to bring some to life on his campus. The protestors were taken aback, and then their leader asked why they were not invited. Redl replied, "If we had invited you, you wouldn't have come." Everyone laughed, they sat down, and we had a most stimulating and informative afternoon, greatly enriched by the contributions of the youths.

Let us hope that our adolescents will do battle with society's dehumanized institutions, and that they will continue to question our beliefs and our values, for implicit in their challenge is their faith in the future and their belief that they can build a better world. History is on their side.

REFERENCES

Adams, M. (1992), *The Young Fogeys.* Toronto Globe and Mail, May 23.

Aristotle (1964), *The Universal Experience of Adolescence*, ed. N. Kiell. Boston: Beacon Press, p. 18–19.

Conger, J. J. (1971), A world they never knew. In: *Daedalus*, 100:1105–1138.

Freud, A. (1965), Dissociality, delinquency, criminality as diagnostic categories in childhood. In: *The Writings of Anna Freud*, Vol. VI. New York: International Universities Press. pp. 182–183.

Friedenberg, E. (1959), *The Vanishing Adolescent.* New York: Dell.

_____ (1965), *Coming of Age in America.* New York: Random House.

Fromm, E. (1947), *Man for Himself.* New York: Rinehart & Company.

Group for the Advancement of Psychiatry Report (1978). *Power and Authority in Adolescence*, Vol. 10, No. 101. New York: Group for the Advancement of Psychiatry.

Kenniston, K. (1965), Social change and youth in America. In: *The Challenge of Youth.* ed. E. Erikson. New York: Anchor Books, pp. 191–222.

_____ (1975), Prologue. In: *Youth: National Society for the Study of Education Yearbook.* Chicago: University of Chicago Press. pp. 3–26.

Lage, G. & Nathan, H. (1991), *Psychotherapy, Adolescents, and Self-Psychology.* Madison, CT: International Universities Press.

Lindner, R. (1956), *Must You Conform?* New York: Grove Press.

Masterson, J. (1967), *The Psychiatric Dilemma of Adolescence.* Boston, MA: Little, Brown.

Mead, M. (1970), *Culture and Commitment*. New York: Natural History Press/Doubleday.

Offer, D. (1987), The mystery of adolescence. In: *Adolescent Psychiatry*, 14:7–27. Chicago: University of Chicago Press.

Toffler, A. (1970), *Future Shock*. New York: Random House.

MAX SUGAR

Media coverage of disasters usually highlights the reactions of children and adults, but little is usually said about the reactions of teenagers. Because the younger child is at greatest physical risk, this perhaps invites our early healing efforts. Usually the adult verbalizes the need for help and seeks it voluntarily unless psychological denial is practiced. Since adolescents generally tend to avoid making their reactions and needs known following a disaster, it is important to learn how they react, what interferes with the expression of their reaction, and what to do for them. These are the foci of this chapter.

Review of Literature

Very few reports of disasters have adolescents as the central issue, and most of the following data were extracted from general assessments. For example, during a blackout in San Francisco, delinquent female juveniles in a group home fought one another violently in the dark (Solomon, 1942). Crawshaw (1963) reported that after a cyclone teens exhibited group excitement, and denial with more conscious anxiety. Two years after the Buffalo Creek flood disaster, the teenagers showed increased juvenile delinquency (Erikson, 1976).

On reviewing the findings of the Buffalo Creek disaster, Gleser, Green, and Winget (1981) noted that two years after the event, the presence of symptoms depended on age, with those aged 12 to 14 having more symptoms than younger children and fewer than adults. The overall severity of symptoms—belligerence, depression, and anxiety—was greatest in the 16- to 20-year-olds. Prior to the flood, there was hypertension in 9% of black males, 2% of white males, 23% of black females, and 8% of white females. However, two years after the flood, 25% of white adolescent females and 41% of white adolescent males had hypertension. These are markedly increased rates for whites, and a reversal of the usual black and white ratio.

Two years after the flood the youngsters were smoking, drinking, racing vehicles, robbing, and brawling in groups. Those aged 12 to 15 years had more belligerence, post-flood, based on separation or death of parent, and 75% of these youngsters had insomnia. There was a 12% increase in delinquency. Females were more disturbed compared with males at every age and had a 9% increase in teen pregnancies. White male and female adolescents were more disturbed than their black counterparts. Four years after the disaster some adolescents showed more impairment than before, and more than 30% suffered debilitating symptoms.

Green et al. (1991) corroborated the findings of Gleser et al. (1981) on young adolescents. They noted increased intrusion, denial, and arousal symptoms compared with children and that the highest total of posttraumatic stress disorder (PTSD) symptoms was in older adolescents. Depending on the mothers' and fathers' severity of symptoms, parental functioning had a significant effect on youngsters, and more so with mothers' severity than fathers'. An irritable or depressed family atmosphere predicted increased PTSD symptoms in the adolescents, but the presence of a life threat was the most significant predictor of PTSD in the youngster.

Using community-based data, pre- and postdisaster, Adams and Adams (1984) found an increase in juvenile bookings, vandalism, and assaults.

Frederick (1985) observed that after a disaster, 60% of those under age 18 had PTSD. Among children 11 to 14 he noted sleep and appetite disruption, rebelliousness, fighting, withdrawal, loss of interest, excessive need for attention, physical and psychosomatic symptoms, and school misbehavior. Those aged 14 to 18 had similar symptoms, as well as amenorrhea or dysmenorrhea, apathy, agitation, decreased interest in the opposite sex; and irresponsible or delinquent behavior.

One and a half years after the threat of a nuclear radiation disaster, which led to evacuation at Three Mile Island, a residual level of anxiety was found in adolescents (Handford et al., 1986). Rigamer (1986) noted increased denial, suspicion, xenophobia, and prejudice along with intellectualization in adolescents in a life-threatening situation. Toubiana et al. (1988) recorded withdrawal, school refusal, and separation anxiety symptoms in adolescents following a school bus disaster.

Yule and Williams (1990) observed that after a shipwreck, ten youngsters aged 11 to 15 reported higher levels of disaster symptoms (of 50% and 75%) when seen separately from parents and teachers, respectively.

Family Considerations

After a cyclone, Crawshaw (1963) found that there was often a family fight and hostility between spouses even when there was no physical damage to the home or injury to its occupants. The overall symptom severity in parents two years after the Buffalo Creek disaster correlated with those of the offspring. The increase in out-of-wedlock pregnancies correlated with the mothers' overall symptom severity and mothers' alcohol abuse. The increase in delinquency related to alcohol abuse for fathers and mothers, alcohol-related imprisonment for fathers and mothers, and depression in fathers. The severity rating of the fathers correlated with that of adolescent sons, and anxiety in sons and daughters. Belligerence in fathers correlated with depression in sons (Gleser et al., 1981).

With violence in the family atmosphere after the Buffalo Creek flood, the children were more impaired. The distress of each family member "tended to feed and grow on that of the other members" (Gleser et al., 1981).

Since adolescents are generally less dependent on others than are young children or the aged, they may seem to be comparatively self-sufficient and less vulnerable to further trauma postdisaster. After a disaster, adults experience a confused state with shock, disruption of their daily lives, and threats to their integrity (physically, socially, and emotionally), which affects their handling of the children. When parents, rescue workers, and physicians have their own posttraumatic difficulties to deal with (or use denial), they may not notice the adolescent's problems (Handford et al., 1986; Sugar, 1988a; Wraith, 1988; Yule and Udwin, 1991).

Factors Contributing to Disaster Effects

Disasters may cause death, leading to bereavement or grief reactions in the survivors; injuries with physical pain or handicap; emotional disturbance; domiciliary displacement; and geographic relocation. All of these contribute to the teenager's emotional response.

A disaster is accompanied by multiple traumatic events, during and afterward, such as intrusions, loss of home, loss of community, and so on, with a consequent upheaval of family life which causes disruption in the youngsters' development (Erikson, 1976; Sugar, 1988b, 1989; Wraith, 1988).

Fifty percent of adolescent refugees from Cambodia had PTSD four years after their Cambodian trauma. They, unlike U.S.-born youngsters, had no substance abuse or oppositional or disruptive behavior (Kinzie et al., 1986; Sack et al., 1986). Different behaviors are manifest to express distress in adolescents, depending on family and cultural factors. The absence of cultural and family models for the Cambodian refugees to abuse substances or to be disruptive or oppositional was apparent in the absence of such among these youngsters.

Adolescents' Responses to Disaster

In adolescents there may be a specific postdisaster clinical presentation along with some varying symptoms. Among immediate nonspecific effects are marked anxiety, brief crying or screaming, confusion with a shocklike state, disorganization, frozen or inhibited movement, apathy, a sense of hopelessness, withdrawal, disturbed appetite, insomnia, separation anxiety, and school refusal.

Nonspecific reactions that may be evident in a few days or weeks after the disaster include insomnia, nightmares, somnambulism, clinging to parents, a lack of personal responsibility, poor school performance, withdrawal, apathy, loss of usual interests including the opposite sex, concentration and attention problems, headaches, nausea, vomiting, loss of appetite and weight, bowel problems, psychosomatic symptoms, hostility, irritability, anxiety, violent behavior, brooding, development of omens with negative predictions, lesser goals, foreshortening of the future, pessimism, guilt about survival (Terr, 1979, 1983; Sugar, 1989), and hypertension (Gleser et al., 1981).

Postdisaster adolescents are at risk for vandalism, malicious mischief, disorderly conduct and assault (Adams and Adams, 1984), brawling, robbery, delinquency, increased use and abuse of alcohol, drugs and tobacco (Erikson, 1976; Gleser et al., 1981). There may be early dissociative reactions (i.e., sudden temporary altered states of consciousness, identity, or motor behavior), and multiple personality organization may occur later.

Specific to the disaster, adolescents may have fears, depression, anxiety, and belligerence (Green et al., 1991); recalling and reexperiencing the disaster with various stimuli; phobias about these with startle (diffuse motor) responses; and risky behavior. There are also distortions and misperceptions in time with sequencing, duration, and time skew. Yule and Williams (1990) and Sugar (1989) have noted intrusive symptoms and amnesia in some adolescents, which is opposite to the findings by Garmezy and Rutter (1985). Yule and Williams (1990) also found flashbacks and avoidance.

Adolescents have increased cognitive ability compared with children and can assess and perceive trauma quite well. The youngsters' responses are due to their own perceptions of the trauma, based on their cognitive, emotional, and physical developmental level. However, the responses may be influenced by family factors. (Gleser et al., 1981; Frederick, 1985; Handford et al., 1986). There is a more extreme or severe reaction in those closer to the disaster; the injured; those whose parents or friends are injured, dead, or missing: those with poor and disorganized living conditions; those relocated geographically or separated from their family; and in response to intrusions by strangers.

Gender Differences

Milne (1977), Ollendick and Hoffman (1983), Dohrenwend et al., (1981), Gleser et al. (1981), Milgram et al., (1988), and Zeidner (1993) report that adolescent girls show more distress than boys. Adolescent boys tend to discharge angry and anxious feelings in a hostile and antisocial fashion, even if this had not been their previous pattern. They use significant denial and experience more difficulty in engaging, and remaining, in therapy compared with girls. Teenage girls also are threatened by revealing their symptoms, and by a sense of lost control (similar to feelings about their menses) that decreases motivation for therapy.

Diagnoses Resulting from Disaster Trauma

Youngsters have variable abilities to cope, and some resilient ones may have no evidence of emotional residua of a disaster. Others may have delayed effects such as continued and repeated frightening dreams of the trauma, dissociative episodes, intrusive thoughts, amnesia, hypervigilance, hyperarousal, fugues, or multiple personality. The connection between the disaster and adolescents' poor academic performance, misconduct, increased numbers of unwed pregnant adolescents, delinquency, vandalism, alcoholism, rowdiness, and substance abuse may be overlooked. Some youngsters may not have any reaction owing to their poor perception of the trauma.

All youngsters in a disaster will not have an observable emotional reaction or PTSD. They may have a generalized anxiety disorder, a depressive disorder, an adjustment disorder, conduct disorder, or other psychiatric diagnosis. The diagnosis of PTSD is a frequent accompaniment of disasters.

PTSD may be seen immediately in some adolescents and last for years after. Their symptoms may not be obviously connected with the disaster and may go unnoticed for many years. Prior individual or family psychopathology compounds the problem (Handford et al., 1986).

Case Examples

CASE EXAMPLE 1

During a disaster that destroyed his home, an 11-year-old male was severely injured. The family was evacuated safely and moved to temporary, cramped quarters, without a phone, in another town. For many months afterward, there were poor arrangements for daily needs, school, recreation, and so on. He complained of backache and neckache. Several months later he still had not resumed school One night while the boy's mother was experiencing an anxiety attack, her mate insisted on sexual intercourse. When she refused and he persisted, she screamed for help and all five children came to the bedroom. When this boy then attacked the father-surrogate with a knife, the father-surrogate took it from him. The mother feared the boy would be killed, but the boy escaped their quarters and ran for the police two-and-a-half blocks away. By the time the police appeared the man had fled with the only set of keys to the apartment after locking the family inside. Later, when he returned, apparently after he had been drinking, they feared he would kill them. When evaluated many weeks later, the youngster had PTSD and a conduct disorder with violent behavior. He was hostile and distrustful, and rejected efforts to engage him in therapy. The mother was interested in the youngster's continued psychiatric treatment, but he refused it.

This case illustrates some of the multiple trauma (dislocation, school and community disruption) after a disaster (Sugar, 1988b) as well as the inappropriate behavior of the father-figure (drinking, violence, denial of his mate's distress) and the disrupted family of an early adolescent with severe emotional disorders.

CASE EXAMPLE 2

This girl, aged 15, whose neck and back were injured in a disaster, had thought intrusion, flashbacks, recurrent thoughts and nightmares about the disaster, an increase in weight and appetite, and an avoidance of stimuli that reminded her of the disaster. She was restless and irritable and fussed with her siblings, emotionally distant from peers, and felt picked on by peers and teachers after the disaster. She had great sensitivity to noise and avoided it (e.g., movies). She showed denial but was aware of her sadness. She pursued repetitive meaningless activities, for example, repeatedly writing her name. Her diagnosis was PTSD. She was uncooperative and hostile about psychotherapy.

CASE EXAMPLE 3

This 13-year-old male injured his neck and jaw in a disaster and was still in a neck brace several months later. He was withdrawn, less talkative and friendly than before the disaster, and insomniac. His daydreaming about the disaster in class led to disciplinary action by teachers. His other symptoms fulfilled criteria for the diagnosis of PTSD, but he was opposed to therapy.

These cases illustrate some of the range of reactions, symptoms, and diagnoses in adolescent victims of disasters.

Developmental Tasks and Disasters

Does experiencing a disaster propel adolescents into a more exaggerated, obviously rebellious, and disorganized reaction to the separation from the infantile objects? Adolescents seem generally to have intrapsychic general disorganization and in response to a disaster this becomes apparent in their symptomatic behavior (Erikson, 1976;

Gleser et al., 1981; Adams and Adams, 1984; Green et al., 1991). The adolescent's ordinary need for groups (Buxbaum, 1946) is evident and exaggerated in the gang formation and group delinquent acts among adolescent victims of disaster. Some of this may be attributed to loss of home, family, community, or routine and may reflect family dysfunction and community disorganization, while some appears to be a response to the survival threat from the disaster. In addition, these acts may be viewed as compounded by generalized and unfocused expressions of anger and revenge at the disaster, losses, feelings of helplessness, and as efforts at mastery. Peer friendships are very important to adolescents, and if there are losses of or injuries to peers, this may increase these reactions.

Blos (1979) observed that when trauma occurs to an adolescent, it confirms the negative polarities of existence —bad, helpless, and so on—which are countered by omnipotent fantasies. In a disaster, when the bad and unpredictable have intruded as actualities that threaten the youngster's survival and against which the family is impotent, then the peer group or gang becomes very important, more so than the usual adolescent groupings. The occurrence of gang delinquency postdisaster is compatible with these developments and is confirmatory of Kernberg's (1984) feeling that their violence "reflects the need to destroy any external reality that interferes with" the illusion of power and omnipotence of the youngster via the group.

Koenig (1964) observed that adolescent Holocaust survivors had chronic identity diffusion, interpersonal difficulties, and poor work values. This indicates arrested or incomplete late adolescent development. Whether this may be the case in other disaster victims is unclear since the Holocaust involved repeated exposure to multiple trauma, death threats, terror, and starvation over many years, whereas disasters are usually of short duration although multiple trauma follow (Sugar, 1988b).

The effects of disaster on long-term adolescent development need further study, since there are no long term individual treatment reports.

Countertransference

Many disasters are currently recorded and some have been recorded since ancient times. But unlike hysteria, which Hippocrates described in antiquity, the effects of disasters on health were not attended to until recent decades. The effects on children were noted later, and those on adolescents are just beginning to be addressed.

There are many man-made and natural disasters annually, but they are not often totaled. For example, between 1971 and 1980, the presidents of the United States declared 326 major natural disasters (e.g., floods, hurricanes) (Gordon, 1982). This excluded industrial and societal disasters such as wars, toxic fumes, airplane crashes, train wrecks, and nuclear accidents. The Federal Emergency Management Agency, the Red Cross, cities, and states have disaster teams that usually provide a good response and care for children and adults. However, little of the care appears to be directed to adolescents. This reduced focus may be seen also in the paucity of reports (medical and psychiatric) on adolescents.

If we turn to events that are more frequent than the major disasters, perhaps they will shed further light on this problem. Fires are the fifth leading cause of fatalities in those under age 19 (Centers for Disease Control, 1990), and there were 4,835 fatalities to all ages in 1986 as a result of fires (U.S. Dept. of Commerce, 1990, p. 85). Many child-adolescent family survivors and neighbors have emotional distress in response to the fires, but these problems are frequently unnoticed (Jones and Ribbe, 1991) although the youths may have PTSD symptoms.

Accidents are the leading cause of death among 15- to 24-year-olds with a rate of 51.3 per 100,000 in 1988, most of which are males by about a 3:1 ratio (U.S. Department of Commerce, 1990). Many of these fatalities are accompanied by alcohol or other drug abuse. There are many survivors whose physical condition is attended to but without much focus on their emotional distress, although they may have a variety of psychiatric diagnoses. What might account for this? Only during infancy does the human undergo more developmental changes than in adolescence, and therefore more attention would be expected for adolescents after a disaster than has been the case. Denial occurs in the adults involved as victims, observers, or helpers, including parents, teachers, relief workers, and physicians. There is often a feeling of helplessness in the helpers as they witness the youngsters' struggle to deal with the disaster effects. These feelings may intrude on adults' ability to assess the needs of the teenager for psychiatric help. Countertransference interferences with observation, guidance, and caretaking seems to be the basis for this denial and inattention (Benedek, 1985; Sugar, 1988a, 1989).

The following case highlights some of these considerations.

CASE EXAMPLE 4

A male in his late teens survived a nighttime two-car accident in which his girlfriend, who was the driver, and the driver of the other car were killed. He had some injuries to his limbs for which he received excellent orthopedic treatment, but no psychiatric assessment was done. About two years after the event, he was persuaded to seek psychiatric treatment.

Although he was intoxicated during the accident, he saw and later recalled all the gruesome details of his girlfriend's demise. He had flashbacks, thought intrusion, and some amnesia. He had poor academics, risk-taking behavior, distrust, aggressivity, unsettled vocational goals and friendships, irritability, loss of appetite, insomnia (early and midsleep), anxiety attacks, and fears of dying with night driving, nightmares, feelings of guilt, numbness, lack of interest, and a foreshortened sense of the future. He noted a change from his having been agreeable and compliant around his parents to his being in a state of constant verbal clashes or silence with them.

Prior to the accident he had severely abused alcohol and had been in three car wrecks in which he was the driver. Continued alcohol abuse led to a brief exposure to Alcoholics Anonymous but without any habit change. He was diagnosed with PTSD and alcohol abuse and entered treatment.

Approaches to Adolescent Disaster Victims

Mild transient feelings of depersonalization and derealization appear to be a normal experience that is particularly common in adolescence (Bernstein and Putnam, 1986). Perhaps the stress of a disaster and the reaction to it are experienced as depersonalization or derealization by adolescents. They may then disavow or deny their symptoms of distress, making them less available for psychotherapy. This may be augmented by a "macho" defense and by denial on the part of parents or teachers.

Since their faith in parents' and their own invincibility has been decreased or nullified by the disaster, there is often a sense of hopelessness with apathy that makes them difficult to engage in an evaluation or therapy. Their anger and wish for revenge for losses and disruptions is quite evident in their symptomatic behavior, but the correlation is easily overlooked.

Eighty-nine percent of untreated refugee Cambodian youngsters had emotional disturbance in their twenties, about six years after the events (48% PTSD and 41% depression) (Kinzie et al., 1989). This is similar to the children of Chowchilla who were also untreated, and showed effects of their trauma four to five years afterward (Terr, 1983). The emotional effects of a disaster may be acute and there may be chronic illness with extensive and lengthy impairment that is highly resistant to change. An extended period, and additional effort, is needed for its treatment.

At the time of writing, the literature on adolescents in disasters is limited to epidemiology, phenomena, assessment, and symptoms. Crisis intervention was focused by Toubiana et al. (1988). Currently, there are only two detailed reports of individual treatment of children postdisaster (Saigh, 1986; Sugar, 1988a) but none of adolescents.

Rigamer (1986) recommends giving adolescents more information than younger children, appealing to their cognitive abilities and experiences, and respecting their defenses. Kiser et al. (1993) found that tenth graders who spoke about their feelings before an anticipated earthquake (which did not occur) had increased symptoms before the anticipated date, but they had a significant decrease in symptoms of stress at the second interview, which took place after that date. If the youngsters' families had prepared them for the quake, the adolescents had more stress symptoms before the anticipated date of the quake and a much larger decrease in symptoms afterward compared to those whose families did not prepare them. Yule and Williams (1990) consider that screening scales are of limited value without detailed individual interviews.

Brief group therapy should be available to all disaster victims immediately after the disaster. This is usually provided by the state or local disaster agencies and may go on for 6 to 12 weeks on a weekly or biweekly basis (Sugar, 1989). This is supported by the observations of Toubiana et al. (1988) that crisis management was useful and that some adolescents responded to such efforts.

Immediate psychiatric attention is in order when risky or dangerous behavior follows a disaster. Psychiatric consultation is needed if the youngster's symptoms continue unabated despite reassurance, support, and medication for several weeks after the disaster.

Yule and Williams (1990) found that group therapy with adolescents postdisaster was helpful. However, after more than a year of treatment in a group, the majority of youngsters still had "significant psychological morbidity." Individual, group, and family therapy (Gleser et al., 1981) should be used as needed along with medication. A parallel parents' therapy group may be helpful.

Anger usually accompanies loss (Bowlby, 1958). Anger is a major component in youngsters' mood, behavior, and symptoms. It also is part of their projection and identification with the aggressor when the disaster is of human origin. Therefore, the adolescents' anger is an early and major issue to be addressed in treatment.

Conclusions

This chapter has reviewed the emotional effects on adolescents involved in a disaster. Symptomatic behavior by adolescents postdisaster often involves group delinquent behavior, substance abuse, and unwed adolescent pregnancy. These may be overlooked as related to the disaster, especially when coupled with the youngsters' denial. The consequences may be societal or legal disapproval, but not often psychiatric assessment or treatment.

Recognition of adolescents' postdisaster denial and symptoms is a major determinant for them to have an evaluation and treatment. A complicating factor is that parents and caregivers, owing to their own distressed posttraumatic state, may have problems in recognizing or supporting adolescents' need for therapy. That these adolescents are not seeking treatment clearly adds to their difficulties in obtaining help. For therapists there may be countertransference problems with these youngsters. Among the areas in need of further observation and study are long-term developmental effects and treatment outcome.

REFERENCES

Adams, P. R. & Adams, G. R. (1984), Mount Saint Helens's ashfall: Evidence for a disaster stress reaction. *Amer. Psychol.*, 39:252–260.
Benedek, E. (1985), Children and disaster: Emerging issues. *Psychiat. Annals*, 15:168–172.

Bernstein, E. M. & Putnam, F. W. (1986), Development, reliability and validity of a dissociation scale. *J. Nerv. Ment. Dis.*, 174:727–735.

Blos, P. (1979), *The Adolescent Passage*. New York: International Universities Press.

Bowlby, J. (1958), The nature of the child's tie to his mother. *Internat. J. Psycho-Anal.*, 39:1–23.

Buxbaum, E. (1945), Transference and group formation in children and adolescents. *The Psychoanalytic Study of the Child*, 1:351–365.

Centers for Disease Control. (1990), Childhood injuries in the United States. *Amer. J. Dis. Child.*, 144:627–646.

Crawshaw, R. (1963), Reaction to disaster. *Arch. Gen. Psychiat.*, 9:157–162.

Dohrenwend, B. P., Dohrenwend, B. S., Warheit, G. J., Bartlett, G. S., Goldstein, R. L., Goldstein, K. & Martin, J. L. (1981), Stress in the community: A report to the President's Commission on the accident at Three Mile Island. *Annals NY Acad. Sci.*, 365:159–174.

Erikson, K. (1976) *Everything in Its Path*. New York: Simon & Schuster.

Frederick, C. J. (1985) Children traumatized by catastrophic situations. In: *Post-Traumatic Stress Disorder in Children*, ed. S. Eth & R. S. Pynoos. Washington, DC: American Psychiatric Press, pp. 73–99.

Garmezy, N. & Rutter, M. (1985), Acute reactions to stress. In: *Child Psychiatry: Modern Approaches,* 2nd ed., ed. M. Rutter & L. Hersov. Oxford: Blackwell.

Gleser, G. C., Green, B. L. & Winget, C. (1981), *Prolonged Psychosocial Effects of Disaster*. New York: Academic Press.

Gordon P. (1982), *Special Statistical Summary—Deaths Injuries and Property Loss by Type of Disaster, 1970–1980* (Report No. A127645). Washington, DC: Federal Emergency Management Agency.

Green, B. L., Korol, M., Grace, M. C., Vary, M. G., Leonard, A. C., Gleser, G. C. & Smitson-Cohen, S. (1991), Children and disaster: age, gender and parental effects on PTSD symptoms. *J. Amer. Acad. Child Adoles. Psychiat.*, 30:945–951.

Handford, H. A., Mayes, S. D., Mattison, R. E., Humphrey, F. J., Bagnato, S., Bixler, E. O. & Kales, J. D. (1986), Child and parent reaction to the Three Mile Island nuclear accident. *J. Amer. Acad. Child Psychiat.*, 25:346.

Jones, R. T. & Ribbe, D. P. (1991), Child, adolescent and adult victims of residential fire. *Behav. Mod.*, 15:560–580.

Kernberg, O. F. (1984), The couch at sea: Psychoanalytic studies of group and organizational leadership. *Internat. J. Group Psychother.*, 34:5–23.

Kinzie, J. D., Sack, W. H., Angell, R. H., Manson, S. & Rath, B. (1986), The psychiatric effects of massive trauma on Cambodian children: I. The children. *J. Amer. Acad. Child Adoles. Psychiat.*, 25:370–376.

Kiser, L., Heston, J., Hickerson, S., Millsap, P., Nunn, W. & Pruitt, D. (1993), Anticipatory stress in children and adolescents. *Amer. J. Psychiat.*, 150:87–92.

Koenig, W. K. (1964), Chronic or persistent identity diffusion. *Amer. J. Psychiat.*, 120:1081–1084.

Milgram, N. A., Toubiana, Y. H., Klingman, A., Raviv, A. & Goldstein, I. (1988), Situational exposure and personal loss in children's acute and chronic stress reactions to a school bus disaster. *J. Traum. Stress*, 1:330–352.

Milne, G. (1977). Cyclone Tracy: II. The effects on Darwin children. *Austral. Psychologist*, 12:55–62.

Ollendick, D. G. & Hoffman, M. (1983). Assessment of psychological reactions in disaster victims. *J. Comm. Psychol.*, 10:157–167.

Rigamer, E. F. (1986), Psychological management of children in a national crisis. *J. Amer. Acad. Child Psychiat.*, 25:364–369.

Sack, W. H., Angell, R. H., Kinzie, J. D. & Rath, B. (1986), The psychiatric effects of massive trauma on Cambodian children: II. The family, the home and school. *J. Amer. Acad. Child Psychiat.*, 25:377–383.

Saigh, P. A. (1986), In vitro flooding in the treatment of a 6-year-old boy's post-traumatic stress disorder. *Behavior Res. Ther.*, 6:685–688.

Solomon, J. C. (1942), Reactions of children to blackouts. *Amer. J. Orthopsychiat.*, 12:361–362.

Sugar, M. (1968), Normal adolescent mourning. *Amer. J. Psychother.*, 32:258–269.

——— (1988a), A preschooler in a disaster. *Amer. J. Psychother.*, 42:619–629.

——— (1988b), The multiple trauma in a disaster. In: *The Child in His Family. Perilous Development: Child Raising and Identity*

Formation Under Stress, ed. E. J. Anthony & C. Chiland. New York: Wiley, pp. 429–442.

———— (1989), Children in a disaster—An overview. *Child Psychiat. Human Develop.*, 19:163–179.

Terr, L. C. (1979), Children of Chowchilla. *The Psychoanalytic Study of the Child*, 35:547–623. New Haven, CT: Yale University Press.

———— (1983), Chowchilla revisited: The effects of psychic trauma four years after a school-bus kidnapping. *Amer. J. Psychiat.*, 140: 1543–1550.

Toubiana, Y. H., Milgram, N. A., Strich, Y. & Edelstein, A. (1988), Crisis intervention in a school community disaster: principles and practices. *J. Commun. Psychol.*, 16:228–240.

U. S. Department of Commerce, Bureau of the Census (1990), *Statistical Abstract of the United States 1990*. Washington, DC: US Government Printing Office, pp. 81, 85.

Wraith, R. (1988), Experiences in children of workers in emergency services and disaster situations. Presented at the international conference on Dealing with Stress and Trauma in Emergency Services, Melbourne, Australia.

Yule, W. & Udwin, O. (1991), Screening child survivors for post-traumatic stress disorders: Experiences from the "Jupiter" sinking. *Brit. J. Clin. Psychol.*, 30:131–138.

———— & Williams, R. M. (1990), Post-traumatic stress reactions in children. *J. Traum. Stress*, 3:279–295.

Zeidner, M. (1993), Coping with disaster: The case of Israeli adolescents under threat of missile attack. *J. Youth Adoles.*, 22:89–108.

5 BREAKING UP OR BREAKING AWAY: THE STRUGGLE AROUND AUTONOMY AND INDIVIDUATION AMONG ADOLESCENT DAUGHTERS OF DIVORCE

ELIZABETH PERL

When Terri angrily walked out in the middle of her psychotherapy session, I felt abandoned, fearful she would not come back, aware of her power to end our relationship. My response can be understood as an identification with Terri's childhood experience of her parent's divorce. From my position in this interaction, I was able to empathize with Terri's sense of vulnerability, but I could also feel the force of her aggression expressed through rejection of me. For a daughter of divorce, the shifting identifications between an active (e.g., abandoner) and a passive (e.g., abandoned one) position become a central problem in the adolescent struggle to separate and individuate.

The developmental press toward individuation in adolescence may feel threatening by virtue of its identification with the marital break-up. Whatever the difficulties underlying the dissolution of the marriage, there is room for the adolescent to project her own issues onto her parents' relationship. Through the eyes of the adolescent, immersed in a struggle to find and assert her autonomy, parental divorce may confirm the fear that the push for individuation can jeopardize any bond. She may imagine that there is no way to be separate without breaking off the relationship in an angry way—dissolving the relationship entirely. The developmentally appropriate process of asserting one's independent identity through rebellion and conflict may be experienced by the adolescent as a threat to her tie with parents, much as the marital conflict jeopardized her parent's ties to each other. When autonomous strivings are confused with aggression, like that expressed by feuding parents, the adolescent may come to fear that attachment prohibits volition.

In this essay, I explore how the marital dissolution colors the adolescent's experience of the interplay between attachment and the assertion of autonomy. In clinical work, the process of attaching to and eventually leaving the therapist becomes a vital part of this interpersonal struggle. There is opportunity for repetition of different aspects of the childhood experience of parental divorce, for expression and exploration of varied identifications, and for creating different experiences with attachment, individuation and separation. I use my work with Terri, a 12-year-old daughter of divorce, to explore the dynamics of attachment and separation in the treatment, which included Terri's aggressive and self-protective pulls to leave me, as well as my need to leave her when I terminated my training at the hospital clinic. I then consider the implications for dealing with termination in treatment of daughters of divorce.

Parental Divorce and Female Separation-Individuation

Parental divorce can complicate, and possibly impede, the process of separation-individuation for adolescent daughters. Disruption in contact with the father has been a focus of concern because of his gender-specific role in facilitating a daughter's separation from her mother. A father is in a unique position both to foster a positive sense of femininity and to promote ease in approaching peer relationships, especially those of a heterosexual nature (Machtlinger, 1981). Triadic interaction can facilitate the process of separation-individuation, both in infancy (Abelin, 1977; Benjamin, 1988) and in adolescence (Blos, 1967). In an intact family, attachment to the father can provide an anchor point outside of the mother's orbit, enabling an adolescent to resist regressive longings for her mother without retreat to sexual, aggressive, or self-destructive acting-out. The bond with father, in adolescence, provides a bridge to attachments outside of the family. A mother and a father can each offer their daughter different, and complementary, experiences with attachment, which fosters the capacity to separate from family and form intimate ties with peers. A father's absence, or at least his separation from mother, disrupts the triadic interplay within the family, thereby increasing the risk of separation-related difficulties among daughters of divorce in adolescence.

From infancy, a mother serves as both the primary object of attachment and the primary object of identification for girls. The female is therefore faced with the paradoxical task of introjecting and identifying with the person from whom she must separate, after years of uninterrupted attachment (Chodorow, 1978; Friedman, 1980). The exclusive nature of the mother–daughter tie extends through childhood; allowing the "two-person relationship of infancy" with mother to remain primary (Chodorow, 1978, p. 96). Other familial and extra-familial relationships supplement rather than supersede the primary bond with the mother.

The press toward individuation may seem particularly threatening to a bond partially based on a sense of sameness. In a process parallel to the infant's struggle to emerge from union with mother, father may serve as an alternate object of attachment, enabling the adolescent to resist regressive longings for mother. When the father is not available during this transition, drugs or sexual promiscuity may be used as an alternative to the more threatening pull to turn to mother for comfort and nurturance (Giovacchini, 1985). The rebellious aspects of these behaviors function to deny the dependent longings. This pseudo-independent stance, with its self-destructive consequences, may gratify the dependent longings by prompting increased parental control that further restricts the adolescent's opportunity for independent activity (Kalter, 1985). The acting-out of adolescent daughters of divorce may represent a response to the father's departure as it interfaces with gender-specific aspects of the course of separation-individuation.

Dissolution of the Marital Bond

What of the developmental impact of the marital dissolution, in and of itself? This question expands the focus from concern with parenting functions to the meaning of the parents' relationship with each other and its dissolution. The changing constellation of family membership initiated by divorce overturns the normative childhood vision of marriage as a permanent bond, calling into question for the child the solidity of all family ties. The illusion of the permanence of marriage is lost, as divorce initiates a series of changes in family membership, some temporary and others enduring (loss of contact with parents; introduction and possible loss of contact with parent's partners and their families; the child's sense of displacement by new family members). Clinical interviews with this group of adolescents have suggested that parental divorce fosters skepticism regarding the capacity of relationships to endure (Wallerstein and Blakeslee, 1990). For these adolescents, the prospect of moving from the family to intimate ties outside may seem less possible and more frightening (Kalter, 1987).

The ability to comprehend the meaning of divorce in terms of the continuity of the family demands an understanding of the distinctions between blood and legal relationships, an awareness of the difference between the marital bond and the bond between parent and child. Understanding of such intangible distinctions in relationships may be beyond the emotional, if not the intellectual, grasp of the child. If a marriage can end, the child may fear that her bond to parents might also be vulnerable. The power and persistence of reunion fantasies (Lohr et al., 1981) speak to a child's need to preserve an idealized view of both her parents and of the marital relationship.

In this context, the adolescent, and perhaps also the parent, may have difficulty differentiating rebellion against parents from the battles between parents that ultimately brought the marital relationship to an end. To the extent that the generational boundary is blurred through parentification of the child or, in the extreme, when the child perceives herself, or is perceived, as a surrogate spouse, adolescent separation takes on overtones of divorce. The offspring is more likely to feel that she is rejecting or abandoning the parent. In a similar vein, the divorced parent may be more likely to feel threatened by conflict or abandoned by the adolescent's press to reject at least some things about the parent in the service of asserting ways that she is different.

Inevitably, rebellion in the service of individuation from parents stimulates anger, disappointment, and disillusionment for both the adolescent and her parents. The struggle for increased autonomy may appear to jeopardize the adolescent's continuing family ties. It may seem impossible for interpersonal differences to be embraced and integrated into the relationship, allowing for separation in the context of a close bond. When separation is equated with a severing of family ties, and when the family is no longer perceived as a steady base for "emotional refueling" (Mahler, 1979a, p. 37), it feels more risky to venture into one's own life and relationships.

The Struggle with Attachment and Autonomy in Treatment

The therapeutic relationship can represent both a step toward separating from family, and a re-creation and extension of the resistance to separation and individuation. A pervasive counter-dependent stance on the part of the adolescent may defend against or remove the attachment as well as the prospect of rejection and loss. Yet a focus on the fear of abandonment, the longing for the lost idealized parent, or the hunger for and fear of attachment, can distract from the underlying struggle for autonomy in the relationship with the therapist. This struggle was central in my work with Terri. Her pattern of walking out in the middle of sessions and her threats to quit treatment or to find a better therapist (the idealized absent parent, perhaps), can be seen as a reenactment of the trauma of parental divorce. Here she dealt with her fear of being left by actively taking on the role of the leaver. Certainly the threat of Terri leaving me, and the actuality of her mini-abandonments, carried meaning in terms of her family history, but also served as an enactment of issues around separation. She exhibited both a conflicted, angry press to launch from me, and a defensive maneuver to avoid the struggle to individuate and achieve autonomy within our relationship.

Terri's parents divorced when she was four years old. Mr. T had been divorced previously but had no children from this first marriage. Mrs. T left Terri and her sister in the custody of their father. Although this was an unusual arrangement, especially at that time, it was consistent with the division of responsibilities prior to the divorce. Mrs. T traveled frequently for her job as a buyer for a department store, while Mr. T, who worked independently as a bookkeeper in the home, assumed primary responsibility for the children. One year later, Mr. T remarried. This marriage, which lasted only two years, was turbulent, in part as a result of the stepmother's emotional volatility. Nevertheless, Terri remembered her stepmother Louise with great fondness and longing. Terri persistently asserted how special her relationship with her stepmother had been, insisting that Louise had been the only one who really cared about and understood her. Terri clung to this notion despite the fact that the stepmother sought no contact with Terri following her divorce.

Mr. T married for a fourth time two years later. Terri disliked and battled with the second stepmother, and she resented the marriage and her new stepsiblings. Terri's idealization of her first stepmother seemed to be based on affection, but it also represented a rebellion against pressures to accept her new stepmother. At the age of 11, Terri requested that she be allowed to live with her biological mother, who had visited her every two to four weeks, and who was in support of such a plan. Terri moved as soon as her father withdrew his initial protests. Although she was initially pleased about being allowed to make the move, Terri began to feel rejected as she saw her father's eventual compliance as a way for him to get rid of her. Whereas the repeated loss of mother figures in Terri's case was somewhat unusual, ongoing shifts in family composition involving multiple losses, which may or may not take the form of remarriage and divorce, are not atypical sequelae of divorce.

Terri was referred to me for treatment after the move to her biological mother's home because of her angry, defiant stance toward her mother. Mrs. T was also troubled by Terri's sexually provocative behavior. She would, for example, parade around in front of the mother's boyfriend in nothing but a nightshirt. Mrs. T suspected that Terri might be sexually active, as she did once catch her slipping away from a party in the arms of a much older boy. I met with Terri twice a week for psychotherapy in the outpatient clinic of a children's psychiatric hospital. This was Terri's first treatment. Although initially I also met in separate individual sessions with her mother and father for parent-guidance work, my discussion here focuses on the dynamics of the individual treatment with Terri.

Conflict regarding autonomy was particularly complex for Terri as a function of her changing position over the course of the multiple divorces. At the time of the original divorce, she was only four years old and must thus be considered a powerless victim of the will of her parents. By the time of the third remarriage, Terri's determination to leave her father and stepmother reflected her own choice to reject her father and stepmother in favor of her biological mother. This represents a shift in Terri's role from that of a young child left by her mother, struggling to deal both with the loss and with the powerlessness of her position, to that of a preadolescent, who uses her power, however limited, to actively reject her reconstituted family, if only to test their commitment to her. In this later move, Terri was dealing with a sense of being abandoned while living out an identification with the parent who leaves. She may have been using the opportunity to reject others as a means of expressing pent-up anger associated with her history of repeated losses. In addition, Terri's sense of autonomy was entangled with aggression: the passive, vulnerable side contained the fear that asserting autonomy would cause the other to leave, whereas the active side contained the inclination to use rejection as a tool of self-assertion.

At the beginning of treatment, Terri came to sessions full of news from her day in school. She would ask me for money to buy snacks or for a mirror to check her makeup. When Terri did not seem to register my failure to meet these requests, I found myself feeling as though I had indeed provided in accord with her wishes. The rigidity of the ready-made idealized transference, fueled by Terri's wish for a nurturant, infallible mother figure, paradoxically left little room for spontaneous giving. My expression of feelings or attempts at play did not seem to register with her. Despite my discomfort, I felt reluctant to challenge her idealization both because of my wish to provide the complete nurturance that she craved, and because of my fear of disrupting our bond.

About five months into the treatment, just prior to the episodes of her walking out of the session, Terri began to retreat to a stance of angry, sullen devaluation. When I would ask her about this change, she would blandly insist that she did not like me, that she had never liked me, and that she really wanted a new "shrink." The shift did not represent a developmental step toward deidealization. Instead, she flipped from a view of me as a wholly satisfying, nurturing figure to one who was useless. Both positions protected her from the disappointment of confronting my real shortcomings as her therapist and her need to provide for herself in ways that I could not. By renouncing her attachment, Terri avoided the painful process of giving up the fantasy that I could meet all her needs.

Terri's angry demands to change therapists, and her devaluation of the treatment, like her wish to leave her stepfamily, seemed to represent an attempt to reject the other so as to fend off being rejected. With her self-protective, hostile-dependent position, she asserted that she had little to lose because our relationship was worthless and therefore expendable. Terri dealt with her fear of powerlessness by identifying with the aggressor, justifying her behavior by assailing the value of the caregiver, parent, or therapist. Each position, that of the vulnerable child left by her mother, and that of the aggressor who exercised control by rejecting, functioned defensively to protect Terri from confronting and dealing with painful feelings associated with the opposing position. The thrill of the power to reject me could be used to deny her sense of vulnerability in the face of separation initiated by myself. At the same time, her tendency to regress to a stance of helplessness served, in part, to avoid confronting her inclination to inflict pain on herself and me by means of rejection.

By identifying with the aggressor, Terri undermined her efforts to achieve autonomy. The push to reject became an end in itself, rather than a means to embrace her own identity and place in the world, apart from caregivers. In this context, Terri's rejecting stance not only served to protect her against feelings of vulnerability, but also represented a means of asserting herself by exerting her will and influence on others. Rather than negotiating to find ways to get her needs met as fully as possible in relationships that were available to her, Terri looked to a relationship that was unavailable. It was less threatening to Terri to reject me, or provoke me to reject her, than to face possible rejection on the basis of her efforts to assert who she was. This counterdependent stance allowed Terri to avoid settling for a situation in which her needs would be met only incompletely in a partially satisfying relationship.

The Clinical Interaction

The first time Terri walked out of a session, we had been in the midst of a conversation about my upcoming vacation. She denied having any feelings about my vacation and insisted that she had learned of my plans from her mother before I had told her myself in the last session. I responded that I thought that I had informed her of my plans before I talked with her mother. Then Terri announced that she was going to the bathroom. She did not return for 15 minutes. Her departure at that moment might be seen as a reaction to my intention to leave her. Terri might also have been escaping painful feelings about losing the attention of her mother, who was becoming increasingly involved with a boyfriend. Like Terri's parents, I was allowing other interests in my life to take me away from her, and she believed that I was not even conscientious about informing her directly of my plans.

When she returned with snacks, evidence that she had made a stop by the candy machine, I found myself looking, perhaps wishfully, for a more positive side to her departure. Perhaps Terri was venturing out into the world. She was getting supplies for herself, demonstrating her self-sufficiency when separated from me, or at least seeking a way to fill herself up. Perhaps she was attempting to show me up by demonstrating that she could do better on her own, wherein her venture could be seen as an autonomous move that was connected, competitively, to our relationship.

I tried to engage with her, joking about her hunt for munchies. Terri failed to acknowledge what I had experienced as the surprise of seeing her return with snacks. She did not join with me in bringing the sense of adventure and fun into our interaction. Instead she stayed angry, and sat silently eating her snack. Had I chosen to focus here on her possible search for the nurturance of the lost idealized parent, her feelings of emptiness, or her fear of making herself vulnerable by turning to me with her needs, I might have been avoiding, her expression of aggression disguised as autonomy. Instead, I said that I felt pushed away by her, that she seemed to want to shut me out from what she had done on her own. I said that I felt like I was intruding on her when I tried to join with her in what she did, but on the other hand I felt that if I tried not to be involved, it made it seem like I opposed her doing things independently.

Terri behaved as though she could not trust that I could support her if her desire conflicted with my own, or simply if her desire was initiated independent of our interaction. It was as if Terri could not assert her independence unless she was free of me. Self-assertion seemed undifferentiated from, or synonymous with, defiance. She related to me as if I were an obstacle, rather than, at least, as an opponent driven by conflicting needs and interests. In this position I found little room to support, appreciate, or even recognize her autonomy as a reflection of her capacity to meet some of her own needs better than I could. Nor could I recognize with her my failure to meet her needs as fully as she would have liked. Terri's rebellion seemed to be engineered to draw me in (even as she ostensibly worked to shut me out), rather than to help me disengage and support more genuine independence.

A second and more threatening departure took place the following month. In this session, Terri told me she had learned from her mother that the time of her second weekly appointment was to change. As with the news of my vacation, Terri acted as though all her information emanated from her mother. I confirmed the change, but I also noted that I had involved Terri in the planning to accommodate this change in her mother's work schedule, which impacted on the mother's ability to drive Terri to her sessions at the previously scheduled time. In the midst of this discussion Terri stormed out of the office, coat in hand, threatening that she would not be coming back. Was Terri acting out because she felt that her input was not considered in her mother's plans? Did Mrs. T's efforts to rearrange the therapy schedule represent to Terri another rejection and devaluation of her importance in her mother's life? Was Terri caught off guard when her stance of indifference could no longer contain feelings of dependence and vulnerability in our relationship? Was she so unable to tolerate any such feelings that she would not return?

Issues of control were dominant both in our interaction and in my countertransference feelings. I felt frustrated by my powerlessness to force Terri to stay in the office and obey the "rules" of psychotherapy, let alone to explore the feelings fueling her actions. I struggled with feelings of inadequacy as a therapist which, in addition to suggesting an identification with Terri's own sense of inadequacy associated with the parental divorce, may have served as an attempt to make sense of my experience of rejection. To the extent that my worth as a therapist seemed to be connected to my ability to impose my will on Terri, at least to keep her in the session, my own autonomy came to be compromised. I guiltily entertained fleeting wishes that Terri would not come back. Although Terri would inevitably return, her departures evoked a sense of the tenuousness of our connection.

In the psychotherapy sessions, unlike her early experience in her family, Terri took control of both the separations and the reunions. Terri's control, however, was largely illusory. It seemed to serve to deny her lack of control over the broader context of separations in the psychotherapy, specifically over the beginnings and endings of the sessions, the scheduling of appointments, my vacations, and perhaps especially the fact that our work would be limited by my two-year commitment to the hospital. Her often precipitous departures at the end the hour, for example, likely served as an attempt to mask this lack of control, as Terri prematurely called the sessions to a halt. In addition to denying her vulnerability, Terri was avoiding any interaction where her needs would be curbed by a limit determined by my own needs.

I became a participant in the dynamics of rejection that were being re-created in our relationship. As the one who was left, I was identified with the role of the innocent victim while Terri took on the role of the aggressor, the one who abandons. My wish to end our relationship may have represented a means to counter my sense of inadequacy and powerlessness. Through my fantasies of escape, I was also taking on the role of the caregiver who would reject Terri. The guilt I experienced in association with my wish for relief from her, together with the reality that I would be leaving her in the future, was attenuated by the blatant nature of Terri's provocations. She created the sense that she alone was responsible for the precarious state of our alliance. Despite the intermittent insecurities I felt about myself as therapist for Terri, I could find reassurance in the belief that the problems in the treatment were rooted in her resistance. In that sense, blaming Terri for my own inclination to abandon her corresponded with Terri's belief that she had caused her mother to leave and that her inadequacies had driven her father to seek out a different family. This belief allowed Terri to preserve some idealization of her parents as caregivers. In the psychotherapy, Terri was protecting me from confronting aspects of my behavior and attitudes that might have represented an abdication of my responsibility as her caregiver. The sense that she was depleting or unlovable was more tolerable to Terri than the possibility that caregivers could be driven to leave because of their own needs. Terri was struggling to preserve a fantasy of the selfless caregiver.

The sense of fragility regarding the treatment alliance seemed to be a reenactment of Terri's experience of the fragility of the ties within her family. The therapeutic relationship seemed to be sustained only by some sort of external coercion (e.g., she claimed that she came to see me only because her mother made her come). Like her parents' marriage, our connection seemed vulnerable to dissolution. The survival of the therapy did not dispel the sense of the fragility of our alliance. To deny the risk that Terri could and might end the treatment would have been to deny the vulnerability of our bond and the pain of the prospect of failure and loss in our relationship. Similarly, a determination on my part that the treatment was of no use to Terri and should be terminated would have been a way of ridding myself of uncertainty regarding the fate of the treatment and my relationship with Terri, and the anxiety about where the blame for failure might lay.

Our capacity to maintain involvement throughout sustained conflict and discontent in the later part of the treatment afforded some opportunity for our relationship to become differentiated from Terri's experience within her family. In the therapeutic context there was room for Terri to protest and reject me without repercussions in terms of my availability or investment in her. I was concerned that my need to leave Terri at the end of my hospital training would be experienced as retaliatory rejection, especially because I was frustrated with and angry about her continued devaluation and rejection of me. Yet, at the same time, I also felt regret about leaving her before she was ready and, despite my anger and hurt, I did not want to abandon her. I believed that Terri still needed a relationship where she could work through her fears of dependence, rejection, and abandonment and move toward better tolerance of attachment.

When I talked with Terri about my need to end my work with her three months prior to my planned departure, Terri expressed only relief. Now she would not have to waste her time in therapy anymore. She was glad, she said, that I would not continue to see her. She would not even consider the idea of transferring to a new therapist in the clinic following my departure. Terri explained that her mother had told her up front that all she was required to do was to finish her work with me; and Mrs. T knew from the start, as did Terri, that I had only 18 months remaining in my two-year training involvement with the hospital. Terri had never mentioned the prospect of my leaving, and no one assumed from the start that I would complete my training at the clinic before Terri was ready to terminate. It is possible, nonetheless, that Terri's shift from positive attachment to devaluation was a way for her to try to protect herself in the face of the limits of my availability. While the risk of potential abandonment would have been an issue for Terri regardless of the circumstances of her treatment, the nature of my transitory tie to the clinic likely exacerbated Terri's sense of vulnerability throughout our work together.

When I began to discuss specifics about my plans to leave, Terri began to walk out of sessions with increasing frequency and in a more casual manner. She explained to me in an offhand tone that she left sessions to wait the time out in the hospital stairwell. This way her mother would think she was using the treatment when she really wasn't. This disclosure was certainly a provocation, an attempt to put in my face that she was outsmarting me, getting nothing from me, and using my time to get her mother off her back. I felt that her disclosure was also admission that she had found a way to make the treatment her own: She felt forced to be there, but she still retained a sense of autonomy and control over her involvement, and a sense of trust that I would not report to her mother her goings and comings. Terri was not yet able to use relationships directly to deal with and modulate her feelings, but she had found for herself a safe place near me, in the stairwell, which seemed to feel to her like a place of her own. I feared that to share my interpretation of her departures, and in particular to recognize her adaptive efforts, would have compromised Terri's experience of acting autonomously. I commented instead on how much she seemed to want to act like there would be no loss in my leaving, either for her or for me, and how she was able to find ways to manage things on her own.

In retrospect, I think that my failure to deal more actively with the fact that I would be ending the treatment unilaterally, before Terri would be ready to leave me, repeated some of the most painful aspects of her history of losses of mother and mother-figures. Although I did talk, well in advance, about my plans to leave, and although I was open to listening to Terri's feelings about the termination, she was not really able to verbalize these feelings, especially given the associated pain and vulnerability. I would connect her anger and her leaving of me to my plans to leave her, but the focus remained more on her behavior, rather than on my contribution to her feelings in our relationship. The pervasive, often relentless nature of her anger contributed to this inclination and perhaps served defensively to protect us from confronting the full impact of my departure. If Terri allowed herself to feel more fully my regret about leaving and the loss involved in ending our relationship, she might have been overwhelmed by feelings of deprivation associated with past losses and with parental ambivalence about their involvement with and responsibility for her. I did not face the fact of my leaving her squarely enough, perhaps because of my guilt and my wish not to be yet another abandoning caregiver. Yes, I was imposing upon Terri another loss over which she had no control. I could do nothing to change or to soften this reality. But to the extent that I shared with Terri my concern about ways that my departure might be repeating painful aspects of her parents' divorce and the fact that I felt and was affected by her anger, this, in and of itself, might have provided some differentiation from her experience of the parental divorce.

Implications for Dealing with Termination

Although the paradox of attachment and separation must be negotiated in any psychotherapy, the accompanying ambivalence will likely be especially intense and complex in work with the adolescent daughter of divorce. The process of forming a therapeutic attachment demands a capacity to tolerate the absence or withdrawal of attachment on the part of the adolescent (Gerson, 1994). The attachment and identification that develop then become the basis for working toward individuation and, ultimately, separation. The process of terminating, to be therapeutic, must encompass a sense of continuing connection, both in terms of an internalized sense of identification and involvement with the other, and in terms of opportunities for continued contact.

Resistance to treatment, particularly to an overt show of dependence on or alliance with the therapist, may take the form of the adolescent's rejecting the goals and currency of psychotherapy, for example, by refusing to disclose, to explore feelings, or by resisting change. Such rejection may be narcissistically injurious and discouraging, challenging the therapist to tolerate a degree of separateness from the adolescent sufficient to be able to sustain independent feelings regarding the value of the treatment, the therapeutic bond, and himself or herself as therapist. There may be an added degree of provocation here, as the adolescent daughter of divorce may press to elicit a repetition of the rejection she may have experienced in association with the parental divorce. The capacity of the therapist to tolerate lack of attachment and to remain invested in the adolescent can allow for attachment based on an acceptance of differences, including even rejection of values most integral to the identity of the other. To the extent that conflict and even experiences of rejection can be accepted as part of, rather than a threat to, the therapeutic relationship, there is opportunity for differentiation from the experience of parental divorce. Therapist and patient sustain an attachment in the face of the adolescent's press to individuate.

A sense of frustration, even despair and hopelessness, which might otherwise cause the therapist to question the efficacy of the treatment, needs to be explored in the context of the meaning and function of the therapeutic relationship for the adolescent. The press to repeat the experience of divorce in a failed treatment relationship can propel termination planning or acquiescence in the patient's wish to quit therapy. Power struggles over the goals of or approach to treatment gain intensity as the survival of the relationship may seem to hang in the balance. Conversely, fear of termination may reflect an unconscious association between loss and unresolved conflict or failure, along with a belief that separation ends the relationship. There is danger of using termination to escape problems in the treatment relationship, to eliminate the risk that the adolescent will unilaterally decide to quit, or to avoid the uncertainty of a more vague sense that the relationship would otherwise be lost.

The termination with Terri, as in her experience with parental divorces, was dictated by my need (my tenure with the clinic coming to its planned end), rather than by her own initiative. As I acknowledged this reality, Terri came face to face with the impact of my needs on our relationship. It was unfortunate, I think, that Terri did not have the opportunity to initiate the termination based on her own sense of readiness. Particularly in Terri's case, with her history of repeated loss of caregivers, it would have been optimal for separation to be internally driven and paced. But with limited funding for treatment, with attrition or dislocation of therapists, this outcome is not uncommon. The loss of another caregiver, however, does not mean that the termination need be a repetition of the parental divorce, nor that the imposition of the needs of the other must be experienced as toxic. The therapist's response to the patient's feelings, and the way they create together their own experience with separation, can allow for differentiation from past experience. With Terri there was a need for her to have room to reject me angrily as her caregiver while I remained invested enough to feel the hurt and still try to care for and about her. Despite the pain involved, my investment in Terri was neither unconditional nor masochistic. Rather, the differentiation from past family relationships derived, in part, from the attempt to absorb anger, pain, and aggression in the context of an attachment, and to verbalize the experience of abandonment rather than to simply act it out.

The opportunity for continued contact after termination can be a means of asserting that separation does not have to end the relationship. With Terri's lack of readiness for termination, it was difficult to explore the possibility of continued involvement. I was, I think, too focused on Terri's continued need for treatment and my inability to provide this for her. My hope was for Terri to stay connected with the clinic and to become involved with another therapist, but such a transition represented for Terri being passed along to the next stepmother, and perhaps there was a healthy aspect to her resistance. Terri's denial of any need for me, along with my countertransference wish to pass along the responsibility, contributed to my failure to discuss with Terri how she might keep in contact with me, whether or not she was to continue in treatment with a different therapist. Terri and I needed to grapple with what different types of contact would have meant to each of us, but if in fact Terri had been able to do this, I think it would have meant that she was closer to being ready to terminate than was actually the case. Short of this, though, I should have at least presented to her ways she could reach me, and I should have explained the limits of my availability, despite the inevitable protest I would have encountered that she would never want to contact me. Had this occurred, the termination would have been less of a disappearance, would have been different from Terri's experience of her parents' marital dissolution, and would have, I think, promoted her ability to consider connecting with a new therapist in the future.

Continuity in therapeutic work following termination results from internalization, from the opportunity for increased autonomy fostered by the disruption in predictable contact with the therapist, and from the sense of availability of the therapist in the patient's current and future life. The feeling on the part of the adolescent that she can look back to the therapist, both by remembering past interactions, and by seeking renewed contact, allows the therapist to function, after termination, as a secure "home base" that can be used for "refueling" (Mahler, 1979b, pp. 124–125). Knowledge of the therapist's availability may, paradoxically, obviate the need for contact, maximizing the adolescent's confidence in her capacity for autonomous functioning.

Although recognizing the therapist's limitations is part of the process of separation-individuation, as was evident with Terri, devaluation can perpetuate an illusion of omnipotence, with the therapist seen as an all-powerful source of oppression and obstruction. In this way Terri was able to deny her attachment and project onto me her own wish not to separate, to be controlled so she could fight the control rather than achieve more genuine individuation. The extreme and absolute nature of the devaluation, perhaps representing, in part, an identification with parental attitudes toward the ex-spouse, functions to justify the need to divorce the therapist, thereby completing the repetition of the parental experience. Abandonment then becomes the only route to autonomy. A goal of treatment would involve an effort by the patient and therapist to recognize the limitations of the therapist and of the psychotherapy and the adolescent's lessening need for the therapist, while appreciating the continued value of their relationship, both before and after termination.

The struggle toward separation is mutual, and the experience will be different for each dyad. For patient and therapist, this process demands an integration of his or her past experience and ongoing sense of self, with the nature of the therapeutic relationship. Much of the value of the psychotherapy may be derived from the capacity of the adolescent and therapist together to create a bond that survives the process of separation and the eventual termination of the work. In contrast with the experience of a divorce, the sense of loss is then sustained in the context of an enduring relationship.

REFERENCES

Abelin, E. (1971). Role of the father in the separation-individuation process. In: *Separation-Individuation*, ed. M. Settlage. New York: International Universities Press.

Benjamin, J. (1988). *The Bonds of Love*. New York: Pantheon.

————— (1991), Father and daughter: Identification with difference—A contribution to gender heterodoxy. *Psychoanal. Dial.*, 1:277–299.

Blos, P. (1967), The second individuation process of adolescence. *The Psychoanalytic Study of the Child*, 22:162–186. New Haven, CT: Yale University Press.

Chodorow, N. (1978), *The Reproduction of Mothering*. Berkeley: University of California Press.

Friedman, G. (1980), The mother-daughter bond. *Contemp. Psychoanal.*, 16:90–97.

Gerson, M. (1994), Standing at the threshold: A psychoanalytic response to Carol Gilligan. *Psychoanal. Psychol.*, 11:491–508.

Giovacchini, P. (1985), Countertransference and the severely disturbed adolescents. *Adolescent Psychiatry*, 12:449–467.

Kalter, N. (1985), Implications of parental divorce for female development. *J. Amer. Acad. Child Psychiat.*, 24:538–544.

————— (1987), Long-term effects of divorce on children: A developmental vulnerability model. *Amer. J. Orthopsychiat.*, 57:587–600.

Lohr, R., Chethik, M., Press, S., & Solyom, A. (1981), Impact of divorce on children: Vicissitudes and therapeutic implications of the reconciliation fantasy. *J. Child Psychother.*, 7:123–136.

Machtlinger, V. J. (1981), The father in psychoanalytic theory. In: *The Role of the Father in Child Development*, 2nd ed., ed. M. Lamb. New York: Wiley.

Mahler, M. (1979a), Mother–child interaction during separation-individuation. In: *The Selected Papers of Margaret S. Mahler, Vol. 2*. New York: Aronson, pp. 35–48.

————— (1979b), On the first three subphases of the separation-individuation process. In: *The Selected Papers of Margaret S. Mahler, Vol. 2*. New York: Aronson, pp. 119–130.

Wallerstein, J. & Blakeslee, S. (1990), *Second Chances*. New York: Ticknor & Fields.

6   PARENT LOSS IN CHILDHOOD
AND ADULT PSYCHOPATHOLOGY

BENJAMIN GARBER

With the publication of Freud's early case histories, psychiatrists have considered childhood experiences to bear a causal relationship to psychiatric morbidity in adult life. The linearity between childhood trauma and adult psychopathology has been well established in clinical practice, so that one of the primary tasks of psychotherapy has been to search for the significant traumatogenic events in a person's life.

Since the loss of a parent in childhood is seen as an all encompassing trauma of unique proportions, it has been considered a prime etiological factor in a wide range of psychopathologic conditions. Such diverse disorders as schizophrenia, sociopathy, neuroses, and depressive disorders have been seen as originating from parent loss in childhood (Tennant, Bebbington, and Hurry, 1981). The psychoanalytic literature in particular suggests that depression in adulthood is the most likely outcome following parental loss (Abraham, 1911; Freud, 1915; Bowlby, 1960). Mental health practitioners have automatically assumed an etiology for parent loss in childhood in the genesis of adult psychopathology. Clinicians have also assumed that childhood parent loss is one of the significant variables in the study of psychic development. As a result of this assumption, researchers have consistently returned to the exploration of such an association.

A number of studies in the 1960s and 1970s confirmed the impression that there is a higher incidence of childhood bereavement in the histories of psychiatric patients compared with the general population (Brown, 1961; Beck, Sethi, and Tuthill, 1963; Birtchnell, 1969, 1971, 1972, 1974, 1975)

Two excellent studies by Brown (1961) and Beck, Sethi, and Tuthill (1963) found significantly higher numbers of depressed patients who had lost a parent within the first sixteen years of life as compared to the general population. Birtchnell (1969, 1971, 1972, 1974, 1975), one of the most prolific researchers in this area, has contributed a number of studies to our understanding of the correlation between parent loss and psychopathology.

Birtchnell (1969) demonstrated that when a sample of early bereaved psychiatric patients was compared with one of early bereaved general population controls, there was an overrepresentation of older siblings of the same sex as the lost parent in the patient group. With a younger sibling to care for, the premature assumption of the parental role may contribute to subsequent psychopathology.

Birtchnell (1971) also concluded that childhood bereavement plays a causal role in a minority of cases of mental illness. In none of the patient groups in this study is the incidence of childhood bereavement greater than double what it is in controls, and in most groups it was found to be much less.

In a later study, Birtchnell (1972) arrived at the following conclusions: 1) only when the death of a parent has occurred before the 10th birthday, significant differences between patient and control groups are found, and 2) an increased incidence of childhood bereavement was found more often among female patients than among males.

Eventually he noted (Birtchnell, 1974) that in his attempts to correlate parent loss in childhood with adult psychopathology, findings are so inconsistent that they cast serious doubt on the use of epidemiological methods in this domain.

Birtchnell (1975) found an association in women between early maternal bereavement and excessive dependency (as demonstrated by the MMPI) and maintained that such findings are an example of the complementarity between statistical and clinical approaches in psychiatric research.

This vacillation between the epidemiological and the clinical is indicative of a basic trend in studying the implications of parent loss for subsequent psychopathology. The two approaches have often yielded different and contradictory results.

In the late 1970s and early 1980s researchers began to question the obvious clinical association between parent loss in childhood and adult psychopathology.

The early studies were conducted by clinicians who may have had a vested interest in demonstrating connections between childhood bereavement and adult psychopathology; however, subsequent studies were carried out by epidemiologists whose views seemed more dispassionate and objective. Whereas early empirical investigations of the relationship between childhood parental loss and adult psychopathologic conditions were plagued by methodologic problems, the last two decades have seen an increasingly large and sophisticated body of work in this area. The latter studies were careful to avoid the earlier inconsistent conclusions and clinical generalizations.

In a lengthy review of the literature Crook and Eliot (1980) conclude that there is no sound base of empirical data to support the theorized relationship between parental death during childhood and adult depression. Studies that have demonstrated a higher incidence of childhood bereavement among depressed patients than among nondepressed subjects have without exception been methodologically flawed.

While there may be some relationship between parental death in childhood and adult depression, the overwhelming etiologic significance attached to the event by many writers is unwarranted.

Tennant, Bebbington, and Hurry (1981) reviewed the literature in an attempt to correlate parental death in childhood and adult depressive disorder. The findings from epidemiologic studies remain confusing. Several studies show no association between parental death and adult morbidity of depression. Other studies show some association, usually of a specific nature, according to the type of loss and the age at the time of the loss. Even in those studies, there was little consistency between their positive findings, either across diagnostic groups or within the same diagnostic category.

Where experimental and control samples were most vigorously matched, no association was found between childhood parental bereavement and depression in later life. Parental death in childhood appears to have little effect on adult depressive morbidity.

These authors believe, however, that parental death in childhood has some effect, albeit weak, on risk of adult depression. The weakness of an effect is consistent with the ease with which the relationships may be confounded by social variables.

Roy (1983), in a large clinical study carried out over six years, matched 300 neurotic depressives with 300 controls. His results showed no significant relationship between either maternal or paternal death before ages 11 or 17 and neurotic depression in either working-class or middle-class patients of either sex.

A study by Ragan (1986) attempted to correlate parental death and adult psychopathology. The author found no association with psychiatric diagnosis among 72 inpatients who had experienced the death of a parent when they were children, compared with 460 other patients in the Chestnut Lodge Follow-Up Study. The patients with childhood parental death did, however, have significantly greater family patholo-gy and impaired social and heterosexual functioning. The main point of this study is that comparisons between patients who had experi-enced parental death in childhood and patients who had not did not yield any significant differences.

These results fail to support the hypotheses that early parental death is a nonspecific risk factor in the development of severe mental illness. However, these findings do not rule out the significance and impor-tance of parental death in specific patients.

An excellent review of the literature by Breier et al. (1988) attempted to determine specific factors in the life of the child that might be significant predictors of adult psychopathology or adaptation. Environmental factors after the loss, such as the quality of the relationship with the surviving parent, were critical in determining who developed affective illness. The quality of childhood adjustment to the loss may be a strong predictor of adult psychiatric illness. A nonsup-portive relationship with the surviving parent in which the child felt burdened by parental emotional needs was a strong predictor of adult psychopathology. Thus, the quality of the relationship with the surviving parent coupled with the parent's healthy adaptation to the loss were critical protective factors in determining the child's well-being later in life. Other factors, however, such as family history of psychiatric disorder, age at the time of parent loss, and reason for loss were not significantly different between subjects with and without adult psychopathology.

The most recent study, by Kendler et al. (1992), found that parental loss was not specific in its effect and was associated with an increased risk for depression, generalized anxiety disorder, panic disorder, and phobias. These results do not support the widely held view that childhood parental loss is more strongly related to depression than to anxiety disorders.

Much of the work on the impact of parental separation has focused exclusively on mother-loss, presuming that maternal separation would be more pathogenic than paternal separation. Kendler et al. (1992) found that, for depression, maternal and paternal separation were associated with the same increase in risk, although, because of larger numbers, only the effects of paternal separation reached statistical significance. Although Kendler et al. (1992) demonstrated an association between early parental loss and adult psychopathology, correlation does not imply causation.

Although most current studies have challenged the association between parent loss and psychopathology, others continue to elaborate the connection. The results of a study by Sklar and Harris (1985) suggest that the loss of a parent in childhood has a broad impact on adult personality. Unlike most previous statistical studies, this one supports the pervasive clinical impression that loss of a parent does have a powerful pathogenic influence.

Harris, Brown, and Biffulco (1986) approach the correlation of depression in adulthood and parent loss on childhood as a function of the lack of parental care. In a sample of women aged 18 to 65, loss of the mother before the age of 17, either by death or by separation of one year or more, was associated with clinical depression in the year of the interview. Loss of father was not associated with current depression. Examination of the caregiving arrangements in childhood suggests that it is a lack of care, as defined in terms of neglect, that accounts for the increased rate of depression. Such a lack of care is more frequently associated with the loss of a mother than the loss of a father.

Carefully conceived, epidemiologically oriented follow-up studies have questioned and forced us to reexamine the notion that parent loss in childhood leads automatically to adult psychopathology.

A number of the reviewed studies indicate no association between parent loss and subsequent psychopathology. Does that mean that the loss of a parent has no effect whatsoever, or that it has at least no clinically discernible impact? Some studies hedge on this question. In those instances where no obvious clinical effect has been demonstrated, one surmises that there are effects, but they are individually variable and their magnitude may be determined by subsequent life events. Although the clinical impact in a large population may not be impressive, on an individual basis the effects of parent loss cannot be ignored.

Clinical Considerations

When therapists are called upon to assess a prospective patient, they assume that a history of parent loss, in childhood or adolescence, has had a severe pathogenic effect on the psychic integrity of the individual.

Consequently, all or most clinical data can be explained and understood within a conceptual framework revolving around the loss of the parent.

The psychoanalytic literature on the impact of bereavement conveys impressive evidence for the correlation between parent loss and subsequent psychopathology. Highly regarded authors such as Fleming and Altschul (1963), Pollock (1961), Wolfenstein (1966, 1969), Nagera (1970), and Furman (1974) project serious long-term consequences for the child's adaptive capacities as a result of parent loss. Pollock (1961) writes that an interference in the integration and structuralization of the ego and superego may result from childhood parent loss. Fleming and Altschul (1963) and Altschul (1968) find arrests in many ego functions, especially in the area of object relations and a failure to resolve developmental conflicts. Wolfenstein (1966) emphasizes a position that those who have lost a parent in childhood more often succumb to mental illness in adulthood than those who have not suffered such a loss. Nagera (1970) speaks of bereavement in childhood as a developmental interference that leads to simultaneous symptom formation and creeping character distortions.

Because these impressions are based on work with both children and adults, they cover a range of observations over the entire developmental spectrum.

Many authors do not consider the death of a parent as necessarily pathogenic and find that under favorable circumstances, children cope with it successfully either by means of mourning or through other adaptive measures (Barnes, 1964; Furman, R. A., 1964; Gauthier, 1965; Wolfenstein 1966, 1969). There are studies of adults who, as children, suffered parental bereavement and made a normal adjustment (Hilgard, Newman, and Fisk, 1966). However, the bulk of the psychiatric and psychoanalytic literature supports the conclusion that the emotional development of the child is impaired as a result of the loss. The degree of impairment depends on a host of internal variables and external circumstances. Which variables are the most significant in helping the child surmount the loss depends on a particular researcher's point of view. Most researchers feel that therapeutic intervention with the child, as well as the adult who has experienced bereavement in childhood, has a beneficial effect. The work of E. Furman (1974) with children and the work of Fleming and Altschul (1963) with adults support this point of view. The therapist who sees children with a range of emotional difficulties feels that whereas the loss of a parent is traumatic, there are a host of traumas far more pathogenic for future adaptation. Consequently, one comes away with the impression that the loss of a parent is traumatic; however, given an approximation of adequate intervention, such a trauma is manageable and workable.

Clinical case studies have been one of the main sources of data regarding the effects of childhood bereavement. These case studies have prompted researchers to attribute etiologic significance to early bereavement for a variety of emotional disorders in later life. Such reports have also been instrumental in focusing on the dynamic issues and subtle nuances of each unique clinical situation.

Some writers focus on a category of disturbances in which childhood bereavement leads to an interference in development and results in arrest, regression, or distortion of the personality. Difficulty in object relationships is most often referred to, but there is diverging opinion as to whether it is caused by arrest or regression and to what level regression proceeds. Some authors stress the effect on the structuralization of the personality or on certain ego functions.

Clinical responses to the loss of a parent can be classified along a time line. Responses are classified as *immediate reactions*, which occur in the initial weeks and months after the death; *intermediate reactions*, which may emerge some years later in childhood or adolescence; and *long-range or sleeper effects*, which may appear in adulthood either as ongoing reactions or as delayed reactions to the loss.

A developmental perspective on parent loss assumes that the personal meanings and implications of a major interpersonal loss will be affected by the individual's level of cognitive and emotional maturity. Whereas adults may grieve intensely for a year or more, children are more likely to express their grief intermittently for a number of years after the death. At successive levels of subsequent development, thoughts and feelings about the loss will typically resurface and need to be reexamined and reresolved.

At certain ages, children are seen as exceptionally vulnerable to the loss of a parent. The impact of bereavement may be greater at some ages or developmental stages than at others. Rutter (1966) and Bowlby (1980) have reported that children under age 5 are more vulnerable to major interpersonal loss than older children. Early adolescence also has been cited as a vulnerable age, as the trauma interferes with the consolidation of identity.

Consequently, there is no ideal time to experience loss, because every developmental level will assume its unique conflicts and resolutions.

In spite of varying clinical presentations and a range of adaptive responses influenced by a number of internal and external factors, how do we account for the pervasive expectation of serious problems in the grieving child? How can we understand the strong tradition of associating adult psychopathology and childhood parental death? There are a number of possible explanations.

Depressed adults who come to us as patients are more likely to think and ruminate about the losses experienced in childhood. The loss of a parent may indeed become a preoccupation and an obsession. Such preoccupations ultimately become explanations. In the work with children and the surviving parent, one finds a history in which life did not exist before the parent's death.

A balanced picture of the parent and circumstances prior to the loss is impossible. Only after the loss has life assumed meaning and color, albeit the predominant colors are black and gray. Such an obsession with the loss may then assume a life of its own and become a metaphor and explanation for subsequent events, whether success or failure.

Another reason for an overemphasis on the loss may be retrospective justification or the need to construct etiologic hypotheses that externalize to past events responsibility for mental illness. This may be done to defend against personal feelings of blame, guilt, and shame. A strong need for retrospective rationalization and closure may be another reason for overdetermining the loss. As therapists and patients, we have an overriding need to render certain that which is unknown and therefore frightening.

However, apart from the aforementioned possibilities, there is a more basic consideration as to why the death of a parent becomes so pivotal in our genetic reconstructions. As concerned professionals, we are stunned and horrified by the events that shape and distort the lives of our patients. We empathize and sympathize with their plight and through vicarious introspection try to imagine the child's experience in losing a parent. In attempting to experience the patient's distress, we feel the worst that can happen to a child, especially a younger one, is the loss of a parent. Consequently, we assume that such a traumatic event is bound to have long-term deleterious effects as anything less is not plausible.

Although it is possible that the loss may bring relief or that replacements may be beneficial, we dismiss such thoughts as heresy. The event seems so horrendous that the idea of compensations has no place in our thinking.

Therapists search with their patients through their remembered histories for pertinent life experiences that may provide the key therapeutic metaphor for understanding and perhaps changing the patient's life. Once the metaphor has been found, the therapy will proceed forward or backward in time. Therapists would agree that one works with whatever reconstructive metaphor offers the most force and explanatory power about the patient's life (Stern, 1985).

When psychopathology is viewed from the clinical point of view, the primary task is to find the narrative point of origin—invariably the key metaphor. Our theories about the actual point of origin tell us only how to conduct the therapeutic search for such a point. One of the major tasks of the therapist is to help the patient find a narrative point of origin as a working model. That such a point is readily available in a case of parent loss may be a partial explanation why therapists are willing and eager to work with such patients as an intensive search is not necessary. Everything can be explained on the basis of the parent's death. The problem with such a ready-made explanation is that other genetic elements contributing to the psychopathology may be ignored.

Developmental Issues

Recent research in developmental psychology has led to a beginning reassessment of basic assumptions about continuities from infancy into adulthood. A corollary questioning has emerged about the special and unique importance of the infantile experience for subsequent development.

Data from early developmental research have challenged long-held assumptions about continuities from infancy. So far, little evidence has been found for predicting continuity from early to later development. For example, the New York Longitudinal Study (Chess, Thomas, and Birch, 1967) gave clear evidence that simple linear prediction from early childhood to later childhood, adolescence, and early adult life is not possible. The work of Kagan (1980) has demonstrated that various competencies in infants and very young children may disappear as a result of environmental failures; however, other competencies appear, which then pursue an independent course. These competencies were not present initially, yet they are present and they may continue or disappear. How or why these occur is not known; however, their appearance under adverse circumstances has been amply demonstrated.

A constructive environment reverses earlier mental deficits so as to bring the individual to an average level of functioning, but this says nothing about the individual's potential or functioning had the adversity not occurred. Nevertheless, the earlier notion that even a bad home is better than a good institution has not been verified. The recent upsurge and social awareness of child abuse supports that position. There is now overwhelming evidence that wider ego deficits need not occur when an early adverse environment is corrected by a later salutary one. Even on the basis of gross outcome measures, we would have to say that correction can occur to a far greater extent than our theories might have predicted.

There is a growing awareness that given a sufficiently decent environment, the child mobilizes self-righting tendencies to catch up after early prolonged adversity. Once again, the key questions remain how and why this occurs. Because there are many variables, we do not understand how people develop competence in situations of deprivation and environmental handicap.

The psychological structures of early childhood are dynamic and undergo consolidation and transformation; many of these may become free of the original experiences that preceded them. A single traumatic episode is unlikely to be pathogenic; after a deflection from a developmental pathway, there is a strong tendency to get back on track. Exactly how this happens we do not know, but we may speculate that parents and children make compensatory adjustments to extreme variations in expectable behavior. These adjustments may confound developmental continuities since different outcomes may result, determined by what compensatory adjustments are employed. Consequently, we need to reconsider the belief in irreversibility of adverse effects from early experience, even with major deprivations. The old model of development as a linear process is inappropriate.

Just as developmental psychologists have raised questions about continuities in infants and children, there has emerged a parallel explosion of research from the other end of the life cycle. Lifespan psychology has generated data showing that active development continues throughout life. From a psychological viewpoint, structural change does not stop at adolescence but continues at a lesser pace into adulthood.

The work of Vaillant (1977) illustrates the evolving psychodynamic changes that may occur in adulthood. One of the key points of his study is that no single childhood factor accounted for happiness or unhappiness at age 50; rather, it seemed to be the sustained emotional environment that appeared to have a lasting influence. Isolated traumatic events do not mold individual lives: what seems important is the continued interaction between the choice of adaptive mechanisms and sustained relationships with other people.

Vaillant concludes that mental health is not static but evolutionary. Little could be observed at age 19 that predicated mental health at 50. As a result, Vaillant postulates developmental discontinuities in adults that are as great as the difference in personality between a 9-year-old and what he becomes at 15.

In this study, as in those of early development, it seems so much easier to account for how things went wrong than for how things went right. We are still at a loss descriptively and dynamically to understand just why things do turn out well in development.

To round out the picture of adulthood as an evolving process, a study by Block (1971) demonstrates that not just emotional but cognitive development continues in adult life and that environmental factors can increase intellectual capacity among adults as well as children.

It is clear that developmental change in adulthood is not simply or continuously determined from the experience of the childhood or adolescent past. The use of the past is selective.

We must realize that developmental thrust is not over in adolescence. There is a continuing dynamic process, and the adult personality continues to undergo structural changes. It may be in fact that the psychology of adult development is as important as is the psychology of early development.

While the recent findings of discontinuities in development may shake the foundations of developmental psychology, the more pertinent and practical question is what impact, if any, will they have on clinical work. The obvious challenge of these early findings is primarily exerted on the genetic point of view, for they cast doubt on explanations of current pathology based on specific childhood traumas. What we reconstruct, and what may be helpful to the patient in reconstructing his history, may be experienced as anchored in a framework of screen memories and "known incidents" in the individual's history. With the current discoveries in developmental discontinuities, even real events may be questioned as to the validity of their traumatic nature and as determinants that may be closely linked to current psychopathological states.

Although such challenging of the genetic point of view, may be unsettling to the clinician, there is a potential positive effect from such theoretical upheaval. Owing to the self-righting tendencies, a single traumatic episode or even a brief early experience is unlikely, by itself, to cause a developmental deflection. If this is valid, then perhaps one can view human adaptation, as well as our therapeutic efforts, in a far more positive light. It is not unusual for the patient who comes with a horrendous childhood history to cloud the therapeutic work with an aura of pessimism. It is as if there is an unconscious need to demonstrate that severe childhood trauma leads to the inevitable crippling psychopathology in the adult. The clinician becomes an unwitting ally in the patient's need to prove that he is a helpless victim of his own traumatic historical past.

I am not implying that early deprivation is good for the developing organism, nor that development is totally discontinuous.

Adverse childhood experiences have effects of at least two kinds. First, they make the individual more vulnerable to later adverse experiences. Second, they make it more likely that he or she will meet with further such experiences. Whereas the earlier adverse experiences are likely to be wholly independent of the agency of the individual concerned, the later ones are likely to be the consequences of his or her own actions, actions that spring from those disturbances of personality to which the earlier experiences have given rise.

Developmental considerations have revealed that there is continuity from infancy but that it is of a different sort than we have imagined.

Integration

As the practitioner attempts to assess the mass of clinical data presented by a patient, a useful organizing principle emerges from an awareness of the work of others, relevant to a particular clinical problem. In an attempt to create order out of chaos, coherence out of confusion, and stability from instability, clinicians pay attention to that research which traces continuity between childhood experience and subsequent adult psychopathology. While such associations offer a sense of comfort to the therapist, and perhaps even suggest an aura of mastery for the patient, questions have arisen about the pervasive applicability of such an orientation.

Psychiatric and psychoanalytic studies reviewed in this presentation have vacillated between the extreme positions of early parent loss resulting in psychopathology to early parent loss being nonpredictive and noncontributory to subsequent clinical findings. This indecision is partly based on a differentiation between the clinical and epidemiologic points of view. It may well be that the results of large epidemiologic studies do not mesh with impressions gathered from individual case reports or small clinical samples. Such discrepancies are based on disparities in sample size and the variety of populations. The individual case report is slanted towards psychopathology since it is the clinician's task to elaborate a particular point of view and a bias to justify his or her efforts.

Other factors, however, may be equally significant contributors to the ongoing debate. Intellectually, we speculate that the child who loses a parent may surmount the trauma effectively, given the proper circumstances. We support such impressions with personal experiences and an accumulating body of research. Emotionally, however, we discard such possibilities because we assume that the loss of a parent is the worst that can happen to a child. Hence, we cannot resist the conclusion that such a trauma is bound to have long-term deleterious effects.

While the linkage of parent loss with various forms of psychopathology is questionable and problematic from a research perspective, the association of parent loss with depression is a viable consideration. On the basis of his clinical observations, Bowlby (1980) has asserted that profound early loss renders individuals highly vulnerable to later depressive disorders, especially with each subsequent loss. Nonetheless, the empirical evidence on early loss and depression remains suggestive at best. A review of controlled studies investigating the association between bereavement during childhood or adolescence and depression during adulthood (Crook and Eliot, 1980) reported that eight of eleven studies found a significantly higher rate of depressive disorders among the bereaved group; childhood loss of a parent increased the risk of depression by a factor of two or three. In seven of eight controlled studies, early loss was correlated with severity of depression.

As research efforts have become more sophisticated and discriminating, a separate line of inquiry has emerged which may indeed become the single most significant predictor of outcome. It has been suggested that not the loss per se but environmental factors after the loss may be more accurate predictors of outcome. The quality of the relationship with the surviving parent may be critical in determining who develops affective illness. A nonsupportive relationship with the surviving parent in which the child felt burdened by the parent's emotional needs was a particularly strong discriminator of adult psychopathology. The quality of the relationship with the surviving parent coupled with the parent's healthy adaptation to the loss of a spouse are critical "protective" factors in determining the child's well-being later in life.

Another significant impression from the work with parents is that a parent whose own parent died in childhood encountered difficulties in parenting but showed minimal disturbances in other areas. The parent encountered serious difficulties in parenting when his or her child's developmental phase coincided with the developmental period when his own parent died.

While such point-for-point correlations may not be constantly predictable, they should alert the clinician to a possibility hitherto not recognized nor appreciated. Traumatic events from childhood, specifically the loss of a parent, may be considered as a general framework that has value for organizing data in the therapeutic situation. However, before drawing conclusions about the impact on the adult of a loss in childhood, it is important to explore the function, role, and meaning of the lost object at various periods in the life course. The lost object may have a far different significance for the child in the early latency versus the late latency or for that matter in mid-adolescence.

In order to be more accurate in our assessments of childhood trauma, we need to be more appreciative of the possibility that both post-early childhood and post-adolescent life span periods that have their own unique developmental contributions and need not be explained solely in terms of earlier developmental achievements or failures (Pollock, 1982).

The need to impose meaning on a patient's life based on our romance with the infant may hamper the understanding and appreciation of the unique contributions of later developmental eras. Whereas the impact of early life events is more gross and global, the impact of later events may be more subtle in the nuances and may require a finer appreciation of the back-and-forth of multiple developmental shifts.

Given the current state of knowledge and the absence of conclusive data, what is one to predict for the future of a child who has experienced the loss of a parent? As a clinician, one is called upon to make such projections. One response would be to plead discontinuities in development and the inability to foresee the relative valences of significant replacement figures. If we assume that the death of a parent is traumatic for the child and if we avoid the extremes of profound clinical psychopathology and a stable adult, then we may consider alternate possibilities.

In dealing with well-functioning adults who were bereaved in childhood, one senses that there persists a recurrent sense of restlessness, drivenness, and vague dissatisfaction with life, with others, and primarily with themselves. There is invariably a persistent feeling that something is not right and that something is missing, which then has to be searched for, replaced, or compensated. Such an individual is on an ongoing quest, a search for something he or she may never find, yet feels compelled to search for at all costs. It may well be the adult's ability to come to terms with such vague and disquieting feelings that will ultimately determine one's stability and adaptation to the loss.

REFERENCES

Abraham, K. (1911), Notes on the psychoanalytic investigation and treatment of manic-depressive insanity and allied conditions. In: *Selected Papers on Psychoanalysis*. London: Hogarth Press, 1927, pp. 137–149.

Altschul, S. (1968), Denial and ego arrest. *J. Amer. Psychoanal. Assn.*, 16:301–317.

Barnes, M. (1964), Reactions to the death of a mother. *The Psychoanalytic Study of the Child*, 19:334–357. New York: International Universities Press.

Beck, A. T., Sethi, B. B. & Tuthill, R. W. (1963), Childhood bereavement and adult depression. *Arch. Gen. Psychiat.*, 9:295–302.

Birtchnell, J. (1969), Parent death in relation to age and parental age at birth in psychiatric patients and general population controls. *Brit. J. Preventive Soc. Med.*, 23:244–262.

—————— (1971), Case-register study of bereavement. *Proceed. Royal Soc. Med.*, 64:279–282.

—————— (1972), Early parent death and psychiatric diagnosis, *Soc. Psychiat.*, 7:202–210.

———— (1974), Is there a scientifically acceptable alternative to the epidemiological study of familial factors in mental illness? *Soc. Sc. Med.*, 8:335–350.

———— (1975), The personality characteristics of early bereaved psychiatric patients. *Soc. Psychiat.*, 10:97–103.

Block, J. (1971), *Lives Through Time*. Berkeley, CA: Bancroft.

Bowlby, J. (1960), Grief and mourning in infancy and early childhood. *The Psychoanalytic Study of the Child*, 15:9–52. New York: International Universities Press.

———— (1977), The making and breaking of affectional bonds, I: Etiology and psychopathology in the light of the attachment theory. *Brit J. Psychiat.*, 130:201–210.

———— (1980), *Loss: Sadness and Depression*, Vol. 3. *Attachment and Loss*. London: Hogarth Press.

———— (1982), Attachment and loss: Retrospect and prospect. *Amer. J. Orthopsychiat.*, 52:664–678.

Breier, A., Kelsoe, J., Kerwin, P., Beller, S., Wolkovortz, O. & Prickar, D. (1988), Early parental loss and development of adult psychopathology *Arch. Gen. Psychiat.*, 45:987–993.

Brown, F. (1961), Depression and childhood bereavement. *J. Ment. Sci.*, 107:754–777.

Chess, S., Thomas, A. & Birch, H. (1967), The plasticity of human development. *J. Amer. Acad. Child Psychiat.*, 6(2):321–331.

Crook, T. & Eliot, J. (1980), Parental death during childhood and adult depression: A critical review of the literature. *Psychol. Bull.*, 87: 252–259.

Fleming, J. & Altschul, S. (1963), Activation of mourning and growth. *Internat. J. Psychoanal.*, 44:419–431.

Freud, A. (1960), Discussion of Dr. John Bowlby's paper. *The Psychoanalytic Study of the Child*, 15:53–62. New York: International Universities Press.

Freud, S. (1915), Mourning and melancholia. *Standard Edition*, 14: 248–258. London: Hogarth Press, 1957.

Furman, E. (1974), *A Child's Parent Dies.*. New Haven, CT: Yale University Press.

Furman, R. A. (1964), Death and the young child: Some preliminary considerations. *The Psychoanalytic Study of the Child*, 19:321–393. New York: International Universities Press.

Gauthier, Y. (1965), The mourning reaction of a ten and one-half year old boy. *The Psychoanalytic Study of the Child*, 20:481–494. New York: International Universities Press.

Harris, T., Brown, G. & Biffulco, A. (1986), Loss of a parent in childhood and adult psychiatric disorder: The role of lack of adequate parental care. *Psychol. Med.*, 16:641–659.

Hilgard, J. R., Newman, M. F. & Fisk, F. (1966), Strength of adult ego following childhood bereavement. *Amer. J. Orthopsychiat.*, 30:788–798.

Kagan, J. (1980), Family experience and the child's development. In: *Annual Progress in Child Psychiatry and Child Development*, ed. S. Chess & A. Thomas. New York: Brunner/Mazel, pp. 21–30.

Kendler, K., Neale, M., Kessler, R., Heath, A. C., & Eaves, L. T. (1992), Childhood parental loss and adult psychopathology in women. *Arch. Gen. Psychiat.*, 49:109–116.

Nagera, H. (1970), Children's reactions to the death of important objects: A developmental approach. *The Psychoanalytic Study of the Child*, 25:360–400. New York: International Universities Press.

Pollock, G. H. (1961), Mourning and adaptation. *Internat. J. Psycho-Anal.*, 42:341–361.

––––––– (1978), Process and affect: Mourning and grief. *Internat. J. Psychoanal.*, 59:255–276.

Ragan, D. V. (1986), Childhood parental death and adult psychopathology. *Amer. J. Psychiat.*, 143:153–157.

Roy, A. (1983), Early parental death and adult depression. *Psychol. Med.*, 13:861–865.

Rutter, M. (1972), *Maternal Deprivation Reassessed*. Harmondsworth, Eng.: Penguin Books.

Sklar, H. & Harris, J. (1985), Effects of parent loss: Interaction with family size and sibling order. *Amer. J. Psychiat.*, 142:708–714.

Stern, D. (1985). *The Interpersonal World of the Infant*. New York: Basic Books.

Tennant, C., Bebbington, D. & Hurry, J. (1981), Parental death in childhood and risk of adult depressive disorders: A review. In: *Annual Progress in Child Psychiatry and Child Development*, ed. S. Chess & A. Thomas. New York: Brunner/Mazel, pp. 238–257.

Vaillant, G. E. (1977), *Adaptation to Life*. Boston: Little, Brown.

Wolfenstein, M. (1966), How is mourning possible? *The Psychoanalytic Study of the Child*, 21:93–123. New York: International Universities Press.

———— (1969), Loss, rage and repetition. *The Psychoanalytic Study of the Child*, 24:432–460. New York: International Universities Press.

7 THOUGHT DISORDERS IN ADOLESCENT SCHIZOPHRENIA: TOWARD AN INTEGRATIVE MODEL

JOHN PORT, MARTIN HARROW,
THOMAS JOBE, AND DARIN DOUGHERTY

Schizophrenia, a disorder that often begins to manifest itself in late adolescence and early adulthood, is characterized by a number of dramatic symptoms. Among the most dramatic are gross reality distortions, of which one of the more important types is thought disorder. This paper focuses on thought disorder in adolescent and early adult schizophrenia, specifically on positive thought disorder and its manifestations in schizophrenia, on its frequency in schizophrenia compared with other major psychotic disorders, on its persistence over time, and on several existing theories of schizophrenic thought disorder. We also advance a formulation concerning possible biological and cognitive factors that may be involved in its pathogenesis.

There are two different types of disturbances in cognition that at various times have been discussed in relation to schizophrenia. One is a disorder involving cognitive deficits, such as impoverished or deficit thinking, and involving concrete thinking (Benjamin, 1944; Goldstein, 1944; Vigotsky, 1962; Chapman and Chapman, 1973; Harrow, Adler, and Hanf, 1974; Andreasen, 1979a, b; Andreasen and Olsen, 1982; Crow et al., 1982; Pogue-Geile and Harrow, 1985; Harrow and Quinlan, 1985). The second type of cognitive disturbance involves strange or idiosyncratic ideas. Some label this latter type as positive thought disorder, although other terms have been used such as bizarre-idiosyncratic thinking and autistic thinking (Shimkunas, Gynther, and Smith, 1967; Chapman and Chapman, 1973; Johnston and Holzman, 1979; Harrow and Quinlan, 1985; Oltmanns et al., 1985; Braff et al., 1988).

Although both concrete thinking and positive thought disorder are found frequently in schizophrenia, in recent times positive thought disorder has been the most frequently studied and appears to be linked to other reality distortions such as delusions. At present the strength of the relationship between positive thought disorder and delusions is controversial; some data suggest that each is a part of a separate factor (Strauss, 1993), and other data suggest that there is a strong relationship between positive thought disorder and delusions (Harrow, Silverstein, and Marengo, 1983; Harrow and Marengo, 1986).

Signs of positive thought disorder in schizophrenia have been found to emerge in routine conversations with schizophrenics, in clinical interviews, and in responses to special tests for which scoring systems have been designed to study positive thought disorder, such as the Rorschach test and the Proverbs Test.

The following is an example of positive thought disorder that ymerged from the clinical interview of a 19-year-old female schizophrenic patient:

> I had a . . . I was . . . first, uh, I found myself constantly trying to find myself, and part of that got me into Alaska where I was fishing. And I enjoyed the work on the boat but some of the implications of that work...I made a lot of free associations about what I was doing, and how that pertained to myself or my image of myself, and when I lost the job on the boat . . . and later that fall my mother called several times and telegrammed—I flew down to her house and found that things that were going on between myself and her were very strange to me.
>
> I felt very frightened about the idea of . . . of . . . of . . . uh . . . of what a supposition my thinking the earth as being a universal woman image could mean as far as being much too heavy a burden for anybody and especially difficult, uh, for me and yet it seemed like a lot of people were on that kind of a merry-go-round—that was becoming increasingly destructive to life and to a sense of home which I liked to feel about being in. [slight pause] Also, I guess I probably felt some fear of being kind of left on my own, without any . . . uh . . . any patterns, really, it didn't make any sense to me. . . . I seemed to be robbed of just the ability to go by my sense and what I thought was natural . . . that seemed to be something too . . . too demanding. Uh, what

I was in was a relationship to someone else. And, uh . . . sometimes I'd feel like I wanted to hold on and stop, uh, that whole cycle, and other times I would feel kind of giddy about being involved in that whole cycle [Harrow and Quinlan, 1985].

Four other examples of positive thought disorder that emerged from responses to the Proverbs Test from our own research group's program of study include the following. An 18-year-old male schizophrenic patient responded to the proverb "Barking dogs seldom bite" with the response. "A bear in a tree is worth two in a zoo." A 19-year-old male schizophrenic patient responded to the proverb "Gold goes in any gate except heaven's" with the response, "Don't trade in for a stash in gold, a pot of gold, but strive for a crown of glory." When questioned further, he continued with, "Don't sell your soul for anything." Another 19-year-old male schizophrenic patient responded to the proverb "Don't swap horses while crossing a stream" with the response, "Stay on your horse or you just might scream, and possibly get a little wet and lose your dream." When questioned further, he continued, "If a guy was with a girl and they were slopping around in the water and she fell in, they might come up ugly and he'd lose his dream. Especially if she liked him." An 18-year-old female schizophrenic patient responded to the proverb "One swallow does not make a summer" with the response, "A summer makes a swallow. In summer time the winds will come. Will come back, I hope."

Does the Strange Speech in Schizophrenia Result from a Language Disorder or a Thought Disorder?

While the examples that we have presented are dramatic ones, they illustrate a problem that has spawned decades of controversy, namely, are these and similar examples of pathological schizophrenic speech due to thought disorder or to a speech or language disorder? Even classic investigators such as Vigotsky (1962) have attempted to address this issue. In more recent times such theorists as Chaika (1982) have proposed that examples of schizophrenic pathology such as those we have presented should be viewed as due to a "speech disorder" rather than to a "thought disorder." We agree that disordered speech and disordered thinking cannot *automatically* be equated with each other, but there is considerable evidence that the disordered speech we see in schizophrenic patients is usually part of a larger pathological picture involving disordered thinking and reality distortions (Lanin-Kettering and Harrow, 1985; Harrow, Prather, and Lanin-Kettering, 1986; Schwartz, 1982).

Looked at in one way, thinking is a theoretical construct that describes a wide range of internal cognitive behaviors rather than an overt behavior such as speech. There is, however, overwhelming evidence for the usefulness of the construct of "thinking," including strong evidence about many of its products and strong and uniform evidence about the results of interference with the process of thinking.

NONVERBAL TESTS ELIMINATE LANGUAGE ISSUES: OBJECT SORTING PARADIGM

When we examine evidence supporting the hypothesis that most schizophrenics have a thought disorder rather than just a speech disorder, one important subset of data emerges from studies in which both disordered verbal and nonverbal behaviors are investigated. An example of evidence indicating that schizophrenics have a thought disorder can be found in their performance on tasks requiring the manipulation of objects or things used in real-life situations. One of the major tasks in this area used successfully by our own research team and by a number of other investigators is the Object-Sorting Test (Goldstein and Scheerer, 1941; Harrow and Quinlan, 1985; Harrow and Marengo, 1986).

When schizophrenics are administered this task, the strange sortings of objects that are observed often result from ideas and thinking that are strange and inappropriate in that particular task, rather than from disordered words or speech (Lanin-Kettering and Harrow, 1985).

Our research provides evidence for a relatively high correlation (For $r = .45$ to $r = .60$) between the use of strange ideas and concepts on the Object-Sorting Test and ratings of thought disorder on more purely verbal tests such as the Proverbs Test (Marengo et al, 1986). These data suggest that some of the underlying factors responsible for disordered behavior on less verbal tests (e.g., the strange ideas, strange concepts, and strange styles of thinking observed in the schizophrenic's object-sorting performance) may be related to the underlying factors responsible for disordered speech and behavior on more verbal tests (e.g., the Proverbs Test).

Both this evidence and other evidence on delusional thinking in schizophrenia fit into a theoretical model described as a nomologic net, which relates various theoretical constructs and observable events to one another (Cronbach and Meehl, 1956). In such a nomologic net, the various types of behaviors and events, with the relationship between them fitting into a theoretical model, can be used as a way of validating a construct or set of constructs (Cronbach and Meehl, 1956). This type of nomological net, involving constructs about schizophrenia and related observations and data on cognition and behavior can lead to rich hypotheses about how different types of schizophrenic psychopathology may or may not be linked.

STRANGE NONVERBAL BEHAVIORS IN NONTEST SITUATIONS

A second and related type of evidence on disordered schizophrenic thinking that fits into the nomologic net just described involves other data indicating that disordered speech is not the only type of strange behavior displayed by schizophrenic patients. Many schizophrenics do strange things and behave in strange ways in nontest situations. The strange behavior of a schizophrenic patient who engages in strange speech is part of a larger cluster of behaviors that can be attributed to a more general tendency to think strangely and to behave inappropriately. If the schizophrenic patient demonstrated only strange speech and strange word usage, there would be no reason to expect some schizophrenic patients to engage in strange posturing or other unusual types of behavior. Here again the formulation that strange speech suggests strange thinking can fit into a construct about schizophrenic disordered thinking that is grounded in a larger nomological net involving various different types of strange behaviors.

STRANGE SCHIZOPHRENIC VERBALIZATIONS OFTEN REFLECT INAPPROPRIATE IDEAS

Further evidence suggesting the presence of thought disorder in schizophrenics can be seen by taking a closer look at the type of strange and inappropriate speech behavior elicited during verbal tests. An analysis of schizophrenic patients' disordered speech on these tests indicates that these patients frequently intermingle personal material (i.e., ideas related to conflicts and issues of personal concern) into speech when it does not fit into the external context of the conversation. This makes the schizophrenic patients' speech appear strange and inappropriate (Harrow and Prosen 1978, 1979; Harrow et al., 1983). In these cases, the disturbance is at the level of ideational relevance associated with thinking rather than at the level of individual words or parts of speech. The disordered verbalizations involved in intermingling are based on a mixing in of ideas and thoughts about personal conflicts at the wrong time.

SCHIZOPHRENICS EXPRESS STRANGE DELUSIONS WITH ADEQUATE LANGUAGES

Another type of evidence that schizophrenics' strange speech is usually due to strange thinking is the data indicating that a large percentage of acute schizophrenic patients have delusions involving grossly false ideas about the world. These grossly false beliefs about the world are usually expressed using adequate syntax and adequate speech, indicating that the schizophrenic thought disorder is at the ideational level and not solely at the verbal level.

Delusions that often represent strange and inappropriate thinking of a less transitory kind are further evidence on the larger nomological net bearing on formulations about strange ideation that we have discussed earlier. Our group has provided strong data indicating that there is a high correlation between the presence of delusional beliefs (which often involve strange and unreal ideas that are presumably related to thinking) and disordered speech (Harrow, Silverstein, and Marengo, 1983; Harrow and Quinlan, 1985; Harrow and Marengo, 1986). The high correlations between these two types of psychopathological phenomena indicate that, among patients who are schizophrenic, those patients who are most delusional are the ones most likely to show speech disorder.

Thought Disorder Is not Limited to Schizophrenia

A large number of studies have been conducted exploring the frequency of thought disorder in adolescent and early adult schizophrenics during the acute phase (Chapman and Chapman, 1973; Johnston and Holzman, 1979; Neale and Oltmanns, 1980; Harrow and Quinlan, 1985; Walker, Harvey, and Perlman, 1988). The research in this area has consistently found a high number of schizophrenics that show thought disorder. These results are not specific to a single test instrument or method of detecting thought disorder; consistent, severe thought disorder in young acute schizophrenics can be demonstrated using the Rorschach test (Rapaport, Gill, and Schafer, 1968; Blatt and Wild, 1976; Harrow and Quinlan, 1985; Holzman, Shenton, and Solovay, 1986), the Proverbs Test (Adler and Harrow, 1974; Marengo and Harrow, 1985; Harrow and Marengo, 1986) and various other assessment techniques, such as structured interviews (Andreasen, 1979a, b; Harvey, 1983; Harvey and Walker, 1987) and preverbalization techniques (Reilly et al., 1975). Thus, for instance, our research program studying late adolescent and young adult patients has found from 80% to 85% of recently hospitalized schizophrenics as showing positive thought disorder during the acute phase (Harrow et al., 1982; Marengo and Harrow, 1985), and other major investigators have also found a similar high percentage of acute schizophrenics showing positive thought disorder (Andreasen, 1979b).

It should be noted that, while a high percentage of early young schizophrenics show overt thought disorder, not all young schizophrenics have severe thought disorder. In any single study one usually finds from 5% to 25% of young schizophrenics without overt signs of thought disorder. In this respect, thought disorder is like other types of reality distortions in schizophrenia, such as delusions: it is found frequently in schizophrenics but not in every schizophrenic.

Originally, on the basis of earlier work by Kraepelin (1919) and by Bleuler (1911), thought disorder was believed to be exclusive to schizophrenia. Bleuler, in particular, saw a disorder in the associative processes, with loose associations as one of the central characteristics of the schizophrenic process. Nonetheless, clinical observers periodically noted that some psychotic patients who were not schizophrenic also showed signs of thought disorder.

Two major studies in the 1970s established conclusively that thought disorder was not unique to schizophrenia. The first of these involved research by Andreasen, who found evidence indicating that bipolar manic patients seemed to manifest as much thought disorder as schizophrenics, and possibly even more thought disorder. Andreasen's research compared schizophrenic with bipolar manic patients, first using the Object Sorting Test (Andreasen and Powers, 1974), then using the patients' verbalizations in interview situations (Andreasen, 1979b). In both situations she found that manic patients manifested as much or more thought disorder than schizophrenics did. Her findings were later confirmed by a number of other investigators (e.g., Harrow et al., 1982, 1986; Harvey, 1983; Harvey, Earle-Boyer, and Wieglus, 1984; Holzman, Shenton, and Solovay, 1986; Shenton, Solovay, and Holzman, 1987). Because these results did not support the earlier view that thought disorder predominates only in schizophrenia, they helped to established a new, more realistic view of schizophrenic thought disorder.

The second wave of studies on schizophrenic thought disorder was our own research indicating that severe thought disorder is frequent in schizophrenia but is not exclusive to schizophrenia or to mania and can be found to a lesser extent in many other types of acute patients (Harrow and Quinlan, 1977). We investigated whether the frequency of thought disorder is greater in acute schizophrenia and acute mania because these patients are psychotic. The data indicate that, although thought disorder is significantly more frequent in schizophrenic and manic patients than in other types of psychotic patients, psychotic patients in general do tend to show more thought disorder than nonpsychotic patients do (Marengo and Harrow, 1985).

In addition, mild levels of thought disorder such as cognitive slips had once been felt by some to be an early sign of schizophrenia. Our research indicates that milder levels of thought pathology, such as cognitive slips, can be found in a variety of different types of disturbed people (Harrow and Quinlan, 1977), including not only those who have schizophrenia, but also those with a variety of other disorders. Indeed, when one looks carefully, one can find cognitive slips in normal people, especially when they feel upset or are under pressure (e.g., political candidates who engage in TV debates).

Thought Disorder in Schizophrenia Tends to Persist or Recur

Earlier views of thought disorder by Bleuler and others were based on the belief that thought disorder persists throughout the schizophrenic patient's lifetime. This viewpoint has been brought into question by recent research. Studies of schizophrenic thought disorder over time do suggest that a number of schizophrenics show either persistent or frequently recurring thought disorder (Harrow and Quinlan, 1985; Harrow and Marengo, 1986; Parnas and Schulsinger, 1986; Harrow et al., 1986; Parnas et al., 1988). The evidence also suggests, however, that after the acute phase of the disorder, many schizophrenics show partial remission of their thought disorder and a number of others show complete remission (Harrow and Quinlan, 1985; Harrow and Marengo, 1986). Thus, the data suggest that thought disorder does not persist in all schizophrenics. Rather thought disorder, as is the case for other types of positive symptoms in schizophrenia such as delusions, (Harrow et al., 1995), shows slower recoverability in schizophrenia and greater persistence than in other types of psychiatric disorders.

In general, recent research on positive symptoms suggests that schizophrenics and most other types of patients who are acutely psychotic are vulnerable to subsequent positive symptoms also. When we look at positive symptoms such as delusions, this vulnerability holds for more than just schizophrenia and includes bipolar psychotic depressives and other types of affective disorders. One can expect that many patients who are acutely psychotic may show subsequent signs of psychosis later in the course of their disorder (Sands and Harrow, 1994; Harrow et al., 1995). Among acutely psychotic patients, schizophrenics are likely to show more severe positive symptoms subsequently, and their subsequent positive symptoms are likely to persist or recur more frequently than they do in other types of patients who are acutely psychotic.

Although positive symptoms in general and thought disorder in particular do not persist in unabated form throughout the schizo-phrenic's lifetime, it is a psychopathology that poses a challenge for them on a longitudinal basis. Schizophrenics are vulnerable to subsequent positive symptoms, including both thought disorder and psychosis. Thus while the old viewpoint that "once crazy, always crazy" has not been supported among all schizophrenic patients, in general schizophrenics do show severe thought disorder during the acute phase as well as during subsequent active psychotic phases. In addition, for a limited number of schizophrenics, thought pathology may become a permanent part of their thinking, and, in its worst form, severe thought disorder may be continuous.

Theories of Schizophrenic Thought Disorder

Various theories about schizophrenic thought disorder have been advanced over the years to try to understand why schizophrenics show thought pathology, and what mechanisms are involved in their positive thought disorder.

BLEULER'S CLASSIC THEORY

In the early part of this century, Bleuler (1911) advanced his views of the central factors in schizophrenia. The two most important features in his systematic view were loss of associations and affective deterioration. For Bleuler, loss of associations (later called thought disorder) was the critical feature of schizophrenia. In his view, loosening of the normal associate links made it more likely that a person's routine stream of conscious thought would be diverted and eventually dominated by the person's inner life. As a result of this loosening of ongoing thought, the patient's wishes, conflicts, and complexes would emerge into the patient's thinking and verbalizations. This constellation of factors was viewed as a major contributor to the patient's psychosis.

VARIOUS PSYCHOANALYTIC THEORIES

Earlier psychoanalytic theories of schizophrenic thought disorder were based on views about a) distinctions between primary-process thinking and thinking based on secondary processes and b) problems concerning the disruption of thinking by previously undischarged affect. These theories emphasize the importance of primary-process thinking involving primitive forms of drive dominating thinking. The frequent use by schizophrenic patients of primitive modes of thought such as condensation and displacement (major concepts derived from psychoanalytic theory) fit into these views about primitive and magical types of thinking. Key psychoanalytically oriented theorists such as Rapaport et al., (1968) conducted experimental studies on thought disorder that helped set a model for later modern research on schizophrenic thought pathology. In addition, when one casts these older theories within a modern framework, some of the psychoanalytic views may offer promising leads about the potential role of failure of inhibition (and the emergence of more primitive drive-dominated thinking or of primary-process material) as one of several important factors in thought disorder. When we turn again to the specific contributions of Rapaport and colleagues, we note that a number of later measures of thought disorder were based on concepts discussed by this group of therapists. This includes the measure of primitive drive dominated thinking and primary-process thinking constructed by Holt (1977).

Holt's earlier system, based on Rapaport's research (using the Rorschach test) and later derivations of Holt's system have been employed in important studies exploring manifestations of primary-process thinking and drive-dominated thinking in adolescents and young adult patients (Silverman, Lapkin, and Rosenbaum, 1962; Harrow et al., 1976). Other formal manuals to conduct studies of primary-process thinking and thought disorder were constructed, also based on Rapaport's work and also using the Rorschach test (Watkins and Stauffacher, 1952; Quinlan, Harrow, and Carlson, 1973).

Again, the importance of Rapaport and colleagues' thinking is apparent when we look at two major ways that are frequently used in modern research to quantify and study schizophrenic thought disorder. The first of these two techniques is an elaborate system for scoring test responses of patients that was developed by Holzman and colleagues (Johnston and Holzman, 1979). The other method involves Exner's (1993) elaborate system to score responses to the Rorschach test along a number of different dimensions. Included among these different dimensions is a set of special scores used to assess disordered thinking and a schizophrenic diagnosis.

Both of these important methods of assessing schizophrenic thought disorder employ the Rorschach technique, and both use Rorschach test behavior to derive scores for patient responses that are based in part, on concepts derived earlier from psychoanalytically oriented research and thinking by Rapaport et al., (1968). Other key measures of assessing schizophrenic thought disorder have been devised that employ methods other than the Rorschach test, such as those of our research group using the Proverbs Test, a test of social comprehension, and the Object Sorting Test (Harrow et al., 1982; Marengo et al., 1985), Andreasen's (1979a, b) important and frequently employed method of assessment using patients' verbalizations in interview situations and many other systems of assessment as well (e.g., Watson, 1967; Chapman and Chapman, 1973; Goldstein, 1987; Rochester and Martin, 1979). While a number of these latter methods have been used profitably in research that has advanced thinking on schizophrenic thought disorder, the earlier psychoanalytically oriented approach employed by Rapaport and colleagues has had considerable impact on views about thought disorder, many of the ideas persisting in research even to the present day.

Much of psychoanalytic theory has tended to emphasize the ego and its role in defending against inner drives and outside stresses. This emphasis has led to views about schizophrenia as involving a boundary disorder. Research studying the link between disordered thinking, potential boundary disturbance, object representation, and schizophrenia has been conducted by Blatt and colleagues (Blatt and Ritzler, 1974; Blatt and Wild, 1976) and by others (Quinlan and Harrow, 1974; Harrow and Quinlan, 1985).

Other ego-analytic views of schizophrenia see schizophrenia as resulting from a weak or defective ego (Bellak, 1966). This theory emphasizes a multitude of different "ego" functions that are weakened in the schizophrenic. In this more general outlook, thought process, reality testing, object relations, and some other ego functions are seen as important dimensions that are disturbed in schizophrenic patients. While this latter type of theory, emphasizing ego functions and potential ego defects, offers a broad view of human functioning and of potential psychopathology, it presents some difficulty by not specifying exactly which of many potential impaired aspects of functioning mark off the schizophrenic as different from other psychotic patients and even from some very disordered nonpsychotic patients.

THEORIES OF A DISORDER IN FAMILY COMMUNICATION

Extensive research has been conducted on potential communication disorders in the parents of schizophrenics. This line of research was initiated by in the 1960s (see Wynne and Singer, 1963; Lidz, Fleck and Cornelison, 1965; Wild et al., 1965) and has continued throughout the last two decades by researchers including our own team (see Wynne et al., 1977; Singer, Wynne, and Toohey, 1978; Falloon et al., 1981; Harrow and Quinlan, 1985; Goldstein, 1987; Romney, 1988). Much of this research has focused on the parents of schizophrenics. In these theories, the adolescent schizophrenic's thought disorder is seen as the result of distortions in communication in the patient's parental home while he or she was growing up.

Within the parental home, disordered styles of communication are thought to be transmitted from the parents to their children, often as a consequence of the disruption of the maintenance of a shared focus of attention within the family. This results in distorted internal representations of reality for the growing child. Thus, the etiology of schizophrenia is viewed as being the result of the distortions in early parent–child interactions, with a particular emphasis on the distorted and irrational communications of the parents. Over the years there has been sharp debate on this thesis. Opponents of the view that parental behavior toward the child who later becomes schizophrenic is involved in the etiology of schizophrenia have challenged the empirical findings and also have noted that genetic transmission of an underlying disorder may account for some or all of the findings in this area. These results and their interpretation are still controversial, but a recent metaanalysis of various empirical findings on this topic by Romney (1990) has provided some support for views about a relationship between disordered thinking and communication in the adolescent schizophrenic's home. Recent research on expressed emotion and relapse of schizophrenic symptoms also supports this earlier work (Flaherty and Jobe, 1992).

Cognition-Based Theories of Schizophrenic Thought Disorder

ATTENTION DEFICIT/STIMULUS PROCESSING DISORDER THEORY

Over the years therapists have emphasized the importance of a disorder in attention, or in stimulus processing, with this disorder seen by some as the basis of many aspects of reality distortion by schizophrenics. A study by McGhie and Chapman (1961; Chapman, 1966), based on phenomenologic reports by a sample of schizophrenics, has fueled interest in these ideas. Their study showed a disorder in attention involving difficulty separating figure from ground, or in attending selectively to the appropriate stimuli (e.g., "Lately it has been hard for me to focus on one thing because I feel myself distracted by every possible object, line, and color within sight."). The particular technique used by McGhie and Chapman, however, and even the interpretation of their findings have been brought into question by a series of studies using similar techniques. These studies have raised the issue of whether the particular type of disorder in selective attention is specific to schizophrenia or can also be found in a variety of other disturbed patients and even in many upset normals (Harrow, Tucker, and Shield, 1972; Freedman and Chapman, 1973; Freedman, 1974; Harrow and Quinlan, 1985).

Since this research, a number of other theorists have advocated the importance of an attentional disorder in schizophrenia, and some have conducted important investigations showing attentional problems and difficulties in stimulus processing in schizophrenics (Cromwell and Dokecki, 1968; Salzinger et al., 1970; Neale and Oltmanns, 1980; Maher, 1983; Neuchterlein and Dawson, 1984; George and Neufeld, 1985; Saccuzzo and Braff, 1986; Harvey et al, 1986; Hemsley, 1987; Harvey, Earle-Boyer, and Levinson, 1988; Harvey et al., 1990; Cornblatt and Keilp, 1994). Since disordered attention could be part of the general deficit found in many severely disturbed patients (Chapman and Chapman, 1973) one of the issues raised by research in this area is whether the attentional disorder found in schizophrenics and many other severely disturbed patients is sufficient to lead to major reality distortions such as thought disorder, delusions, and hallucinations.

While we are focused on adolescent and young-adult schizophrenics in the current report, it should be noted that there also has been important research studying attentional disorder in high-risk children, and these programs have also found evidence of attentional disorders (Asarnow et al., 1978; Erlenmeyer-Kimling and Cornblatt, 1978; Cornblatt et al., 1985). At times, however, in the study of adolescent and other schizophrenics there have been issues about the specificity of some of the theoretical formulations, since attention covers a very broad band of functions, inasmuch as there are different types of attentional problems and attention.

Some of the mentioned investigators and other theorists have proposed a strong link between a schizophrenic patient's difficulties in attending selectively and other key aspects of attention and thought disorder (Walker et al., 1988). Related hypotheses have involved difficulties in short-term memory and a potential link between a disorder in short-term memory and thought disorder (Koh, 1978; Maher, 1983; Cornblatt et al., 1985; George and Neufeld, 1985; Ragin and Oltmanns, 1987; Harvey et al., 1988; Manschreck et al., 1991). The formulations concerning a link between an impairment in short-term memory and schizophrenia hold considerable promise, since short-term memory, or *working memory*, may serve very broad and important functions in cognition, cutting across attention and other major aspects of information processing. Recent research by Goldman-Rakic (1987), studying monkeys, indicated the importance of short-term memory and attempted to locate sites for short-term memory. Issues about top-down versus bottom-up cognition (and even whether all cognition may be bottom up) (Hinton and Anderson, 1989; Koch, 1993) can be resolved, in part, by research on short-term memory. In general, research on the specific nature of the cognitive processes that occur in short-term memory and on its location can be extremely promising. Indeed, it is quite possible, perhaps even probable, that there is not one site for short-term memory or working memory, but rather a set of different sites in the brain, each serving short-term memory functions.

BROADBENT'S PIGEON-HOLING THEORY

Broadbent (1977) proposed a cognitive mechanism for information organization he termed "pigeon-holing." He described a kind of attention that "selects some of the possible interpretations that a man may hold about the world and eliminates others as candidates for use in the particular situation" (p. 110). Pigeon-holing works by 1) integrating information from the present context and past experience of similar contexts and 2) biasing both the interpretations of current sensory input and the preparation of responses to that input in relation to the expected probabilities of events as derived from that integration (Broadbent, 1977). From a modern neurocomputational view, pigeon-holing may represent a synthesis of top-down and bottom-up processes.

This system may become dysfunctional in schizophrenia, wherein inappropriate responses to sensory input are manifested as cognitive symptoms of schizophrenia. While this theory (and Broadbent's (1984) later modifications of it) emphasizes the connection between the present context and past experience in the cognitive process, it does not elaborate further in regard to the anatomy of these connections. This model, however, has had an important influence on later British theorists, such as Frith (1987; Frith and Done, 1988) and Hemsley (1987) and has also influenced some American theorists. Broadbent's views include basic mechanisms in cognition and are important in considering positive symptoms in general, in that they emphasize the role of contextual influences and subject biasing on perception.

CALLAWAY'S DYSFUNCTIONAL
INFORMATION PROCESSING THEORY

Callaway and Naghdi (1982), concentrating on dysfunctional information processing in schizophrenia, attempt to differentiate the specific components as follows: controlled versus automatic, serial versus parallel, and limited channel capacity versus unlimited channel capacity. Conscious information processing includes among its many components motor reaction times to external stimuli; automatic information processing includes EEG alpha wave blocking following visual stimuli. Channel capacity is closely related to distinctions between serial and parallel processes. Serial cognitive processing, often conscious, exhibits limited channel capacity, whereas automatic parallel cognitive processes often exhibit unlimited channel capacity. This terminology is somewhat analogous to electrical circuitry, where serial circuits are more susceptible to resistance and cannot conduct as much as the parallel circuits can. Using these constructs, Callaway presents evidence that schizophrenics have deficiencies in conscious serial information-processing circuits that have limited channel capacity. It is suggested that schizophrenics may have normal or supernormal ability in automatic parallel circuits with unlimited channel capacity. Recent work with the stroop test assessing schizophrenics tends to support this variability according to the area of functioning (Carter, Robertson, and Nordahl, 1992).

Callaway and Naghdi (1983) especially emphasize that this predisposition to premature overload of conscious serial cognitive circuitry correlates with clinical observations. As he states,

> Clinical observation of schizophrenics is consistent with the evidence that sluggish modality switching, vulnerability to backward masking, and slow, simple reaction times can be modified by training. Nonremitted schizophrenics may appear normal in certain situations. Practice, absence of ambiguity, clear external cues as to appropriate behavior, and a calm, rested state are factors that seem to promote normal functioning in the nonremitted schizophrenic. These factors spare the limited channel capacity processes and allow them to operate more efficiently [pp. 339–347].

Callaway concentrates on the mechanics of faulty information processing after first acknowledging findings from other workers on thought processes in schizophrenics. He provides a sound descriptive theory of how cognitive wiring may go awry in the schizophrenic, but does not delve into specific neuroanatomical correlates. Later, theorists such as Hoffman (1987) will utilize connectionist neural network analysis to expound on this cognitive overload theory of schizophrenia.

HEMSLEY'S WEAKENING OF
MEMORY INFLUENCES THEORY

Hemsley (1987; Gray et al., 1991) has proposed that schizophrenia arises from a "weakening of the influences of stored memory of the regularities of previous input on current perception" (p. 182). In Hemsley's proposal, a major factor in schizophrenic psychopathology is a weakening of the influence of past experience on the interpretation of current perceptual input or on the selection of which environmental stimuli to attend and respond to. As with many other theories of schizophrenic psychopathology, Hemsley focuses on disordered information processing. Hemsley's views are consistent with mismatches produced by a poor synthesis of top-down and bottom-up signalling.

While Broadbent (1977) concentrated on organizational difficulties and Callaway and Naghdi (1982) on overloaded circuitry, Hemsley concentrates on this weakened influence of stored memories on current stimuli. As Hemsley (1987) states: "Schizophrenics are less able to make use of the redundancy and patterning of sensory input to reduce information processing demands" (p. 181). In this manner, Hemsley employs Broadbent's idea of disordered connections between present context and past experience.

FRITH'S STIMULUS VS. WILLED INTENTION THEORY

Frith's (1987; Frith and Done, 1988) neuropsychological model, attempting to explain the positive symptoms of schizophrenia takes into account the role of internally generated goals and plans. He distinguishes between two forms of intention, stimulus intention and willed intention. In stimulus intention, an individual receives a stimuli then "in consultation with long term memory the subject decides what implications the stimulus has for action" (p. 439). He believes this process remains intact in the schizophrenic. Willed intention "starts with the subject having a plan or goal, in consultation with long term memory, the subject decides what action is appropriate to this goal" (p. 439). Frith's distinction between stimulus intention and willed intention is important. Our view, which utilizes concepts such as intermingling (Harrow and Prosen, 1978, 1979; Harrow et al., 1983), emphasizes the importance of internally generated goals and wishes, with the note that frequently behavior and thinking is based as much or more on internal stimuli, thinking, and plans as on external stimuli. Frith codifies this in a formal way with his concept of "willed intentions."

Frith and Done (1988) also hypothesized a "monitor" in the CNS that integrates stimulus intention and willed intention. The importance of monitoring in routine everyday thinking, and the view that monitoring failure results in thought disorder and psychosis (or view), was emphasized years ago by Cohen, Nachmani and Rosenberg (1974) and has been further examined by a number of recent theorists (Harrow and Miller, 1980; Harrow, Ratenbury, and Stoll, 1988; Benson and Stuss, 1989; Harrow, Lanin-Kettering and Miller, 1989; McGrath, 1991). This "monitor" serves two functions. "First, it can detect mismatch between intentions and actions at a very early stage, thus permitting rapid error detection." Second, it "maintains the distinction between willed intentions and stimulus intentions" (Frith and Done, 1988, p, 439) The authors hypothesized that the connection between willed intention and the monitor was disrupted in schizophrenia. In this scenario, willed intentions unchecked by the monitors would manifest themselves as inappropriate actions or positive symptoms in the schizophrenic; furthermore the schizophrenic would not recognize the inappropriateness of the actions.

Frith and Done combine information-processing dysfunction theory with a circuit schema in a model that goes into somewhat more depth than Hemsley's. They describe the various components involved in information processing. They also give a specific schema describing how these components interact with one another. Finally, they explain how a specific interruption in this wiring schema may manifest itself as faulty information processing.

HARROW AND COLLEAGUES' THEORY INVOLVING INTERMINGLING AND A MONITORING DISORDER

In our previous research studying potential mechanisms involved in disordered schizophrenic thinking and delusional ideation, we proposed a model of thought disorder (Harrow and Quinlan, 1985; Harrow, Lanin-Kettering, and Miller, 1989). This model emphasizes the role of heightened cognitive arousal or an overactive or overstimulated central nervous system (CNS) during periods of increased stress or upset, with diminished inhibitory function, in thought disordered and schizophrenia patients at the acute or active phase of disorder. With the heightened cognitive arousal (probably associated with abnormal neuromodulatory activity, that is, increased aminergic and/or serotonergic activity (Oades, 1985: Seeman et al., 1993: Koyama, Jodo, and Kayama, 1994), four factors begin to emerge. These four factors, outlined in greater detail later, are: a) in response selection, there is more diffuse activation, including activation of only partially relevant sets of nodes (that is, dendrites and/or cell bodies; b) intermingling of personal concerns, conflicts, and wishes; c) disorganization-confusion; and d) impaired monitoring and impaired perspective as a consequence of the ineffective use of long-term memory (LTM).

We suggest that under normal, nonaroused conditions, people (including normals) respond to questions by the activation of specific and relevant (or best fit) interconnected sets of nodes (or neural networks). The increased cognitive arousal is associated with a change in the "gain" (e.g., a change in the excitatory threshold for stimulation that leads to the firing of neurons in a particular brain region). Under these conditions of heightened cognitive arousal, during response selection there is a disruption of the "normal" activation of the best fit or most relevant set of nodes (or most relevant and specific neural network) with activation becoming *more diffuse* and *less specific*. The reduction in inhibitory activity and the more diffuse activation would play a role in the coactivation of only partially relevant, and even irrelevant, sets of nodes during response selection (Harrow, 1994a, b). Some, and at times many, of these less relevant interconnected nodes which are activated and intermingled into conscious thinking involve representations of personal concerns, conflicts, and wishes that are inappropriate to the immediate external context. One might expect mild to moderate cognitive disruption in normals and considerably more for vulnerable people. Thus a schizophrenia patient's own wishes and concerns would become strongly intermingled into his or her thinking and behavior, at times in a direct manner and at times in a jumbled up way (Adler and Harrow, 1974; Harrow and Prosen, 1977, 1978; Harrow et al., 1983).

Under such conditions of acute upset and heightened cognitive arousal, monitoring is also impaired. A number of different types of monitoring have been defined. We call one particular type of monitoring "perspective," the form involved in checking and controlling one's moment-by-moment thinking and behavior to maintain normative ytandards of contextual appropriateness (Harrow and Miller, 1980; Harrow et al,, 1988; Harrow et al., 1989). We have proposed that adequate perspective-monitoring is heavily dependent on the effective use of standards of appropriateness stored in long-term memory (Harrow et al., 1989; Harrow and Silverstein, 1991).

In this formulation, adequate perspective serves the function of a metacognitive control process helping to guide message planning and behavior on a moment-to-moment basis. This type of monitoring is based on the continuing ongoing integration and the effective use in one's thinking of stored standards of normative appropriate behavior from long-term memory (Harrow et al., 1989).

Monitoring as a metacognitive control process can be seen as multistep with greater and greater "fine-tuning" as the process occurs. For example, an intention may be generated as it is simultaneously compared with a past experience similar to the current one. A response is then selected; this is tuning at a fairly gross level. As a response is taken to completion there are many almost instantaneous checks of the response (e.g., how it is progressing and what type of feedback is being received) that provide ever-increasing fine tuning (Dougherty and Jobe, 1994).

The maintenance of contextually appropriate thinking and behavior is dependent on this type of moment-to-moment monitoring. Although effective monitoring is based on standards of behavior stored in long-term memory, our experimental evidence suggests that, even in strange and inappropriate behavior by schizophrenic patients, long-term memory is basically intact, and often can be used to judge the adequacy of other patients' thinking and behavior with some effectiveness (Harrow and Miller, 1980; Harrow et al., 1989). We have suggested that, nonetheless, during acute stages of disorder, schizophrenic patients have difficulties in the using of these stored standards of contextual behavior adequately in monitoring their own thinking and behavior (Harrow et al., 1989; Harrow and Silverstein, 1991).

Biologically Based and Computer-Based Theories of Schizophrenia

The theories outlined in this section are biologically based, computer based, or both. The convergence of neurobiology and computer sciences, (e.g., computational neuroscience) has been promoted by increasing agreement that long-term memory is represented by degrees of synaptic strength throughout the brain. Much of the excitement in these fields centers around a search for various ways in which factors associated with synapses can be used to explain cognitive phenomena.

GRAY'S INTEGRATIVE THEORY

Major aspects of Hemsley's formulation and some aspects of Frith's formulation have been incorporated into a larger and more multidimensional neuropsychological model of schizophrenia by Gray et al. (1991). This comprehensive theory was influenced by earlier research on anxiety by Gray (1982) as well as the work of Swerdlow and Koob (1987). It tries to incorporate findings from brain-behavior studies and to integrate cognitive, biological, neurological, and neurochemical research. The theory attempts to correlate aspects of neurocognition with specific neuroanatomical locations.

Gray and colleagues argue that a motor program is composed of a sequence of steps released as sequential output units in which each step can be altered depending on environmental reward cues. Error feedback leads to program modification during execution. If there is a breakdown in the error feedback process, viewed as a kind of output monitoring, schizophrenic symptoms result. The caudate system is viewed as a content register for an entire motor program assembled and relayed from the cortex. The accumbens system operates as a switching device permitting the switch from one step to the next and may interrupt the program in midexecution. The amygdala surveys positive and negative reinforcement associated with each step in the program and relays this information to the accumbens system. Through the subicular pathway to the accumbens, the septohippocampal system relays mismatches between the expected outcome and the actual outcome of each motor step. In this way, momentary corrections are made in the execution of the motor program though its connections with the caudate system, accumbens, thalamus, amygdala, cingulate, and entorhinal areas. The prefrontal cortex coordinates the sequential execution of the program, modulating the final moment by moment self-correction or self-monitoring processes that fine tune and integrate the output.

Gray's model is one of the most comprehensive theories of schizophrenia ever proposed. The weakness of this approach, similar to all exclusive circuit approaches, is that each module is essentially a black-box in which inhibitory and excitatory synaptic events determine the output. Exactly what is represented or how computations occur is not specified, however. The strength of Gray's model lies in circuit specificity drawn from Swerdlow and Koob's (1987) motor program implementation. They state that a motor program is maintained by a postulated pattern of activity in striatal, thalamic and cortical neurons resulting in excitatory activity in Loops I and II. Striatal circuity is further regulated by extensive lateral inhibition. Episodic (not tonic) dopaminergic inputs interrupt firing at the termination of Loop III. Loops I to III provide a sequencing process that determines the duration of each step in the motor program and permits input modification. Theta rhythm determines temporal sequencing at about 100 msec but the temporal window can be expanded or contracted depending on the amount of accumbens activity.

COHEN AND SERVAN-SCHREIBER'S DOPAMINE GAIN MODEL

Cohen and Servan-Schreiber (1992, 1993) model negative symptoms by altering the gain parameter in a pattern recognizing, non-Hopfield network. Gain is defined as a multiplier of the total activation of a nerve cell after multiplying each input by its respective synaptic weight and adding up the resultant total activation. Thus gain can be represented as the slope of the input–output logistic function of a neuron. Cohen and Servan-Schreiber argue that the gain parameter is controlled by dopamine neuron modulation. By reducing the gain parameter in context modules purported to be located in the prefrontal cortex, they show a close correlation between performance of their network model and schizophrenic patients on the Stroop task, continuous performance task, and stimulus disambiguation task.

Their model is more consistent with a neurodevelopmental impairment in mesocortical dopamine function postulated by Weinberger than with current views of the therapeutic function of neuroleptic suppression of dopamine function. Weinberger's hypothesis of a limbic disinhibition due to diminished dopamine activity in the dorsolateral frontal cortex provides a role for limbic dopamine suppression to have a therapeutic effect. In combination with the gain model of Cohen and Servan-Schreiber (1992, 1993) and Weinberger's (1986, 1987) views, one could account for negative symptoms as being generated by frontal lobe dysfunction and positive symptoms as being due to limbic hyperactivity. Indeed, the interactive effect between frontal and limbic systems could be a constant feature in brain models of schizophrenia.

WEINBERGER: A NEURODEVELOPMENTAL MODEL OF SCHIZOPHRENIA

Weinberger (1986, 1987) has constructed a theory of the emergence of schizophrenia in adolescents and young adults, based on a developmental model. In his model, nonspecific brain pathology is viewed as present at birth or relatively early in development, with this brain pathology, or "lesion," not manifesting itself overtly in a gross way during early development. Later symptom development is linked to the normal maturation of brain areas affected by the early "lesion." There is a particular focus in his theory on the dorsolateral prefrontal cortex. Weinberger's theory can account for differential dopamine function. His view is that a neurodevelopmental lesion (as yet unidentified) leads to diminished mesocortical activity that limits the ability of the frontal lobes to deal with stress. The stress-related decompensation reaches a peak during adolescence, when the individual has to face the major challenge of independence. As a result, the mesolimbic system becomes hyperactive, and psychotic behavior ensues. Neuroleptics suppress the limbic hyperexcitability.

HOFFMAN'S NEURAL NETWORK/PARASITIC FOCUS MODEL

Circuit models are important because they specify anatomic areas (i.e, accumbens, prefrontal cortex, caudate nucleus, etc.) that can be experimentally tested in both humans and animals. Because they specify how output is sequenced, shaped and corrected by feedback processes, circuit models can explain hierarchical processes and time windows within which processing takes place. Neural network models, on the other hand, add three important dimensions. First, they allow for representation of perceptual or conceptual stimuli. Second, they can account for learning by various algorithms, that is, back-propagation. Third, they are computable in that they can take in input, learn it, and specify output.

Hoffman (1987) experimented with a type of neural network model devised by Hopfield to imitate such features of human cognition as generalization, pattern recognition, and optimization problem solving.

The physical parameters of this network type include total connectivity between neuronal elements or nodes, symmetry of connection weight change, totally distributed representation, and a back-propagation learning algorithms. Using computer simulation, Hoffman found results suggesting that this kind of network behaves in a manner a) strongly analogous to schizophrenic positive symptoms if it is overloaded with memory, and b) strongly analogous to manic speech discourse if it is noise overloaded. These emergent network pathologies were discovered in his computer simulations, not predicted, thus giving increased strength to his work. Also, the engrams most likely to be configured into loose associations were very different from each other (had the greatest Hamming distances from each other), distinguishing schizophrenic "logic" from the kinds of errors produced by aphasic patients. Hoffman also modeled delusions by showing that abnormal engram configurations would eventually come to dominate output by "top-down" processing, by biasing nodes that were receiving input. He termed these areas "parasitic foci" because, once heated up by a certain level of activity, they would bias other nodes in the network and further distort perception and cognition. Hopfield nets will generate these kinds of pathologies if they are overloaded with normal memory or if enough connections between nodes are eliminated so that the normal amount of memory begins to constitute an overload.

Hoffman and McGlashan (1993) proposed a comprehensive theory of schizophrenia resulting from abnormal pruning of Hopfield net synapses leading to a memory overload under conditions of normal stimulus exposure. By combining neural network architecture with a circuit model, they showed how hypothesized parasitic foci could decouple essential coordinated processing between cortical areas, possibly leading to several heretofore unexplained neurobiological features of schizophrenic patients such as diffuse cortical atrophy, delusions, and thought insertion (Krystal et al., 1994).

Current Neurobiological Evidence for Schizophrenia

Many of the theories presented thus far are not based in neurobiology, a field that is rapidly defining the underpinnings of both normal and disordered cognition. At this point, we will summarize some of the current neurobiological findings, then present our formulation of schizophrenic thought disorder, based, in part, on the potential underlying neurobiology and also utilizing our concepts of intermingling personal material and impaired monitoring. The general trend is a movement away from reliance on receptor deficit concepts to synaptic deficits to explain schizophrenic symptoms.

EVIDENCE OF DISCRETE BRAIN LESIONS

In the past two decades, mounting evidence has led some in the field to believe that schizophrenia results from some sort of anatomical brain defect. Thus, as noted earlier, Weinberger (1986) believes that schizophrenia results from primary fixed congenital/perinatal "lesions" that do not manifest clinical symptoms until early adulthood as neural systems come "online" to "express the defect." Others believe that such defects develop slowly over several years until symptoms become apparent (Benes, 1989; Benes and Bird, 1987).

A plethora of imaging studies (CT, MR, PET) have found evidence of changes in ventricular size in chronic schizophrenics and possibly in other types of schizophrenics (e.g., Cleghorn, Ziporsky, and List, 1991; Johnstone et al., 1976; Pfefferbaum and Zipursky, 1991; Sedvall, 1992; Weinberger et al.,1979; Weinberger, Wagner, and Wyatt, 1983). Recent autopsy studies of schizophrenic brains have provided preliminary evidence of possible circuitry defects in several different cortical areas, including dorsolateral prefrontal cortex (Benes, Davidson, and Bird, 1986), anterior cingulate cortex (Benes and Bird, 1987), entorhinal cortex (Jakob and Beckman, 1986), the parahippo- campal gyrus (Bogerts, Meertz, and Schonfeldt-Bausch, 1985; Brown et al., 1986), and the hippocampus (Kovel and Scheibel, 1984; Bogerts et al., 1985). These areas are known to involve portions of the limbic system (Benes, Majoch, and Bird, 1987).

THE ETIOLOGY OF THESE LESIONS IS UNKNOWN

Although current research has focused primarily on the possible localization of anatomical defects, a number of investigators have explored the etiology of these lesions. Weinberger (1986) proposes that some of these lesions could result from various pre- or perinatal insults (either alone or in combination), such as hereditary encephalopathy, infection, perinatal trauma, toxin exposure, hypoxia, and the like. Benes (1989) proposes that the lesions result from a process of slow neural degeneration. Others have suggested that abnormal synaptic pruning during adolescence might generate potential lesions (Feinberg,

1982/83; Hoffman and Dobscha, 1989). Further questions remain. Are the potential lesions primarily cellular losses, or are they reactive cellular losses secondary to other causes such as destruction of fiber tracts? Do they occur acutely with a short time course, or chronically over many years? Exactly which cortical circuits are affected?

MYELINATION DEFECTS MAY CAUSE LESIONS

Often overlooked are the axonal interconnections between different cortical and subcortical areas. A defect in myelination (either primary, i.e., congenital/toxic problem in myelin formation, or secondary, i.e., breakdown of previously formed myelin) could lead to functional disconnections between different regions, with these disconnections perhaps playing a role in schizophrenic symptoms (Kohler, Heilmeyer, and Volk, 1988). The completion of the majority of myelination overlaps temporally with the onset of schizophrenia in many adolescent and young adult schizophrenics. The prefrontal tracts and the corpus callosum are the last tracts to myelinate and may provide clues to the neurodevelopmental lesions of schizophrenics (Magaro and Page, 1983).

Unfortunately, insufficient research on the normal myelination sequence has been conducted to date. In a landmark paper, Yakovlev and Lecours (1967) performed a qualitative study examining brains ranging in age from the fourth fetal month to six decades, but they point out that only a few cerebra were examined in the age range of the first and second decades. This type of critical gap has limited the exploration of cycles of myelination, particularly in the telencephalic and cortical regions. Since then, most autopsy studies of myelination have been performed on infants up to two years of age (Rorke and Riggs, 1969; Richardson, 1982; Brody et al., 1987; Kinney et al., 1988). In general, cortical and subcortical circuitry is myelinated by the age of 10, with the exceptions of portions of the reticular formation and intracortical association fibers (Yakovlev and Lecours, 1967). Even though the Yakovlev collection was deficient in brains from people in adolescence and early adulthood, Benes (1989) attempted to examine qualitatively the myelination sequence of certain "limbic" structures in a small number of brains in the collection. She found that during the late adolescent periods myelination of the subicular and presubicula regions increases dramatically, thus enhancing communication to the hippocampus.

SOME PSYCHOLOGICAL MANIFESTATIONS OF
DEMYELINATING DISEASES

While it is not known if myelination defects play a role in the etiology of schizophrenia, many symptoms of schizophrenia can be observed in the disease metachromatic leukodystrophy (MLD) (Fluharty, 1990; Baumann et al., 1991; Hyde, Ziegler, and Weinberger, 1992; Hoffman and McGlashan, 1994). MLD is a rare inherited disorder of the nervous system caused by a deficiency in the enzyme arylsulfatase A, leading to the accumulation of sulfatides in the central and peripheral nervous systems and subsequent demyelination of axons and peripheral nerves. MLD can present clinically at any age, and at most ages its occurrence is not strongly associated with severe positive symptoms. For patients in whom it first appears in adolescence or early adulthood, and for whom the myelination problems occur in the frontal region of the cortex, symptoms mimicking schizophrenia can appear, namely, psychosis, thought disorder, delusions, and auditory hallucinations. It is possible that the secondary demyelination seen in this disease interrupts critical pathways between the anatomical regions described earlier, leading to schizophrenic symptoms.

In MLD, however, it is not clear which tracts are destroyed and in what order. Demyelination typically begins in the frontal lobes, primarily involving the periventricular white matter and corpus callosum; the arcuate fibers are generally spared. As the disease progresses, demyelination spreads throughout the forebrain; psychotic symptoms eventually diminish only to be replaced by dementia and sensorimotor losses. We can speculate that perhaps the mesocortical DA links or subiculo-accumbens links or both are somehow compromised, leading to schizophrenic symptoms in other demyelinating diseases (Parker, 1956; Feinstein, duBoulay, and Ron, 1992; Mahler, 1992; Koch, 1996). It is also possible that other portions of limbic circuitry are affected as well (Hauw et al., 1992). In addition, the axons still remain intact. Thus, the defect leads to more of a "dysfunctional connectivity of frontal cortex" (Hyde et al., 1992) than to an anatomical connectivity problem.

Changes in Synaptic Pruning as One Possible
Mechanism in Cognitive Abnormalities

A growing body of evidence about synaptogenesis shows that during neurodevelopment in humans (Huttenlocher et al., 1982;

145

Huttenlocher and Courten, 1987) and in monkeys (Rakic et al., 1986), synaptic density increases dramatically to a maximum level at age 2–3 years in humans (age 2–4 months in monkeys), only to be "pruned" back to reach adult levels by age 15–20 years in humans (age 3–4 years old monkeys). The questions remain a) whether aberrations in synaptic density lead to disruption in cognition, and b) whether this type of cognitive abnormality is related to thought disorder and psychosis. While a link between changes in synaptic density and abnormal thinking has not yet been definitively established, hypotheses in this area present promising leads.

In general, Feinberg (1982/83) has proposed that "the human develops virtually all potentially useful neuronal interconnections in the first years of life since it cannot be specified in advance which connections will actually be needed. . . . At the end of childhood, when the kinds of neuronal connections required for adaptation have been determined by the individual's interactions with his environment, little-used connections are eliminated" (p. 329). One possibility is that schizophrenia "results from deranged synaptic pruning during adolescence, [i.e.] the abnormality is due to the elimination of too many or too few synapses or from the wrong ones" (p. 327). Hoffman and Dobscha (1989) also have proposed that problems in pruning are involved in schizophrenia. Feinberg's theory may account for the subtle lesions observed with schizophrenia, but he leaves the mechanism of such faulty elimination unanswered and proposes a sudden pruning process for which evidence is lacking.

Under normal conditions, how are synapses selected for preservation or destruction? A generally accepted theory, first proposed by Hebb (1949), states that "when an axon of cell A is near enough to excite a cell B and repeatedly or persistently takes part in firing it, some growth process or metabolic change takes place in one or both cells such that A's efficiency as one of the cells firing B is increased." This theory implicitly states that increases in synaptic strength are dependent on concurrent activity in the presynaptic and postsynaptic cells. There is early experimental evidence supporting Hebbian learning in humans; long-term potentiation (LTP) and long-term depression (LTD) have been amply documented in CA1 pyramidal cells in the hippocampus (Kelso, Ganong, and Brown, 1986; Zador, Koch, and Brown, 1990)

Hebb's (1949) formulation requires inputs to be concurrent, or contiguous, in time in order to strengthen existing synapses; those

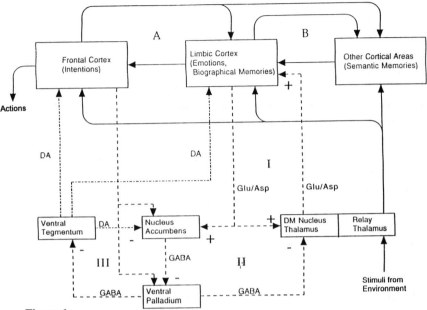

Figure 1

which are not strengthened are gradually eliminated. If some neurological event occurred such that normal inputs could not be concurrent, then supposedly the synapses driven by those inputs would not be strengthened and eventually might be eliminated. In effect, synapses that would be valuable for later adaptation might be inappropriately eliminated, if "normal" inputs could not be strengthened because of a disorder in timing.

It is possible that defects in the myelination of inputs to a given cortical area (e.g., hippocampus or DLPFC) could affect the conductivity of input axons such that one or more inputs that normally arrive concurrently on a given cell would be delayed (conduction velocity is dramatically reduced in unmyelinated axons relative to myelinated ones) (Honer et al., 1987). During normal development, the myelination sequence may proceed in a balanced fashion such that inputs are delivered to given areas concurrently. A possibility is that a defect in the ordered sequence of myelination might delay inputs in an unbalanced fashion, possibly leading to a lack of Hebbian synaptic strengthening. In other words, waves of information that arrive at a given neuron at the same time would be properly reinforced; waves that arrived at different times ("out of sync" with each other due to dysmyelination) would not be reinforced, eventually leading to the improper elimination of the synapses that transmitted the waves of information to that cell.

Figure 1 is a synthesis of the foregoing views and those of other theorists concerning structures involved in cognitive processing. Loop A describes frontal-limbic interaction in which memory accessible to the limbic area (biographical, event-related memory) is activated by thalamic afference, and this partially integrated material (stimulus material plus stored memory) provides excitatory drive to the pre-frontal cortex. The prefrontal cortex then responds with additional stored memory and also inhibitory drive to the limbic structures. This loop will damp itself out if the PFC signal is strong enough to constrain adequately the limbic structures. The strength of the PFC signal is, in turn, influenced by several factors, among which are dopaminergic gain control (high gain) and the synaptic density of the PFC. The ability of the limbic structures to override PFC inhibition is dependent on dopaminergic gain control (high gain), afferent input, synaptic density, and possibly other factors.

A feed-forward escape with disinhibited continuous cycling would occur if an underpruned limbic system overrode an overpruned PFC. If Hebbian processes influence the extent of pruning, then the combination of regional under- and overpruning is possible and more likely than just unidirectional pruning abnormalities. Some break on this override could occur if the gain in the PFC were increased to compensate for the low synaptic density in the overpruned PFC and/or gain were decreased in limbic structures to compensate for high synaptic density in the underpruned limbic system. Most neuroleptics, which block D2 receptors, probably effectively decrease gain by blocking or diminishing the effectiveness of the mesolimbic dopamine system but have the negative side effect of blocking the mesocortical system and thereby impair function in the PFC (Jobe et al., 1994). The ability of the PFC as well as the limbic cortex to self-stimulate and sustain itself through subcortical mechanisms appears to be facilitated by the dopamine D1 receptor. The ability of the PFC and limbic cortex to "turn-itself-off" (i.e., inhibit itself), appears to be blocked by the dopamine D2 receptor. High-potency neuroleptics operate to block D2 receptors preferentially over D1. As a result, high-potency neuroleptics have the effect of increasing the ability of both the PFC and limbic cortex to turn themselves off (Walker, 1994) without significantly reducing the ability of these cortical areas to turn themselves on, or excite themselves. The effect is to move the PFC and the limbic cortex back into balance with each other.

A testable hypothesis is that in a normally pruned synaptic situation, during periods of emotional upset or severe stress, the limbic system may temporarily override the PFC. As a result personal material from stored memory (Harrow et al., 1983; Harrow et al., 1989) (which is normally inhibited by the PFC) will emerge into overt behavior, partly because of the dominance of parts of the limbic system over the PFC (Neumann et al., 1988). Without emotional upset or severe stress, or without heightened cognitive arousal, the psychotogenic threshold would not be reached because the synaptic densities of the PFC and limbic areas are balanced. They, in effect, act as filters for one another. Normals may exceed this "psychotogenic" threshold briefly during periods of severe emotional upset, as a result of heightened cognitive arousal possibly associated with excessive adrenergic activity, but recover quickly because an imbalance in their synaptic densities is not accentuating the disturbance.

We propose that the limbic system provides some or much of the essential "top-down" information flow to the cortex and specifically to the cortical association areas. The limbic system is usually not thought of as the origin of top-down processes. Traditional use of the concept of top-down in the cognitive neuroscience literature refers to hierarchical processes that are rule or symbol driven from one *control* brain source, rather than being based only on the interaction of small partial effects from distributed brain regions. Top-down is here viewed as input that derives from the integration of computations completed in other parts of the brain that are used to match input signals from the outside world (afference) in a comparator fashion. A signal is then generated from this "matching" process that is sent to the prefrontal cortex, which computes an "intention" signal. The intention signal, which serves partly as a "set" and provides goal-direction, is relayed to the limbic system and acts as a constraining and partly inhibitory force. This inhibitory presence modulates limbic top-down output to the rest of the cortex. We propose that during periods of acute stress or heightened cognitive arousal the feedforward cycle of activity between the limbic and frontal systems may become so strong that it escapes the inhibitory factors that typically constrain it (Jobe et al., 1994). Under these conditions, poorly modulated and, for some, unrealistic ideas are more likely to emerge from among multiple competing ideas, partly because the bottom-up afference will no longer adequately "match" the top-down input. The mismatches that result could be experienced as "coming from the outside world." In other words, the subjective internal representation of reality can be distorted by recurrent and iterative processes that lead to faulty activation of long-term memory. There are many possible ways in which strange ideas and reality distortions may arise. This constellation constitutes one possible pathway which should be investigated further.

PRUNING PROBLEMS AND THE POTENTIAL LINK TO POSITIVE SYMPTOMS

One possibility is that there is a disparity in synaptic density between prefrontal and limbic areas so that the psychotogenic threshold can be exceeded more readily by a lower level of emotional upset or stress. A feed-forward, free-running cycle of activity could develop in which the PFC might not damp out limbic activity, and the limbic feed to the rest of the cortex would be excessive. This excessive limbic top-down feed to other cortical areas could distort their processing. The comparator process will be unduly biased toward top-down limbic feed such that bottom-up matching thalamic afference could be overridden by biasing toward an intermingling of personalized intrusions. Delusions and hallucinations could result when the top-down signal totally dominates the bottom-up signal.

On the other hand, monitoring, which is based on the effective use of long-term memory (Harrow et al., 1989), can become impaired as a result of several different constellations. One of these involves situations in which top-down signals are just strong enough to prevent bottom-up afference signals from acting as an appropriate constraint on output production. This process is represented by loop B in Figure 1. That constellation could disrupt cognition. It is not a certainty that this particular type of cognitive disruption would lead to the positive symptoms we see in schizophrenia, but it is at least one possibility that deserves further consideration. Thus, limbic top-down dominance could lead to cognitive abnormalities because the pruning disparity between PFC and limbic areas that has preceded output to the rest of the cortex has distorted matching signals. The resulting cognitive abnormalities could lead to severe thought disorder, although this is a hypothesis that needs testing.

If the foregoing model is carried to its logical conclusion, some patients with thought pathology will have a mixture of both types of pruning abnormalities, creating disparities between the limbic and frontal cortex, possibly in a mosaic, or patchlike, distribution. Unfortunately, this mixture of low and high synaptic density would make the experimental validation by synapse counting more difficult, since large-area samples with patches of abnormally low or high synaptic density might be averaged out. The confusion that has resulted from the premature identification of neuroanatomic aberrance and cognitive aberrance, however, could fit in with the type of model just described. This model raises the possibility of both under- and overpruning at the neuroanatomic level such that a combination of these deficits, manifested as a pruning disparity between frontal and limbic areas, is involved in the substrate that is identified with cognitive aberrance. (Benes et al., 1994). We can again note that this model does not rely solely on a unidirectional pruning abnormality involving only one brain region but, rather, involves the interaction of several regions (David, 1993, 1994). The model combines features of the comparator concept, the intention generator concept, connectionistic neural networks, and neuromodulatory circuits, with these contributing cognitively—especially during periods of stress or heightened cognitive arousal, possibly associated with increased central adrenergic activity—to an intermingling of personal material in an inappropriate fashion. This constellation can lead to potential disorganization and may contribute to an impairment in monitoring involving the ineffective use of long-term memory, which would normally be used to provide adequate contextual material. It is our belief that the integration of the dysmyelination model with potential cognitive mechanisms involved in psychopathology can provide a heuristic framework for future thinking and research.

We should note that there are many possible ways that the positive symptoms of schizophrenia may arise, and the dysmyelination model is only one of them. Thus the model of abnormalities in synaptic pruning presents one possible mechanism in terms of a cognitive disruption and possibly in terms of subsequent positive symptoms as a consequence of this type of cognitive disruption.

We emphasize the potential bridge between cognitive disruption and both thought disorder and positive symptoms, because cognitive disruption is not an automatic pathway to the type of severe cognitive aberrations and reality distortions seen in the positive symptoms in schizophrenia. Thus, one would have to tread cautiously in attempting to establish a link between biological events and the type of cognitive abnormalities that can lead to the positive symptoms of schizophrenia. Nevertheless, the potential link between abnormalities in synaptic pruning and the type of cognitive disruption we have discussed above should at least be investigated to determine whether or not it is one of several possible pathways involved in positive symptoms in schizophrenia.

REFERENCES

Adler, D. & Harrow, M. (1974), Idiosyncratic thinking and personally overinvolved thinking in schizophrenic patients during partial recovery. *Comp. Psychiat.*, 15:57–67.

Andreasen, N. C. (1979a), Thought, language, and communication disorders: I. Clinical assessment, definition of terms, and evaluations of their reliability. *Arch. Gen. Psychiat.*, 36:1315–1321.

—————— (1979b), Thought, language, and communication disorders: II. Diagnostic significance. *Arch. Gen. Psychiat.*, 36:1325–1331.

—————— & Olsen, S. (1982), Negative vs. positive schizophrenia. *Arch. Gen. Psychiat.*, 39:789–794.

—————— & Powers, P. S. (1974), Overinclusion thinking in mania and schizophrenia. *Brit. J. Psychiat.*, 125:452–456.

Asarnow, R. F., Steffy, R. A., MacCrimmon, D .J. & Cleghorn, J. M. (1978), An attentional assessment of foster children at risk for schizophrenia. In: *The Nature of Schizophrenia*. ed. C. Wynne, R.L. Cromwell & S. Matthysse. New York: Wiley, pp. 339–358.

Baumann, N., Masson, M., Carreau, V., LeFevre, M., Herschkowith, N. & Turpin, J. C. (1991), Adult forms of metachromatic leukodystrophy: clinical and biochemical approach. *Develop. Neurosci.*, 13:211–215.

Bellak, L. (1966), The schizophrenic syndrome: A further elaboration of the unified theory of schizoprenia. In: *Schizophrenia: A Review of the Syndrome*. ed. L. Bellak & L. Loeb. New York: Grune & Stratton, pp. 3–63.

Benes, F .M. (1989), Myelination of cortical-hippocampal relays during late adolescence. *Schizophren. Bull.*, 15:585–593.

—————— & Bird, E. D. (1987), An analysis of the arrangement of neurons in the cingulate cortex of schizophrenic patients. *Arch. Gen. Psychiat.*, 44:608–616.

—————— Davidson, J. & Bird, E. D. (1986), Quantitative cytoarchitectural studies of the cerebral cortex of schizophrenics. *Arch. Gen. Psychiat.*, 43:31–35.

_____ Majocha, R. & Bird, E. D. (1987), Increased vertical axon counts in cingulate cortex of schizophrenics. *Arch. Gen. Psychiat.*, 44:1011–1021.

_____ Turtle, M., Yusuf, K. & Farol, P. (1994), Myelination of a key relay zone in the hippocampal formation occurs in the human brain during childhood, adolescence and adulthood. *Arch. Gen. Psychiat.*, 51:477–485.

Benjamin, J. D. (1944), A method for distinguishing and evaluating formal thinking disorders in schizophrenia, In: *Language and Thought in Schizophrenia*, ed. J. Kasanin. New York: Norton, pp. 65–88.

Benson, D. F. & Stuss, D. T. (1990), Frontal lobe influences on delusions: A clinical perspective. *Schizophren. Bull.*, 16:403–411.

Blatt, S.J. & Ritzler, B. A. (1974), Thought disorder and boundary disturbances in psychosis. *J. Consult. Clin. Psychol.*, 42:370–381.

_____ & Wild, C. (1976), *Schizophrenia: A Developmental Approach*. New York: Academic Press.

Bleuler, E. (1911), *Dementia Praecox, or the Group of Schizophrenias*, trans. J. Zinkin. New York: International Universities Press.

Bogerts, B., Meertz, E. & Schonfeldt-Bausch, R. (1985), Basal ganglia and limbic system pathology in schizophrenia: A morphometric study of brain volume and shrinkage. *Arch. Gen. Psychiat.*, 42:784–791.

Braff, D. L., Glick, I. D., Johnson, M. H. & Ziscook, S. (1988), The clinical significance of thought disorder across time in psychiatric patients. *J. Nerv. Mental Dise.*, 176:213–220.

Broadbent, D. E. (1977), The hidden preattentive processes. *Amer. Psychol.*, 32:109–118.

_____ (1984), The Maltese cross: A new systematic model for memory. *Behav. Brain Sci.*, 7:55–94.

Brody, B. A., Kinney, H. C., Kloman, A. S. & Gilles, F. H. (1987), Sequence of central nervous system myelination in human infancy: I. An autopsy study of myelination. *J. Neuropathol. Experiment. Neurol.*, 46:283–301.

Brown, R., Colter, N., Nicholas-Corsellis, J. A., Crow, T. J., Frith, C.D., Jagoe, R., Johnstone, E. C. & Marsh, L. (1986), Postmortem evidence of structural brain changes in schizophrenia. *Arch. Gen. Psychiat.*, 43:36–42.

Callaway, E. & Naghdi, S. (1982), An information processing model for schizophrenia. *Arch. Gen. Psychiat.*, 39:339–347.

Carter, C. S., Robertson, L. C. & Nordahl, T. E. (1992), Abnormal processing of irrelevant information in chronic schizophrenia: Selective enhancement of stroop facilitation. *Psychiat. Res.*, 41:137–146.

Chaika, E. (1982), Thought disorder or speech disorder in schizophrenia? *Schizophren. Bull.*, 8:587–591.

Chapman, J. (1966), The early symptoms of schizophrenia. *Brit. J. Psychiat.*, 112:225–251.

Chapman, L. J. & Chapman, J. P. (1973), *Disordered Thought in Schizophrenia*. Englewood Cliffs, NJ: Prentice Hall.

Cleghorn, J. M., Zipursky, R. B. & List, S. J. (1991), Structural and functional brain imaging in schizophrenia. *J. Psychiat. Neurosci.*, 16:53–74.

Cohen, B., Nachmani, G. & Rosenberg, S. (1974), Referent communication disturbances in acute schizophrenia. *J. Abn. Psychol.*, 83:1–13.

Cohen, J. D. & Servan-Schreiber, D. (1992), Context, cortex, and dopamine: A connectionist approach to behavior and biology in schizophrenia. *Psychol. Rev.*, 99:45–77.

———— & ———— (1993), A theory of dopamine function and its role in cognitive deficits in schizophrenia. *Schizophren. Bull.*, 19:85–104.

Cornblatt, B. A. & Keilp, J. G. (1994), Impaired attention, genetics, and the pathophysiology of schizophrenia. *Schizophren. Bull.*, 20:31–46.

———— Lenzenweger, M., Dworkin, R. & Erlenmeyer-Kimling, L. (1985), Positive and negative schizophrenic symptoms, attention and information processing. *Schizophren. Bull.*, 11:397–408.

Cromwell, R. L. & Dokecki, P. R. (1968), Schizophrenic language: A disattention interpretation. In: *Developments in Applied Psycholinguistics Research*, ed. S. Rosenburg & J.H. Koplin. New York: Macmillan, pp. 209–260.

Cronbach, L. J. & Meehl, P. E. (1956), Construct validity in psychological tests. *Psycholog. Bull.*, 32:281–302.

Crow, T. J., Cross, A. J., Johnson, E. C. & Owen, F. (1982), Two syndromes in schizophrenia and their pathogenesis. In: Schizophrenia as a Brain Disease,. ed. F. A. Henn & H. A. Nasrallah. New York: Oxford University Press, pp. 196–234.

David, A. S. (1993), Callosal transfer in schizophrenia: Too much or too little? *J. Abn. Psychol.*, 102:573–579.

_____ (1994), Dysmodularity: A neurocognitive model for schizophrenia. *Schizophren. Bull.*, 120:249–255.

Dougherty, D. & Jobe, T. H. (1994), Neurobiology of Monitoring in Schizophrenia. Unpublished manuscript.

Erlenmeyer-Kimling, L. & Cornblatt, B. (1978), Attentional measures in a study of children at high risk for schizophrenia. *J. Psychiat. Res.*, 14:93–98.

Exner, J. E. (1993), *The Rorschach, Vol. 1.* New York: Wiley.

Falloon, I. R. E., Boyd, J. L., McGill, C. W., Stang, J. S. & Moss, H. B. (1981), Family management training in the community care of schizophrenia. In: *New Developments in Intervention with Families of Schizophrenics*, ed. M. J. Goldstein. San Francisco: Josey-Bass pp. 61–77.

Feinberg, I. (1982/83), Schizophrenia: Caused by a fault in programmed synaptic elimination during adolescence? *J. Psychiat. Res.*, 17:319–334.

Feinstein, A., du Boulay, G. & Ron, M. A. (1992), Psychotic illness in multiple sclerosis: A clinical and magnetic resonance imaging study. *Brit. J. Psychiat.*, 161:680–685.

Flaherty, J. A. & Jobe, T. H. (1990), Gender expressed emotion and outcome in schizophrenia. *Current Opin. Psychiat.*, 31:23–28.

Fluharty, A. L. (1990), The relationship of the metachromatic leukodystrophies to neuropsychiatric disorders. *Molec. & Chem. Neuropathol.*, 13:81–94.

Freedman, B. J. (1973), Early subjective experience in schizophrenic episodes. *J. Abn. Psychol.*, 82:46–54.

_____ & Chapman, L. J. (1974), The subjective experience of perceptual and disturbances in schizophrenia. *Arch. Gen. Psychiat.*, 30:333–340.

Frith, C. D. (1987), The positive and negative symptoms of schizophrenia reflect impairments in the perception and initiation of action. *Psycholog. Med.*, 17:631–648.

_____ & Done, D. J. (1988), Towards a neuropsychology of schizophrenia. *Brit. J. Psychiat.*, 153:437–443.

George, L. & Neufeld, R. W. J. (1985), Cognition and symptomatology in schizophrenia. *Schizophren. Bull.*, 11:264–285.

Goldman-Rakic, P. S. (1987), Circuitry of the prefrontal cortex and the regulation of behavior by representational knowledge. In: *Handbook of Physiology.*, ed. F. Plum. Bethesda, MD: American Physiological Society, pp. 373–417.

Goldstein, K. (1944), Methodological approach to the study of schizophrenic thought disorder, In: *Language and Thought in Schizophrenia*, ed. J. Kasanin, New York: Norton, pp. 17–39.

———— & Scheerer, M. (1941), Abstract and concrete behavior, and experimental study with special tests. *Psycholog. Monogr.*, 53:No. 2. Whole No. 239.

Goldstein, M. J. (1987), Family interaction patterns that antedate the onset of schizophrenia and related disorders: A further analysis of data from a longitudinal perspective study. In: *Understanding Major Mental Disorders*, ed. K. Hahlweg & M. J. Goldstein. New York: Family Process Press, pp. 11–32.

Gray, J. A. (1982), *The neuropsychology of anxiety.* Oxford: Oxford University Press.

———— Feldon, J., Rawlins, J. N. P., Hemsley, D. R. & Smith, A. D. (1991) The neuropsychology of schizophrenia. *Behav. & Brain Sci.*, 14:1–84.

Harrow, M. (1994a), What factors are involved in the vulnerability of schizophrenics to delusions and thought disorder? Presented at International Symposium on Body-Mind Problems, Osaka, Japan, October 5–7.

———— (1994b), Delusions and thought disorder: what cognitive mechanisms are involved? Presented at Frontiers in Neuropsychiatry: Third Annual Conference on Clinical Practice in Neuropsychiatry, Chicago, December 9–10.

———— Adler, D. & Hanf, E. (1974), Abstract and concrete thinking in schizophrenia during the prechronic phases. *Arch. Gen. Psychiat.*, 31:27–33.

———— Grossman, L. W., Silversein, M. L. & Meltzer, H. Y. (1982), Thought pathology in manic and schizophrenic patients: At hospital admission and seven weeks later. *Arch. Gen. Psychiat.*, 39:665–671.

———— Grossman, L. W., Silverstein, M. L., Meltzer, H.Y. & Kettering, R.L. (1986), A longitudinal study of thought disorder in manic patients. *Arch. Gen. Psychiat.*, 43:781–785.

———— Lanin-Kettering, I. & Miller, J. G. (1989), Impaired perspective and thought pathology in schizophrenic and psychotic disorders. *Schizophren. Bull.*, 15:605–623.

———— ———— Prosen, M. & Miller, J. G. (1983), Disordered thinking in schizophrenia: Intermingling and loss of set. *Schizophren. Bull.*, 9:354–367.

_____ MacDonald, A. W., Sands, J. R. & Silverstein, M. (1995), Vulnerability to delusions over time in schizophrenia, schizoaffective and bipolar and unipolar affective disorders: A multi-followup assessment, *Schizophren. Bull.* 21:95–109

_____ & Marengo, J. (1986), Schizophrenic thought disorder at follow-up. *Schizophren. Bull.*, 12:373–393.

_____ & Miller, J. G. (1980), Schizophrenic thought disorders and impaired perspective. *J. Abn .Psychol.*, 89:717–727.

_____ Pather, P. & Lanin-Kettering, I. (1986), Is schizophrenia a semiotic disorder? Replies to Harrod. *Schizophren. Bull.*, 12:15–19.

_____ & Prosen, M. (1978), Intermingling and disordered logic as influences on schizophrenic "thought disorders." *Arch. Gen. Psychiat.*, 136:1213–1218.

_____ & _____ (1979), Schizophrenic thought disorders: Bizarre associations and intermingling. *Amer. J. Psychiat.*, 136:293–296.

_____ & Quinlan, D. (1977), Is disordered thinking unique to schizophrenia? *Arch. Gen. Psychiat.*, 34:15–21.

_____ & _____ (1985), *Disordered Thinking and Schizophrenic Psychopathology.* New York: Gardner Press.

_____ _____ Wallington, S. & Prickett, L., Jr. (1976), Primitive drive dominated thinking: Relationship to acute schizophrenia and sociopathy. *J. Personal. Assess*, 40:31–41.

_____ Rattenbury, F. & Stoll, F. (1988), Schizophrenic delusions: An analysis of their persisting of related premorbid ideas, and of three major diagnosis. In: *Delusional Beliefs*, ed. T. Oltmanns & B. Ma. New York: Wiley, pp. 184–211.

_____ & Silverstein, M. (1991), The role of long-term memory (LTM) and monitoring in schizophrenia: Multiple Functions. *Behav. & Brain Sci.*, 14:30–31.

_____ _____ & Marengo, J. (1983), Disorder thinking: Does it identify nuclear schizophrenia? *Arch. Gen. Psychol.*, 40:765–771.

_____ Tucker, G. J. & Shield, R. (1972), Stimulus overinclusion in schizophrenic disorders. *Arch. Gen. Psychiat.*, 27:40–45.

Harvey, P. D. (1983), Speech competence in manic and schizophrenic psychosis: The association between clinically rated thought disorder and cohesion and reference performance. *J. Abn. Psychol.*, 92:368–377.

_____ Docherty, N. M., Serper, M. R. & Rasmussen, M. (1990), Cognitive deficits and thought disorder: II. An 8-month follow-up study. *Schizophren. Bull.*, 16:147–156.

_____ Earle-Boyer, E. A. & Levinson, J. C. (1988), Cognitive deficits and thought disorder. A retest study, *Schizophren. Bull.*, 14:57–66.

_____ _____ & Wielgus, M. A. (1984), The consistency of thought disorder in mania and schizophrenia: An assessment of acute psychotics. *J. Nerv. Mental Dis.*, 172:458–463.

_____ _____ _____ & Levinson, J. C. (1986), Encoding, memory, and thought disorder in schizophrenia and mania. *Schizophren. Bull.*, 12:252–261.

_____ & Walker, E. F., ed. (1987), *Positive and Negative Symptoms of Psychosis*. Hillsdale, NJ: Lawrence Erlbaum Associates, pp. 68–93

Hauw, J. J., Delaère, P., Seilhean, D., Cornu, P. & Associates. (1992), Morphology of demyelination in the human central nervous system. *J. Neuroimmunol.*, 40:139–152.

Hebb, D. O. (1949), *The Organization of Behavior*. New York: Wiley.

Hemsley, D. R. (1987), An experimental psychological model for schizophrenia. In: *Search for the Causes of Schizophrenia*, ed. H. Hafner, W. F. Gattaz & W. Janzavik. New York: Springer, pp.179–188.

Hinton, G. E. & Anderson, J. A. (1989), *Parallel Models of Associating Activity*. Hillsdale, NJ: Lawrence Erlbaum Associates.

Hoffman, R. E. (1987), Computer simulations of neural information processing and the schizophrenia-mania dichotony. *Arch. Gen. Psychiat.*, 44:178–188.

_____ & Dobscha, S. K. (1989), Cortical pruning and the development of schizophrenia: A computer model. *Schizophren. Bull.*, 15:477–490.

_____ & McGlashan, T. H. (1993), Parallel distributed processing and the emergence of schizophrenic symptoms. *Schizophren. Bull.*, 19:119–140.

Holt, R. R. (1977), A method for assessing primary process manifestations and their control in Rorschach responses. In: *Rorschach Psychology*, ed. M. A. Rickers-Ovsiankina. Huntington, NY: Krieger, pp. 375–420.

Holzman, P., Shenton, M. E. & Solovay, M. R. (1986), Quality of thought disorder in differential diagnosis. *Schizophren. Bull.*, 12:360–372.

Honer, W. G., Hurwitz, T., Li, D. K. B., Palmer, M. & Paty, D. W. (1987), Temporal lobe involvement in multiple sclerosis patients with psychiatric disorders. *Arch. Neurol.*, 44:187–190.

Huttenlocher, P. R, C. de Courten, L., Garey, J., van der Loos, H., (1982). Synaptogenesis in human visual cortex-evidence for synapse elimination during normal development. *Neuroscience Letters.* 33:247–252.

—————— & —————— (1987), The development of synapses in the striate cortex of man. *Human Neurobiol.*, 6:1–9.

Hyde, T. M., Ziegler, J. C. & Weinberger, D. R. (1992), Psychiatric disturbances in metachromatic leukodystrophy. *Arch. Neurol.*, 49:401–406.

Jakob, H. & Beckmann, H. (1986), Prenatal developmental disturbances in limbic allocortex in schizophrenics. *J. Neural Trans.*, 65:303–326.

Jobe, T. H., Harrow, M. H., Martin, E. M., Whitfield, H. J. & Sands, J. R. (1994), Schizophrenic deficits: Neuroleptics and the prefrontal cortex. *Schizophren. Bull.*, 20:413–416.

Johnston, M. H. & Holzman, P. S. (1979), *Assessing Schizophrenic Thinking.* San Francisco, CA: Jossey-Bass.

Johnstone, E. C., Crow, T. J., Frith, C. D., Husband, J. & Kreel, L. (1976), Cerebral ventricular size and cognitive impairment in chronic schizophrenia. *Lancet*, 2:924–926,.

Kelso, S. R., Ganong, A. H. & Brown, T. H. (1986), Hebbian synapses in hippocampus. *Proceedings of the National Academy of Sciences USA*, 83:5326–5330.

Kinney, H. C., Brody, B. A., Kloman, A. S. & Gilles, F. H. (1988), Sequence of central nervous system myelination in human infancy: II. Patterns of myelination in autopsied infants. *J. Neuropathol. and Experiment. Neurol.*, 47:217–234.

Koch, C. (1993), Computational approaches to cognition: The bottom-up view. *Current Opin. Neurobiol.*, 3:203–208.

Koch, M. (1996), The septohippocampal system is involved in prepulse inhibition of the acoustic startle response in rats. *Behavior. Neurosci.*, 110:468–477.

Koh, S. D. (1978), Remembering of verbal materials by schizophrenic young adults. In: *Language and Cognition in Schizophrenia.* ed. S. Schwart. Hillsdale, NJ: Lawrence Erlbaum Associates.

Kohler, J., Heilmeyer, H. & Volk, B. (1988), Multiple sclerosis presenting as chronic atypical psychosis. *J.Neurol, Neurosurg, Psychiat.*, 51:281–284.

Kovel, J. A. & Scheibel, A. B. (1984), A neurohistological correlate of schizophrenia. *Biolog. Psychiat.*, 19:1601–1621.

Koyama, Y., Jodo, E. & Kayama, Y. (1994), Sensory responsiveness of "broad-spike" neurons in the laterodorsal tegmental nucleus, locus ceruleus and dorsal raphe of awake rats: Implications for cholinergic and monoaminergic neuron-specific responses. *Neurosci.*, 63:1021–1031.

Kraepelin, E. (1919), *Dementia Praecox and Paraphrenia.* Edinburgh: E. & S. Livingston.

Krystal, J. H., Karper, L. P., Seibyl, J. P., Freeman, G. K., Delaney, R., Bremner, J. D., Heninger, G. R., Bower, M. B. & Charney, D. S., (1994), Subanesthetic effects of the noncompetitive NMDA antagonist, ketamine, in humans: Psychotomimetic, perceptual, cognitive, and neuroendocrine responses. *Arch. Gen. Psychiat.*, 51:199–214.

Lanin-Kettering, I. & Harrow, M. (1985), The thought behind the words: A view of schizophrenic speech and thinking disorders. *Schizophren. Bull.*, 11:1–7.

Lidz, T., Fleck, S. & Cornelison, A. (1965), *Schizophrenia and the Family.* New York: International Universities Press.

Magaro, P. A. & Page, J. (1983), Brain disconnection, schizophrenia, and paranoia. *J. Nerv. Mental Dis.*, 171:133–140.

Maher, B. A. (1983), A tentative model of schizophrenic utterance. In: *Progress is Experimental Personality Research,* ed. B. A. Maher. New York: Academic Press.

Mahler, M. E. (1992), Behavioral manifestations associated with multiple sclerosis. *Psychiatric Clinics of North America*, 15:427–438.

Manschreck, T. C., Maher, B. A., Celada, M. T., Schneyer, M. & Fernandez, R. (1991), Object chaining and thought disorder in schizophrenic speech. *Psycholog. Med.*, 21:443–446.

Marengo, J. & Harrow, M. (1985), Thought disorder: A function of schizophrenia, mania, or psychosis? *J. Nerv. Mental Dis.*, 173:35–41.

——— ——— Lanin-Kettering, I. & Wilson, A. (1986), Evaluating bizarre-idiosyncratic thinking. *Schizophren. Bull.*, 12:497–511.

McGrath, J. (1991), Ordering thoughts on thought disorder. *Brit. J. Psychiat.*, 158:307–316.

McGhie, A. & Chapman, J. (1961), Disorders of attention and perception in early schizophrenia. *Brit. J. Med. Psychol.*, 34:103–116.

Neale, J. M. & Oltmanns, T. F. (1980), *Schizophrenia*, New York: Wiley.

Neuchterlein, K. H. & Dawson, M. E. (1984), Information processing and attentional functioning in the developmental course of schizophrenic disorders. *Schizophren. Bull.*, 10:160–203.

Neumann, P. E., Mehler, M. F., Horoupian, D. S. & Merriam, A. E. (1988) Atypical psychosis with disseminated subpial demyelination. *Arch. Neurol.*, 45:634–636.

Oades, R. D. (1985), The role of noradrenaline in tuning and dopamine in switching between signals in the CNS. *Neurosci. Behav. Rev.*, 9:261–282.

Oltmanns, T. F., Murphy, R., Berenbaum, H. & Dunlop, S. R. (1985), Rating verbal communication impairment in schizophrenia and affective disorders. *Schizophren. Bull.*, 11:292–299.

Parker, N. (1956), Disseminated sclerosis presenting as schizophrenia. *Med. J. Australia*, 1:405–407.

Parnas, J., Orgensen, A., Teasdale, T. W., Schulsinger, F. & Mednick, S. A. (1988), Temporal course of symptoms and social functioning in relapsing schizophrenics: A 6-year follow-up. *Comprehen. Psychiat.*, 29:361–371.

———— & Schulsinger, H. (1986), Continuity of formal thought disorder from childhood to adulthood in a high-risk sample. *Acta Psychiat. Scanda.*, 74:246–251.

Pfefferbaum, A. & Zipursky, R. B. (1991), Neuroimaging studies of schizophrenia. *Schizophren. Res.*, 4:193–208.

Pogue-Geile, M. F. & Harrow, M. (1985), Negative symptoms in schizophrenia: Their longitudinal course and prognostic significance. *Schizophren. Bull.*, 11:427–439,

Quinlan, D.M. & Harrow, M. (1974), Boundary disturbances in schizophrenia. *J. Abn. Psychol.*, 83:533–541.

———— ———— & Carlson, K. (1973), Manual for assessment of deviant responses on the Rorschach. ASIS/NAPS #02211, pp. 1–28, Microfiche Publications, New York.

Ragin, A. B. & Oltmanns, T. F. (1987), Communicability and thought disorder in schizophrenics and other diagnostic groups: A follow-up study. *Brit. J. Psychiat.*, 150:494–500.

Rakic, P., Bourgeois, J., Eckenhoff, M.F., Zecevic, N. & Goldman-Rakic, P. S. (1986), Concurrent overproduction of synapses in diverse regions of the primate cerebral cortex. *Science*, 232:232–235.

Rapaport, D., Gill, M. & Schafer, R. (1968), *Diagnostic Psychological Testing*, ed. R.R. Holt. New York: International Universities Press.

Reilly, F., Harrow, M., Tucker, G. J., Quinlan, D. M. & Siegal. A. (1975), Looseness of associations in acute schizophrenia. *Brit. J. Psychiat.*, 127:240–246.

Richardson, E. P. (1982), Myelination in the human central nervous system. In: *Histology and Histopathology of the Nervous System.* ed. W. Haymaker & R. D. Adams. Springfield, IL: Charles C. Thomas, pp.146–173.

Rochester, S. & Martin, J. (1979). *Crazy Talk.* New York: Plenum Press.

Romney, D. M. (1988), Thought disorder among the relatives of schizophrenics: A reaction to Callahan and Saccuzzo. *J. Nerv. Mental Dis.*, 176:364–367.

———— (1990), Thought disorder in the relatives of schizophrenics. A meta-analytic review of selected publicized studies. *J. Nerv. Mental Dis.*, 178:481–486.

Rorke, L. B. & Riggs, H. E. (1969), *Myelination of the Brain in the Newborn.* Philadelphia, PA: Lippincott.

Saccuzzo, D. P. & Braff, D. L. (1986), Information processing abnormalities: Trait-and state-dependent components. *Schizophren. Bull.*, 12:447–459.

Salzinger, K., Portnoy, S. S., Pisoni, D. & Felman, P. (1970), The immediacy hypothesis and response-produced stimuli in schizophrenic speech. *J. Abn. Psychol.*. 76:258–264.

Sands, J.R. & Harrow, M. (1994), Psychotic unipolar depression at follow-up: Factors related to psychosis in the affective disorders. *Amer. J. Psychiat.*, 151:995–1000.

Schwartz, S. (1982), Is there a schizophrenic language? *Behav. Brain Sci.*, 5:579–626.

Sedvall, G. (1992), The current status of PET scanning with respect to schizophrenia. *Neuropsychopharm.*, 7:41–54.

Seeman, P., Guan, H. C., Hubert, H. M. & Tol, V. (1993), Dopamine D4 receptors elevated in schizophrenia. *Nature*, 365:441–445.

Shenton, M. E., Solovay, M. R. & Holzman, P. S. (1987), Comparison studies of thought disorders: II. Schizoaffective disorder. *Arch. Gen. Psychiat.*, 44:21–30.

Shimkunas, A. M., Gynther, M. D. & Smith, K. (1967), Schizophrenic responses to the Proverbs Test: Abstract, concrete, or autistic? *J. Abn. Psychol.*, 72:128–133.

Silverman, L., Lapkin, B. & Rosenbaum, I. Manifestations of primary thinking in schizophrenia. *J. Proj. Tech.* 26:117–127.

Singer, M. T., Wynne, L. C. & Toohey, M. L. (1978), Communications disorders and the families of schizophrenics. In : *The Nature of Schizophrenia*, ed. L. C. Wynne, R. L. Cromwell & S. Matthysse. New York: Wiley.

Strauss, M. E. (1993), Relations of symptoms to cognitive deficits in schizophrenia. *Schizophren. Bull.*, 19:215–233.

Swerdlow, N. R. & Koob, G. F. (1987), Dopamine, schizophrenia, mania, and depression: towards a unified hypothesis of cortico-striato-pallido-thalamic function. *Behav. Brain Sci.*, 10:197–245.

Vigotsky, L.S. (1962), *Thought and Language*, ed. G. Vaskar (trans. E. Hangman). New York: Wiley.

Walker, E. F. (1994), Developmentally moderated expressions of the neuropathology underlying schizophrenia. *Schizophren. Bull.*, 20:453–480.

———— Harvey, P. D. & Perlmann, D. (1988), The positive/negative symptom distinction in psychosis: A replication and extension of previous findings. *J. Nerv. Mental Dis.*, 176:359–36.

Watkins, J. G. & Stauffacher, J. C. (1952), An index of pathological thinking in the Rorschach. *J. Proj. Tech.*, 16:276–286.

Watson, C. G. (1967), Interrelationships of six overinclusion measures. *J. Consult. Psychol.*, 31:517–520.

Weinberger, D. R. (1986), The pathogenesis of schizophrenia: A neurodevelopmental theory. In: *Handbook of Schizophrenia, Vol. 1*, ed. H. A. Nasrallah & D. R. Weinberger. Amsterdam: Elsevier, pp. 397–406.

———— (1987), Implications of normal brain development for the pathogenesis of schizophrenia. *Arch. Gen. Psychiat.*, 44:660–669.

———— Torrey, E. F., Neophyides, A. N. & Wyatt, R. J. (1979), Structural abnormalities in the cerebral cortex of chronic schizophrenic patients. *Arch. Gen. Psychiat.*, 36:935–939.

_____ Wagner, R. L. & Wyatt, R. J. (1983), Neuropathological studies of schizophrenia: A selective review. *Schizophren. Bull.*, 9:193–211.

Wild, C., Singer, M., Rosman, B., Ricci, J. & Lidz, T. (1965), Measuring disordered styles of thinking using the object sorting test on parents of schizophrenic patients. *Arch. Gen. Psychiat.*, 13:471–476.

Wynne, L. C. & Singer, M. (1963), Thought disorder and family relations of schizophrenia: I. A research strategy. *Arch. Gen. Psychiat.*, 9:191–198.

_____ Bartko, J. J. & Toohey, M. L. (1977), Schizophrenics and their families: Research on parental communication. In: *Developments in Psychiatric Research*, ed. J. R. Tanner. London: Hodder & Stoughton.

Yakovlev, P. I. & Lecours, A. R. (1967), The myelogenetic cycles of regional maturation of the brain. In: *Regional Development of the Brain in Early Life*, ed. A. Minkowski. Oxford: Blackwell, pp. 3–70.

Zador, A., Koch, C. & Brown, T. H. (1990), Biophysical model of a Hebbian synapse. *Proceedings of the National Academy of Sciences USA*, 87:6718–6722.

8 THE FAMILY PERCEPTIONS OF YOUNG ADULTS WITH PUTATIVE RISK FOR SCHIZOPHRENIA

LINDA M. PEROSA, ROBERT SIMONS, AND SANDRA L. PEROSA

During the past decade, researchers investigating subjects who are at a higher than average statistical risk of developing schizophrenic disorders have followed two pathways. Traditionally, they have identified individuals as at-risk for becoming schizophrenic using genetic criteria, such as having one or two schizophrenic parents or a schizophrenic sibling. Compared to a risk of 1% in the general population, children of one schizophrenic parent have a lifetime risk 12%, whereas children of two schizophrenic parents have the exceptionally high risk of 25% to 40% for developing schizophrenia (Gottesman and Shields, 1976; Erlenmeyer-Kinding et al., 1982; Gotterman, McGuffin, and Farmer, 1987). The risk increases to 45% for those with an identical twin with the illness.

But because 80% of people who develop schizophrenia do not have a first-degree relative with the illness, findings from genetic-risk samples may not always generalize to the larger set of preschizophrenic individuals. Recognition of this limitation has led some researchers to follow the complementary strategy of locating subjects with heightened risk for schizophrenia through psychometric criteria, and there is a growing body of evidence that young adults with high scores on the *Perceptual Aberration* (Chapman, Chapman, and Raulin, 1978) or *Physical Anhedonia* (Chapman, Chapman, and Raulin, 1976) scales may constitute such a subject group. The evidence for the link between high questionnaire scores and risk status for future psychosis has come from both cross-sectional and prospective research.

The cross-sectional evidence has taken a variety of forms. Evidence of schizophrenia-like thought disorder, for example, was found in both perceptual aberration subjects (i.e., those who scored two standard deviations above the mean on the *Perceptual Aberration scale*) and anhedonic (i.e., subjects who scored two standard deviations above the mean on the *Physical Anhedonia Scale*) during Rorschach testing (Edell and Chapman, 1979) and psychotic or psychotic-like experiences were reported for perceptual aberration subjects during a structured psychiatric interview (Chapman, Edell, and Chapman, 1980). Both subject groups reported more social withdrawal than did controls. Moreover, laboratory-based behavioral assessment revealed a pattern of social-skill deficits among anhedonic subjects (Haberman et al., 1979; Beckfield, 1985). Cognitive slippage (i.e., the loosening of associations between ideas during Rorschach testing) in subjects with perceptual aberrations was reported by Allen and colleagues (1987) and Martin and Chapman (1982). In addition, both perceptual aberration (Perlstein, Fiorito et al., 1989; Simons and Giardina, 1992) and anhedonic subjects (Simons, 1981; Josiassen et al., 1985; Simons, MacMillan, and Ireland, 1982; Simons and Russo, 1987) have produced schizophrenia-like responses during a variety of psychophysiological assessment procedures.

The longitudinal data have come primarily from the Chapmans' research project involving the prospective study of a large number of undergraduate subjects recruited from a large Midwestern university and evaluated extensively both at two years and 10 years subsequent to their enrollment in the project. At two years, three of the subjects from the perceptual aberration group ($n = 161$) had been diagnosed with psychotic disorders, whereas no subjects from either the physical anhedonia ($n = 67$) or the control group ($n = 144$) had received similar diagnoses (Chapman and Chapman, 1985). Of the three subjects who developed a psychotic disorder, one became schizophrenic, one was diagnosed with paranoid disorder, and one was diagnosed with bipolar affective disorder. Thus, at two years, the at-risk status of subjects with perceptual aberrations was supported, but the risk was not specific to schizophrenia. There was no evidence at two years that subjects with physical anhedonia had a greater risk for psychosis than control subjects.

More recently, preliminary data from the 10-year follow-up of this cohort group has become available (Chapman et al., in press). Again, perceptual aberration subjects stand at a much higher risk for developing a psychotic disorder than control subjects (5.3% versus 0.1%), whereas the high-risk status of subjects with physical anhedonia was still not confirmed. As in the two-year data, high perceptual aberration scores did not pose a risk that was specific to schizophrenia. Rather, the risk for scoring high on the *Perceptual Aberration Scale* was that these individuals tended to develop a psychosis more broadly defined; six of the ten psychotic subjects had clear schizophrenia features, one was delusional, and three suffered from bipolar affective disorder.

Recently Asarnow (1988) reviewed the results of 24 major longitudinal studies aimed at identifying environmental factors and individual vulnerabilities deemed important to the development of schizophrenia. These studies compared young people judged to be at high risk—because they were the offspring of one or two parents with schizophrenia—with control groups considered to be low risk. She organized the factors that were found to be important in these studies into a developmental psychopathology perspective to produce a sequence of patterns for five periods of life: infancy, early childhood, middle childhood, adolescence, and early adulthood. Asarnow concluded that the evidence supports the contention that whatever genetic factors and personal attributes might be present, the risk (especially in adolescence and young adulthood) is compounded by a family environment characterized by communication deviance (CD), that is, peculiarities of language used by the speaker that leave the listener confused; expressed emotion (EE), that is, emotional overinvolvement, hostility, or criticism; and a negative affective climate or style (AS), that is, personal criticism, guilt inducement, and intrusiveness displayed by the parent toward the adolescent.

In contrast to the line of research examining offspring of schizophrenic parents, there has been very little focus on the family dynamics of the psychometrically determined at-risk group. In the only paper we located that specifically targets the family environments of physical anhedonia subjects and perceptual aberration subjects for investigation, Edell (1985) found significant differences between the recollections of both groups and a control group on the *Childhood Experience Scale* (CES; Frank and Paris, 1981) and the *Kvebaek Family Sculpture Technique* (KFST; Kvebaek, Cromwell, and Fourmier, 1980). Although both groups reported less overall approval from their mothers compared with controls, the anhedonics (compared to controls and perceptual aberrators) described their mothers as more disinterested, particularly toward their dependent behaviors during childhood. The childhood environment of perceptual aberrators (compared to controls and anhedonics) was typified by more criticism by their mothers (rather than disinterest), especially toward their

167

dependent behaviors. Their fathers were described as more critical, especially toward their independent behaviors. Hence, the perceptual aberrators saw themselves as having been criticized for being dependent and for being independent, an apparent "double-bind" situation.

What is unclear is how the family variables of personal criticism and mixed messages, which are limited to parent–child interactions, fit into the larger context of total family system functioning. How, for example, do dynamics within the spousal dyad relate to what occurs between mother and child and father and child? How do the parent–child relationships described as too loosely joined (i.e., a disinterested parental response to a child's dependent demands) or too tightly joined emotionally (i.e., an overly intrusive parent) fit into the family structural schema of the rigid triad?

The purpose of the present study was to investigate the family perceptions of a sample of psychometrically determined young adults likely to be at risk for schizophrenia. In this study, current perceptions rather than recollections of early childhood are highlighted in order to extend Edell's (1985) findings to ongoing events and to link them to a family model associated with a rich array of therapeutic interventions.

MINUCHIN'S STRUCTURAL FAMILY MODEL

One such model of family functioning has been developed by Minuchin (1974; Minuchin, Rosman, and Baker, 1978). According to this model, family structure is revealed in the boundaries that define relationships between members; that is, by the unspoken rules that govern who is permitted to participate, what role is allowed, and who is to be in charge when members interact. Boundaries are healthiest when roles are clearly defined and there exists a free exchange of nurturance and opinion. Relationships that present developmental risks for children and adolescents include those in which boundaries are enmeshed—where the flow of thought and feeling is so intrusive that the process of individuation is hindered (Minuchin et al., 1978). In contrast, relationships that are disengaged pose dangers because of excessive autonomy and isolation.

Wood and her colleagues (Wood and Talmon, 1983; Wood, 1985; Wood et al., 1989) have clarified the notion of boundaries by distinguishing between Proximity, or systemwide interpersonal boundaries (i.e., the degree of sharing of time together, emotions, thoughts, conversations, and decision making among family members), and Generational Hierarchy, or the relative strength or weakness of the boundary placing parents in charge of children. Family problems occur when the boundaries separating the parent subsystem from children are crossed and dysfunctional alliances form.

Dysfunctional alignments or rigid triads occur when parents seek to submerge or deflect marital conflict through the child. In triangulation, parents place competing demands on the child for support against the other parent. In parent–child coalitions, one parent consistently sides with the child against the other parent, and in detouring, the parents define the child as the source of family problems either by defining him or her as bad (scapegoating) or by overprotecting the child because he or she is weak or sick.

Thus transactions reflecting overinvolved and enmeshed relationships in Minuchin's (1974) model are similar to the intrusive and guilt-inducing statements between parent and child appearing in the expressed emotions (EE) and negative affective style (AS) codes. Cross-generational triads present situations similar to the double-bind events described in Edell's study. Moreover, the disengaged boundaries and estranged relationships in Minuchin's model mirror the hostile and critical remarks indicative of expressed emotion (EE) and negative affective style (AS) as well as feelings of rejection by participants in Edell's study.

Given these similarities among Minuchin's model, Edell's findings and the family communication codes, we hypothesized that young adults who scored in the extreme range on the *Perceptual Aberration* and/or *Physical Anhedonia* scales, when compared to normal controls, would describe their home environment as more disengaged overall. In addition, they would be more likely to feel that they are involved in some form of a rigid triadic alliance that cuts across inter-generational boundaries.

Method

PARTICIPANTS

The participants were 117 (58 female) Caucasian undergraduates selected from 991 students enrolled in an introductory psychology course at a Middle-Atlantic state university. The 991 students completed a set of screening questionnaires at the beginning of the semester. Individual participants in the current study were assigned to the Perceptual Aberration group (n = 32, 19 female) or the Physical Anhedonia group (n = 32, 12 female) group if their score on the *Perceptual Aberration* or *Physical Anhedonia* Scale exceeded two standard deviations above the mean of the 991 students initially tested. Participants were assigned to the control group (n = 53, 27 female) if their scores fell below one-half standard deviation above the mean on both scales. Two individuals scored above the plus=two standard deviation cutoff on both questionnaires. One declined to participate in the present research project and the second was excluded based on other questionnaire performance (see below). These criteria for selecting participants were the same as those followed by the Chapmans in their longitudinal study of undergraduates.

Ninety-five (78%) of the 117 students were reared in an intact family; 19 reported being in a single-parent home (5 in which one parent had died); and 7 lived with a stepparent. Chi-square analyses revealed that this distribution of students into family types did not differ between anhedonia and perceptual aberration subjects [X^2 (I) = .25, *ns*] nor did families of anhedonia and perceptual aberration subjects differ in type from the families of control subjects [X^2 (l) = .05, *ns*].

Potential participants were excluded from the study if they endorsed any of three locally constructed infrequency or lie items during the initial screening, All of these subjects in the final sample received course credit for their participation in the research project.

MEASURE

At-risk status for developing schizophrenia was assessed by the *Perceptual Aberration* and *Physical Anhedonia* scales. The *Perceptual Aberration Scale* (Chapman et al., 1978) contains 35 true–false items such as "Sometimes I've had the feeling that I am united with an object near me," which refer to distortions in the perception of one's own body. Other items refer to other kinds of perceptual changes, including insensitivity to sights and sounds. Coefficient alpha reliability for the scale is reported to be .90 and test–retest reliabilities with a six-week interval are .75.

The *Physical Anhedonia Scale* (Chapman et al., 1976) is composed of 61 true–false items that assess a pervasive inability to experience pleasure. A sample item reads: "The beauty of sunsets is greatly overrated." Internal consistency estimates (alpha) for the scale are .80 and test–retest reliabilities with six weeks intervening are .79.

Both the *Perceptual Aberration Scale* and the *Physical Anhedonia Scale* have been used in numerous studies to identify psychosis-proneness in college students (see Chapman and Chapman, 1985). The correlation between the two scales is slightly negative, suggesting that the two scales may identify different schizotypes or two distinctly different groups of psychosis-prone young adults.

Family structural dynamics were assessed by the *Structural Family Interaction Scale-Revised* (SFIS-R; Perosa and Perosa, 1990). The SFIS-R is based on a factor analysis of the *Structural Family Interaction Scale* (SFIS) (Perosa, Hansen, and Perosa, 1981) and is designed to measure Minuchin's structural model of family functioning. It contains 83 items, which are answered on a four-point Likert scale of agreement ranging from "very true" to "very false."

Two scales on the SFIS-R assess overall family dynamics. The Enmeshment/Disengagement (E/D) scale reflects the degree of support, responsiveness, and sense of differentiation family members experience in relation to boundaries. Flexibility/Rigidity (FL/R) measures the degree to which the family is able to change as conditions warrant in response to demands associated with the growth of autonomy or to situational stress impacting on the family. These scales are thought to assess Wood's concept of Proximity or systemwide interpersonal boundaries.

Three scales are used to assess Wood's concept of Generational Hierarchy. First, the Parent Coalition/Cross-Generational Triads (PC/CGT) scale reflects the degree to which boundaries between parents and child are crossed to form rigid triadic patterns of communication (i.e., triangulation, parent–child coalition, and detouring) as a way parents avoid dealing with and resolving marital difficulties between themselves. The two remaining scales profile the quality of the relationships the child has with each parent separately. The Mother–Child Cohesion/Estrangement (MCC/E) and the Father–Child Cohesion/Estrangement (FCC/E) scales mirror the degree to which the mother and father respectively provide nurturance and resolve differences with the child so that both parent and child feel close to each other.

Alpha coefficients for the scales range from .71 to .93. Test–retest estimates on a college sample tested at four-week intervals range from .80 to .92 and interscale correlations are moderate (.32 to .61).

The original SFIS (1981) has differentiated perceptions of family interaction of problem-free adolescents from those with learning disabilities (Perosa and Perosa, 1982), anorectic and bulimic adolescents (Kramer, 1983), emotionally disturbed youths (Walrath, 1984), and those with suicidal ideation (Mitchell and Rosenthal, 1992). The revised version has been found to be the best discriminator of incest families from another clinical family control group and a nonclinical family control group (Utech, 1989).

PROCEDURES

Participants were invited to the research room in small groups. Upon arrival they were administered the *Structural Family Interaction Scale-Revised* (SFIS-R) and a personal data sheet.

Because Wood and her colleagues (Wood, 1985; Wood et al., 1989) argue that the concepts of Proximity and Generational Hierarchy are orthogonal, each concept was subjected to multivariate analysis of variance (MANOVA) with a priori univariate contrasts constructed to test the effects of group membership. The first contrast tested for differences between anhedonic and perceptual aberration subjects, and the second contrast tested for differences between the combined group of anhedonic and perceptual aberration subjects and the control group. Proximity was measured by the Enmeshment/Disengagement (E/D) and the Flexibility/Rigidity (FL/R) scores, whereas Generational Hierarchy consisted of the Parent Coalition/Cross-Generational Triads (PC/CGT), the Mother–Child Cohesion/Estrangement (MCC/E), and the Father–Child Cohesion/Estrangement (FCC/E) scores.

Results

Table 1 contains the data for the whole group initially screened as well as the data from each of the three samples resulting from the selection criteria described previously. Both the data for the initial group screened and the individual sample are in line with those of other laboratories (J. Chapman, personal communication, 1992) engaged in the longitudinal study of similarly chosen undergraduate subjects. It is also noteworthy that both the *Perceptual Aberration* and *Physical Anhedonia* scores from the selected samples meet or exceed the scores that schizophrenic subjects achieve on the same questionnaires

TABLE 1
MEAN PERCEPTUAL ABERRATION AND PHYSICAL ANHEDONIA SCORES FOR ALL
STUDENTS INITIALLY SCREENED AND FOR EACH OF THE THREE SUBJECT GROUPS

Questionnaire	All Screened (N = 991) M SD	Perceptual Aberrators (n = 32) M	Physical Anhedonics (n = 32) M	Controls (n = 32) M
Perceptual Aberration	6.73 (5.72)	21.38	7.14	4.82
Physical Anhedonia	11.18 (6.27)	10.87	26.84	9.59

(e.g., Chapman et al., 1978; Schuck et al., 1984; Clementz et al., 1991; Berenbaum and Oltmanns, 1992; Katsanis et al., 1990).

The data for the five SFIS-R subscales are contained in Table 2. As the table suggests, when anhedonic and perceptual aberration subjects were compared to each other, no differences approached significance (Contrast 1; all F's < 1, $p > .05$).

When the combined anhedonic and perceptual aberration subjects were compared to controls, however, significant group differences did emerge for some variables (Contrast 2). Because the MANOVA F was not significant [F (2,117) = 2.80, $p < .10$] for Proximity [i.e., the

TABLE 2
GROUP MEANS AND MULTIVARIATE ANALYSIS OF VARIANCE RESULTS FOR GENERATIONAL
HIERARCHY DIMENSIONS OF FAMILY STRUCTURE

Variable	Perceptual Aberrators M	Physical Anhedonia M	Controls M	Contrast 2; Comparison E Test (df = 1,118)
Family Structure Generational Hierarchy				
PC/CGT	23.8	22.8	20.9	4.90*
FCC/E	20.1	20.1	17.5	3.97*
MCC/E	16.8	16.2	14.5	4.95*

Note. N = 121. SFIS-R = *Structural Family Interaction Scale-Revised*, PC/CGT = Parent Coalition/Cross-Generational Triads, FCC/E = Father–Child Cohesion/Estrangement, MCC/E = Mother–Child Cohesion/Estrangement. Higher scores on PC/CGT indicate more cross-generational triads, on FCC/E more estrangement between father and child, and MCC/E more estrangement between mother and child.
Comparison F test results are given for the anhedonic and perceptual aberration groups combined versus the control group.
*$p < .05$.

Enmeshment/Disengagement (E/D) and Flexibility/Rigidity (FL/R) subscales], we did not consider the univariate tests for these scales. Significant differences were found between the psychometrically determined at-risk group and control subjects on the scales representing Generational Hierarchy [MANOVA F (3,116) = 2.78, $p < .05$]. The univariate contrasts between the at-risk and control subjects indicate that compared to control subjects, anhedonic and perceptual aberration subjects reported more rigid cross-generational triads [F (1,118) = 4.90, $p < .05$], and greater estrangement from both their mothers [F (1,118) = 3.97, $p < .051$, and their fathers F (1,118) = 4.95, $p < .05$].

Discussion

The findings from this study support the conclusions reached by Edell (1985) that the psychometrically determined at-risk group of young adults perceive their family environment more negatively than control subjects. In particular, their reported experiences with parents are more conflictual and are marked by a stronger sense of involvement in some form of cross-generational alliance. Though Edell found some differences in the family perceptions of physical aberrators from those of participants with physical anhedonia (e.g., the former reporting more disinterest and the later more criticism from parents), these differences were not apparent in the present study. That is, anhedonic and perceptual aberration subjects reported equally negative perceptions of their family environments.

Given these findings, it must now be determined whether these differences in the family perceptions of psychometrically determined at-risk for schizophrenia young adults from those of participants not at risk are detrimental to the psychological well-being of the subjects or whether they represent adaptive family responses to an emotionally and socially withdrawn family member (see Coyne and Anderson, 1988, for a similar debate over the functional or dysfunctional role played by the family in maintaining problematic behaviors associated with brittle diabetes in adolescents). It is important to note here that, although the differences in family perceptions between the at-risk and symptom free young adults are significant, the scores for both groups fell within the normal range of Minuchin's theoretical model. For example, in spite of the fact that at-risk participants saw more cross-generational alliances and estrangement from parents in their homes compared to the control group, they reported more cohesiveness overall than complete lack of involvement or caring in family relationships. Apparently, whatever conflicts and disagreements between parent and young adults do exist in these families, the family members are not left feeling isolated or totally cut off from each other. This may augur well for these subjects because Burman and colleagues (1987) have found that, among children with schizophrenic parents, those who went on to become schizophrenic themselves perceived their family relationships *very* negatively, whereas those offspring who remained compensated (i.e., with no mental illness or with schizotypal personality disorder) retained perceptions of their families that were either closer to or within normal limits.

On the other hand, as indicated at the outset, longitudinal data on these at-risk subjects substantiate the risk for severe psychopathology for the perceptual aberrators. For example, at the 25-month follow-up, it was noted that 22% of perceptual aberrators had sought professional counseling compared to only 7% of the control group. Ten% of perceptual aberration subjects reported experiencing psychotic symptoms during this two-year period while no such reports were obtained from control subjects (Chapman and Chapman, 1985). By the 10-year follow-up, with subjects *only midway through the risk period* (Slater and Cowie, 1971), over 5% of the perceptual aberration subjects had received diagnoses of psychosis, while this was true of less than 1% of the control subjects (Chapman et al., in press). Two additional perceptual aberration subjects had died by suicide during this 10-year period and over twice as many perceptual aberration subjects reported psychosis in one or more first- or second-degree relatives than did control subjects. Interestingly, at both the two- and 10-year follow-up, there were no differences on symptom-related measures between control subjects and subjects with high physical anhedonia scores. Whether these differences between the perceptual aberration and physical anhedonia groups will continue in the future is unknown.

This different clinical picture of the two types of putatively psychosis-prone subjects is curious given the similarity of their family perceptions on the SFIS-R (but not on the family measures used in Edell's study). One possible explanation for this discrepancy is that the SFIS-R may not be as sensitive to the family dimensions that were measured by the *Childhood Experience Scale* (CES) that was administered by Edell. Although the SFIS-R scales measuring cross-generational triads, and mother-child and father-child estrangement contain some items tapping feelings of parental support, disinterest, or disapproval, no scale exclusively measures parental support, disinterest, or criticism for a set of independent behaviors or for a group of dependent behaviors displayed by the subjects (as does the CES).

Nor is the SFIS-R designed to elicit information from early childhood recollections. It is possible that feelings of parental disinterest or criticism experienced in childhood by anhedonics and perceptual aberrators become transformed in young adulthood into more general feelings of estrangement from parents. Because adolescence is a stage of development characterized by more overt and covert conflict with parents, compared with childhood, current family perceptions held by the subjects in this study may reflect these types of interactions. According to Minuchin (1974), the most salient features of family functioning at the launching stage of the family life cycle are whether boundaries are clear among members, whether conflict is expressed and resolved, and whether the young adult is able to experience some individuation from parents. These dynamics are the focus of the SFIS-R (but not of the CES).

In sum, the differences in family dynamics between the perceptual aberration and physical anhedonia groups and control subjects reported in the present study may reflect the push and pull on the part of family members struggling to help maturing, yet potentially decompensating, young adults to manage the strains associated with the launching stage of the family life cycle. Differences between the two groups of psychosis-prone subjects, not evident in their report of family environment but inferred from the clinical data at follow-up, seem to suggest that this push and pull has different consequences for perceptual aberration and anhedonic subjects. Further research is needed to pinpoint the exact nature of the families' attempts to assist the struggling young adults and to identify any facilitative family interventions that counseling might provide.

Although the findings from this study are not clear-cut, when placed in context with the earlier work by Edell (1985) and the emerging body of evidence summarized by Asarnow (1988), they do alert the clinician to pay attention to family factors while treating at-risk young adults. The pattern of unresolved conflict (indicating hostility, criticism, and rejection), or overly involved relations (reflecting intrusive and guilt-inducing statements) between parent(s) and child, along with some form of rigid cross-generational alliance, appear to pose the greatest danger.

When helping young adults confront developmental tasks associated with the process of psychologically leaving home, clinicians need to be sensitive not only to the pressures that family system dynamics impose on the choices and behaviors clients display but also to the parallels between parent–adolescent relations and the counselor–client relationship (Oles and Bronstein, 1989; Pistole, 1989; Nichols and Schwartz, 1991). Because individuation is critical at this stage of development the clinician should help these clients explore who they are and what they value as they face choices in terms of career, interpersonal relationships, and lifestyle. As Asarnow's (1988) review suggests, at-risk young adults may be in need of social skills training that emphasizes reflective listening, communicating feelings, or assertiveness training. Whether the clinician works solely with the young adult to model and teach these skills or relies on a group counseling format to reinforce them, there is evidence accruing from the UCLA High Risk Project (see Strachan et al., 1989) that behaviors elicited by the young adult toward the parent can perhaps change the nature of their systemic interaction. For example, Strachan et al. (1989) have shown that parental EE is an index not only of the parents' behaviors toward the patient but also of the patients' behaviors toward the parents. Low EE attitudes are associated with neutral non-critical behavior in parents and frequent use of autonomous statements by patients. The relationship between the two sets of behaviors is reciprocal. If the clinician is trained in family therapy and works with the family, he or she can draw upon numerous techniques used by Minuchin and others to mark boundaries and encourage new communication patterns in the home. Perhaps interventions borrowed from psychoeducation programs or the teaching of parenting skills also might prove beneficial in promoting healthy boundaries between parent and child.

REFERENCES

Allen, J. J., Chapman, L. J., Chapman, J. P., Vuchetich, J. P. & Frost, L. A. (1987), Prediction of psychotic-like symptoms in hypothetically psychosis-prone college students. *J. Abn. Psychol.*, 96:83–88.

Asarnow, J. (1988), Children at risk for schizophrenia: Converging lines of evidence. *Schizophren. Bull.*, 14:613–631.

Beckfield, D. F. (1985), Interpersonal competence among college men hypothesized to be at-risk for schizophrenia. *J. Abn. Psychol.,* 94:397–404.

Berenbaum, H. & Oltmanns, T. (1992), Emotional experience and expression in schizophrenia and depression. *J. Abn. Psychol.,* 101:37–44.

Burman, B., Mednick, S. A., Machon, R. A., Parnas, J. & Schulsinger, F. (1987), Children at high risk for schizophrenia: Parent and offspring perceptions of family relationships. *J. Abn. Psychol.,* 96:364–366.

Chapman, L. J. & Chapman, J. P. (1985), Psychosis proneness. In: *Controversies in Schizophrenia,* ed. M. New York: Guilford, pp. 157–174).

_____ _____ Kwapil, T.R., Eckbiad, M. & Zinser, M.C. (in press). Putatively psychosis-prone subjects ten years later. *J. Abn. Psychol..*

_____ _____ & Raulin, M. L. (1976), Scales for physical and social anhedonia. *J. Abn. Psychol.,* 85:374–382.

_____ _____ & Raulin, M. L. (1978), Body-image aberration in schizophrenia. *J. Abn. Psychol.,* 87:399–407.

_____ Edell, W. S. & Chapman, J. P. (1980), Physical anhedonia, perceptual aberration, and psychosis proneness. *Schizophren. Bull.,* 6:639–653.

Clementz, B., Grove, W. M., Katsanis, J. & Iacono, W. G. (1991), Psychometric detection of schizotypy: Perceptual aberration and physical anhedonia in relatives of schizophrenics. *J. Abn. Psychol.,* 100:607–612.

Coyne, J. C. & Anderson, B. J. (1988), The psychosomatic family reconsidered: Diabetes in context. *J. Marr. Fam. Ther.,* 14:113–123.

Edell, W. S. (1985), Parental perception and psychosis proneness in college students. Paper presented at the 93rd annual meeting of the American Psychological Association, Los Angeles.

_____ & Chapman, L. J. (1979), Anhedonia, perceptual aberration, and the Rorschach. *J. Consult. Clin. Psychol.,* 47:337–384.

Erienmeyer-Kimling, L., Cornblatt, B., Friedman, D., Marcuie, Y., Rutschmann, J., Simmens, S. & Devi, S. (1982), Neurological, electro-physiological and attentional deviations in children at risk for schizophrenia. In: *Schizophrenia as a Brain Disease,* ed. F.

Henn and H. Nasrallah. New York: Oxford University Press, pp. 61–98.

Frank, H. & Paris, J. (1981), Recollections of family experience in borderline patients. *Arch. Gen. Psychiat.*, 38:1031–1034.

Gotterman, I., McGuffin, P. & Farmer, E. (1987), Clinical genetics as clues to the "real" genetics of schizophrenia. *Schizophren. Bull.*, 13:23–47.

Gottesman, 1. I. & Shields, J. (1976), Genetics of schizophrenia: Critical review of recent adoption, twin and family studies. *Schizophren. Bull.*, 2:360–401.

Haberman, M. C., Chapman, L. J., Numbers, J. S. & McFall, R. M. (1979), Relation of social competence to scores on two scales of psychosis proneness. *J. Abn. Psychol.*, 88:675–677.

Josiassen, R. C., Shagass, C., Roemer, R. A. & Straumanis, J. J. (1985), Attention-related effects on somatosensory evoked potentials in college students at risk for psychopathology. *J. Abn. Psychol.*, 95:507–518.

Katsanis, J., Iacono, W. G., Beiser, M & Lacey, L. (1992), Clinical correlates of anhedonia and perceptual aberration in first-episode patients with schizophrenia and affective disorder. *J. Abn. Psychol.*, 101:184–191.

Kramer, S. (1983), Bulimia and related eating disorders: A family systems perspective. Unpublished dissertation: California School of Professional Psychology.

Kvebaek, D., Cromwell, R. & Fourmier, D. (1980), The Kvebaek Family Sculpture Technique: A diagnostic and research tool in family therapy. Jonesboro, TN: Pilgrimage.

Martin, E. M. & Chapman, L. J. (1982), Communication effectiveness in psychosis-prone college students. *J. Abn. Psychol.*, 91:420–425.

Minuchin, S., (1974), *Families and family therapy.* Cambridge, MA: Harvard University Press.

_____ Rosman, B. & Baker, L. (1978), *Psychosomatic Families: Anorexia Nervosa in Context.* Cambridge, MA: Harvard University Press.

Mitchell, M. & Rosenthal, D. (1992), Suicidal adolescents: Family dynamics and the effects of lethality and hopelessness. *J. Youth Adoles.*, 21:23–33.

Nichols, M. & Schwartz, R. (1991), *Family Therapy: Concepts and Methods.* Needham Heights, MA: Allyn & Bacon.

Oles, T. & Bronstein, L. (1989), Bring the family "in": A family systems perspective on student adjustment to college. *J. Coll. Student Psychother.,* 4:35–44.

Perlstein, W. M., Fiorito, E., Simons, R. F. & Graham, F. K. (1989), Prestimulation effects on reflex blink and EPs in normal and schizotypal subjects. *Psychophysiol.,* 26:S48 (Abstract).

Perosa, L., Hansen, J. & Perosa, S. (1981), Development of the Structural Family Interaction Scale. *Fam. Ther.,* 14(1):43–51.

_____ & Perosa, S., (1982), Structural interaction patterns in families with a learning disabled child. *Fam. Ther.,* 2:175–188.

_____ _____ (1990), The revision and validation of the structural family interaction scale. Paper presented at the American Psychological Association Convention, Boston.

Pistole, C. (1989.), Attachment: Implications for counselors. *J. Counsel. Devel.,* 68:190–193.

Schuck, J., Leventhal, D., Rothstein, H. & Irizarry, V. (1984), Physical anhedonia and schizophrenia. *J. Abn. Psychol.* 93:342–344.

Simons, R. F. (1981), Electrodermal and cardiac orienting in psychometrically defined high-risk subjects. *Psychiat. Res.,* 4:47–356.

_____ & Giardina, M. T. (1992), Reflex modification in psychosis prone young adults. *Psychophysiol.,* 29:9–17.

_____ MacMillan, F. W., Ill & Ireland, F. B. (1982), Anticipatory pleasure deficit in subjects reporting physical anhedonia: Slow cortical evidence. *Biol. Psychol.,* 14:297–310.

_____ & Russo, K. R. (1987), Event-related potentials and continuous performance in subjects with physical anhedonia or perceptual aberrations. *J. Psychophys.,* 4:401–410.

Slater, E. & Cowie, V. (1971), *The Genetics of Mental Disorders.* Oxford: Oxford University Press.

Strachan, A., Feingold, D., Goldstein, M. & Neuchterlein, K. (1989), Is expressed emotion and index of a transactional process? II. Patient's coping style. *Fam. Proc.,* 28:169–181.

Utech, W. (1989), A comparison of clinical and non-clinical samples using the concepts of individual personality, family structure, family of origin perception, sexuality, and adjustment/adaptability to determine family risk for father-daughter incest. Unpublished doctoral dissertation, Purdue University.

Walrath, R. (1984), Measures of enmeshment and disengagement in normal and disturbed families. Unpublished doctoral dissertation, Nova University.

Wood, B. (1985), Proximity and hierarchy: Orthogonal dimensions of family interconnectedness. *Fam. Proc.*, 24:487–507.

_____ & Talmon, M. (1983), Family boundaries in transition: A search for alternatives. *Fam. Proc.*, 22:347–357.

_____ Watkins, J., Boyle, J., Nogueira, J., Zimonds, E. & Carroll, L. (1989), The "Psychosomatic Family" Model: An empirical and theoretical analysis. *Fam. Proc.*, 28:399–417.

9 ADOLESCENT MOOD DISORDERS

LYNN E. PONTON

The topic of adolescent affective disorders is fascinating as well as complex. Although research in child and adolescent affective disorders has been slow, it is now rapidly growing. To understand why this research has been delayed, it is necessary to comprehend why it has been difficult for psychiatrists and others to recognize that children and adolescents might get depressed. First and foremost, depression has been regarded as a very severe illness, and it has been difficult to accept that degree of psychopathology in young people, particularly in children (Ponton and Phillips, 1983). Freudian theories contributed to this by promoting the concept that the superego has to be developed in order to experience guilt and associated melancholia, thereby concluding that it is impossible for depression to take place in children before such development has occurred (Freud, 1917). These ideas were prevalent in the 1960s, an era during which psychanalytic precepts held significant weight.

During the past 20 years, much time has been spent on the recognition and detection of depressive symptoms and syndromes in children and adolescents. Research investigations in this area are clarifying the diagnostic process, and it is becoming apparent that children and adolescents manifest some of the same depressive symptoms that adults display. They do have, however, unique ways of showing the disturbance, and the observer must be trained to ask a series of questions that will confirm or disconfirm the diagnosis.

The need for diagnostic criteria specific to children and adolescents can be understood as a second factor limiting our knowledge in this area. David Shaffer (1985) notes both the importance and the limitations of such diagnostic criteria when he states that many researchers have taken as fact that *DSM-III-R* (American Psychiatric Association, 1987) and now *DSM-IV* (American Psychiatric Association, 1994) adult criteria can be directly applied to the child and adolescent age group. These criteria have been very important to research, but adult criteria should not be unequivocally accepted by clinicians working with children and adolescents until further testing allows a determination of their applicability to this group.

A third factor that has limited our knowledge of adolescent depression is that researchers and clinicians have been dissuaded from undertaking projects by the suspected complexity of the field, a complexity that has not been disproved by the research efforts of the past ten years. Children and adolescents undergo very rapid developmental changes responding to hormonal, cognitive, psychological, and social factors. Even with the difficulty of prematurely accepting the *DSM* criteria as applicable to children and adolescents, a sizable number of useful studies have been conducted in the past decade.

This chapter opens with a definition of this complex area, integrates a discussion of research advances in adolescent affective disorders with clinical applications, lists diagnostic criteria, discusses the individual diagnostic categories, and ends with a section on suicide and suicide prevention.

Conceptualization of Adolescent Depression and Related Affective Disorders

In the literature, the term *child and adolescent depression* is used in many different capacities. Some grasp of the multiple uses of this term will aid our understanding. Adrien Angold (1988) expanded on the definitions of Carlson and Cantwell (1980a, b) who delineated differences among depressive symptoms, syndromes, and disorders in children and adolescents. Angold describes seven different uses of the term *depression*. First, he notes that the term is used to describe the low end of the spectrum of fluctuations of normal mood. Second, *depression* is used as a description of unhappiness, sadness, or psychic pain felt as a response to an unpleasant event. Third, *depression* describes a continuing, stable anhedonic state characterizing a specific individual. Fourth, *depression* refers to a symptom that denotes pathological low or sad mood. Psychiatrists commonly use the term for this purpose. Fifth, *depression* refers to a syndrome, a constellation of symptoms regularly found to occur together. Sixth, *depression* refers to a disease, a relatively well-defined disorder that has been shown to have regularly recurring psychopathological correlates, clear genetic basis, a distinctive etiology, physical pathology, and shared prognosis.

Angold also notes a seventh use of the term *depression* to refer to a chronic disability that children or adolescents may manifest. The multiple definitions of the term indicate the importance of its careful use. Although the term is often used by clinicians in a general, even cavalier fashion when speaking with other clinicians, it is particularly important that it be understood and defined when applied to patients. The depression terminology will be expanded below in the section on affective disorders, a group of disorders categorized by the unifying characteristic of abnormal mood.

The theoretical understanding of affective disorders in children and adolescents reflects some of the same confusion as with the term *depression*. No integrated theory demonstrates why children and adolescents manifest affective symptoms and syndromes, only a patchwork theory, pieced together from both clinical and research efforts. A part of this working theory has emerged from the work of Seligman and Peterson (1986) on learned helplessness combined with Beck's work with colleagues (1979) on cognitive determinants. Further understanding has developed from genetic studies such as those conducted by Myrna Weissman and her colleagues (1984). Other theoretical aspects are related to knowledge gained about risk factors such as trauma, loss, and homelessness.

For the purpose of this eassay, *affective disorders* are defined as a collection of disorders associated with abnormal mood states (*mood* refers to a prolonged emotion that colors the psychic life of an individual); however, this definition continues to evolve as new disorders gain description and definition.

Research Advances

Ongoing research in adolescent affective disorders falls into six major areas: diagnostic criteria, scale development, epidemiology, neuroendocrine advances, genetic studies, and clinical medication trials.

DIAGNOSTIC CRITERIA

Understanding and evaluating nosology and diagnosis are important; one cannot study anything without a basic idea of what it is. Slow progress in this area has impaired advances in the understanding of adolescent affective disorders.

Replicable research diagnostic criteria have been and continue to be developed so that ideas can be shared by different groups of researchers and clinicians. The criteria that have been utilized with children include those of Weinberg and colleagues (1973), a second set developed by Poznanski, Cook, and Caroll, (1979), and now the general acceptance of the *DSM-III-R* (American Psychiatric Association, 1987) and *DSM-IV* (American Psychiatric Association, 1994) criteria. The work of Ryan et al. (1987) on criteria helped define a clinical difference between childhood and adolescent depression. They found that prepubertal children with depression displayed a more depressed appearance, increased somatic complaints, psychomotor agitation, separation anxiety, phobias, and hallucinations; whereas adolescents had greater anhedonia, expressed hopelessness, hypersomnia, weight change, use of drugs and alcohol, and lethality of suicide attempts, but not, interestingly enough, greater suicidal ideation or intent. The different symptom pictures for the two age groups helps to define better how depression changes with development—a gradual progression from behavioral symptoms to cognitive and, finally, melancholic symptoms.

SCALES

Several tools have been helpful in confirming and testing the diagnoses and in defining criteria. While useful in research, they can also be used with clinical interviews, school reports, parental histories, and other measures to evaluate an adolescent clinically for depressive illnesses. Three scales, a child depressive index by Kovacs (1981), a modified version of the Beck symptom checklist (Beck et al., 1961) for use with adolescents (Ambrosini et al., 1991), and the Hamilton Child Depressive Scale (Hamilton, 1960) all have relatively good reliability and are easy to administer.

The KIDDIE schedule for affective disorders (KIDDIE-SADS) (Costello and Angold, 1988) is a structured interview format that has value for evaluating depression. Another example of a child and adolescent interview scale is the DISC (Diagnostic Interview Scale for Children) developed by Costello and Edelbroch (1983). These interviews are valued research tools but are generally too extensive for clinical work. The Achenbach Child Behavior Checklist (Achenbach and Edelbrock, 1978) and the Conners scale (Conners, 1973) for evaluating hyperactivity continue to be clinically concise and useful.

Fristad, Weller, and Weller (1991) have adapted the Mania Rating Scale for use with children and believe it may have some applicability in differentiating symptoms of mania from those of hyperactivity. Many of these scales are valuable in research populations but have only limited applicability in the clinical setting. Roberts, Lewisohn, and Seeley (1991) stress the importance of using multiple measures combining scales, structured interviews, and clinical assessment for case evaluation. Multiple measures can serve to increase the reliability of a clinical diagnosis.

EPIDEMIOLOGY

Kashani (1987) surveyed the prevalence of affective disorders, examining 150 adolescents in a community-based study, finding the prevalence of major depressive and dysthymic disorders to be 4.7% and 3.3% respectively, similar to the data of Rutter (Rutter, Tizard, and Whitmore, 1970) in the Isle of Wight study, which found the prevalence of depressive syndrome to be 4.1% in the 10- to 11-year-old age group and 4% among the 14- to 15-year-olds. Not all studies reflect this degree of consistency.

Garrison et al. (1992) investigated the prevalence of major depressive disorder and dysthymia in a population of 12- to 14-year-olds, finding a greater prevalence of 9.04% in males and 8.90% in females for major depressive disorder. The prevalence of dysthymia was 7.98% in males and 5% in females. Previous investigations have noted a higher rate of major depression in adolescent females than adolescent males, consistent with the higher rate of major depressive disorder reported in adult females. The discrepancy can be partially explained by the method of report employed in the study. Garrison et al. (1992) utilized the KIDDIE-SADS and noted that mean scale scores were higher in adolescent females, but their conclusions regarding prevalence were based on a summary of mother and child symptom reports, demonstrating how the method of inquiry can affect results.

Carlson and Cantwell (1980a, b) studied a group of children admitted to the Outpatient Child Clinic at UCLA and noted that 60% of the children who came to the clinic had depressive symptoms. Only 24% of that population met the diagnostic criteria utilized. They also noted that only 75% of those defined as having a depressive disorder had the symptom of depressed affect. This illustrates a difficulty in the clinical diagnosis of depressive illness; a continuum of symptoms in children. It also suggests that many more children manifest depressive symptoms than show the full syndrome picture of a depressive illness.

A number of risk factors have also been investigated. Increasing age is associated with an increasing prevalence and manifestation of melancholic symptoms, related to the transition from childhood to adolescence. Whether adolescents suffer more from depressive illness than do adults is controversial, and further research is needed to clarify this picture. Rutter (1985) also noted that in boys aged 14 to 15, depressive feelings were more highly associated with puberty than with age per se, illustrating the importance of assessing pubertal status when examining the depressed adolescent.

David Shaffer (1985) has examined the "cohort effect" and delineates the idea that children born in subsequent decades in depressed families manifest increased amounts of depression or suicidality. Other high-risk groups include adolescents who have lost a parent to suicide, children who have experienced physical or sexual abuse, and children who have suffered loss of a parent by separation or death. Weissman et al. (1984) examined the relatives of depressed parents and found a significantly increased risk for children and adolescents of parents with depressive disorders, indicating that approximately 40% of children of parents with affective disorders will manifest some affective pathology. A genetic argument is supported by evidence that 67% of monozygotic twins reared apart both manifest depressive illness, compared with 76% for monozygotic twins living together and 19% for dizygotic twins living together (Tsung, 1978). There is also a wide range of psychosocial research presently being conducted on disordered family functioning and its relationship to depression. Currently, both psychosocial and genetic factors are considered to play an important role in the communication of depressive illness to the next generation.

Strober et al. (1988, 1990) have also demonstrated that we have to be concerned about the period during which a child or adolescent manifests symptoms. Adolescents with bipolar illness with symptoms in childhood could be distinguished from adolescents with bipolar illness with no premorbid childhood psychiatric abnormalities because they have an increased number of relatives with bipolar illness and a poorer response to lithium treatments. This type of study further helps us to distinguish between child and adolescent presentations and also clarifies the different manifestations that are seen with each of the age groups.

Lastly, studies of comorbidity are growing. Rutter et al. (1970) found that conduct disorder and depressive illness are often found together and that 42% of children with antisocial disorders have associated affective disturbance. Puig-Antich (1982) reported that when children are treated with antidepressants for an affective disorder, their conduct disturbance often improves: Puig-Antich and Weston (1983) found high rates of separation anxiety disorder in children who met symptomatic criteria for depressive disorder. Carlson and Cantwell (1980a) found that one-third of children and adolescents with anorexia nervosa and bulimia nervosa met *DSM-III* (American Psychiatric Association, 1987) criteria for a major depressive disorder and many also had a positive family history of depression. Hysteria, headaches, enuresis, and inflammatory bowel disease have all been found associated with depressive disorder. Alcoholism and substance abuse also are associated with depressive disorders in adolescents (Shaffer, 1985).

Fergusson, Horwood, and Lynskey (1993) recently examined a cohort of 15-year-olds in New Zealand and found that mood disorders were most frequently found comorbid with anxiety disorders, whereas substance use and disruptive behavior disorders clustered together.

NEUROENDOCRINE RESEARCH

This fourth domain of research is dominated by the work of one investigator, Puig-Antich (Puig-Antich et al., 1984), and his study of biological markers. He recognized both that stress activates the hypothalamic anterior pituitary adrenal cortical axis and that a number of neuroendocrine abnormalities could be discovered in the child and adolescent population with depressive illness. He experimented with the dexamethasone suppression test and found that cortisol levels were not suppressed with 0.5 mg. of dexamethasone in 71% of prepubertal *DSM-III*-diagnosed depressed children and adolescents, while 92% of the nonendogenous depressed individuals had suppression of cortisol levels. Unfortunately, the dexamethasone suppression test has been disappointing in the child and adolescent population and, at present, is not appropriate for clinical use. Second, Puig-Antich (Puig-Antich et al., 1981) noted that the growth hormone response to insulin-induced hypoglycemia is blunted in the active stage of prepubertal depression.

It remains unchanged on recovery and may be a marker for predisposition to the illness. Adolescents with a suicidal plan account for a significant proportion of those with blunted growth hormone response. These tests vary with nutrition and body weight, but one can conclude that the neuroendocrine axis of adolescents is altered by depressive illness. Lastly, Puig-Antich et al. (1984) failed to find changes in the sleep pattern of the prepubertal depressed child, in contrast to the patterns that have been observed with adults.

In summary, biological markers have not yet indicated a consistent profile that can be used to investigate the many diagnoses in adolescents, even though the neuroendocrine axes are altered.

GENETIC STUDIES

Application of the methods of genetic epidemiology is a promising pathway to an understanding of how genes work. This approach is particularly important for diseases such as mood disorders, characterized by moderate degrees of heritability and the lack of direct correspondence between underlying vulnerability factors and the ultimate expression of the disease (Merikangas, 1993). An ideal population to study and follow would be children of parents with affective disorders wherein prevention and treatment efforts could be instituted at an early point. Todd et al. (1993) examined an extended family grouping targeted as high risk because they had several children identified as having affective disorders and compared them with a normal control extended family grouping. The high frequency of affective disorders among the family members of the childhood-onset affective disorder probands identifies families with a higher incidence than the family of adult-onset probands, making them both more high risk and more appropriate for genetic analyses. A second pilot study conducted by Todd, Reich, and Reich (1994) found that when compared with controls, children and adolescents of an adult affective disorder proband had no differences in demographic variables, IQ, school achievement, or temperamental or family characteristics, but there were increases in affective and disruptive disorders, making them ideal targets for treatment and prevention efforts.

CLINICAL TRIALS

A sixth area of research, clinical trials, has also been somewhat disappointing but is expanding rapidly. Tricyclic antidepressants, selective serotonin re-uptake inhibitors, lithium, and carbamazepine have been the medications most frequently used. Some of these studies indicate a positive result such as reported in Carlson's study (1983), where 53% of adolescents with a unipolar depressive disorder responded well to antidepressants, but only 8% of those with a bipolar disorder responded. Angold (1988) is more candid when he notes that the published treatment studies have been exceedingly disappointing. Efficacy of tricyclic antidepressants has never been convincingly demonstrated in adequate control, double-blind placebo trials. Lithium, however, has greater efficacy in a clear diagnosis of bipolar disorder in an adolescent.

Diagnosis and Treatment of Depressive Disorders in Adolescents

In the *DSM-III-R* (American Psychiatric Association, 1987) and the *DSM-IV* (American Psychiatric Association, 1994), mood disorders are divided into disorders related to a single episode (e.g., manic, depressed, or hypomanic), bipolar disorders and depressive disorders (unipolar), and two disorders based on etiology and mood disorder. The two combined disorders include mood disorder associated with a general medical condition, and mood disorder and substance abuse. *Episodes* are described as distinct periods (one week for mania, two weeks for depression), in contrast to *disorders*, which are described as clinical courses, although disorders may consist of only one episode when there is a greater degree of certainty ruling out other illnesses (e.g., schizo-affective). The essential feature of a *bipolar disorder* is the presence of more than one manic or hypomanic episode. The essential feature of a *depressive disorder* is the presence of one or more periods of depression without an existing history of manic or hypomanic episodes. An adolescent with a major depressive disease must have at least five of the following symptoms present for a two-week period, and the symptom must represent a change from previous functioning and cause significant distress or impairment in functioning. The symptoms include a depressed mood that lasts most of the day, decreased pleasure, daily sleep disturbance, daily complaints of fatigue, a significant change in activity level, decreased self-esteem and the presence of guilt, difficulties with schoolwork such as a diminished ability to concentrate, recurrent suicidal thoughts and/or a plan or attempt, and weight loss or a failure to maintain weight gains as

191

measured by normal growth curves. At least one of the symptoms must be a severely depressed or irritable mood, and/or the loss of interest or pleasure. These symptoms must have persisted for longer than a month, although in clinical work with children and adolescents, it is not unusual to discover that the symptoms have been present for much longer.

Certain factors must also be ruled out in order to make this diagnosis. An organic factor must not have initiated or maintained the disorder, and the disturbance cannot be a normal grief reaction. Another alternative diagnosis in the differential is *adjustment disorder with depressed mood*, which is distinguished from the above-mentioned syndrome by the presence of a stressor to which the disease is attributable. *Separation anxiety disorder* also shows similar symptoms but is related to the loss of a caregiver to whom the child or adolescent is attached, and it is more frequently seen in children. One must also exclude the diagnoses of *learning disability with a depressed mood*, and *psychosis with depression* unless the clinical picture also meets the full criteria for either of these diagnoses. Physical illnesses such as renal disease, Crohn's disease, and leukemia may also be present with a concomitant depression. Dysthymic disorder, which will be discussed below, should also be considered in the differential.

Although the *DSM-III-R* does not make many accommodations to children and adolescents, it does remark that in adolescence, negativistic or antisocial behavior and the use of alcohol or drugs may be present and may justify the additional diagnoses of *oppositional defiant disorder, conduct disorder,* or *substance abuse or dependence.* In adolescents, feelings of wanting to leave home or not being understood and approved of, restlessness, grouchiness, and aggression are common. Shaffer (1985) notes the isolation that is often marked in adolescents who complete suicide, a feature highlighted by the *DSM-III-R*. Increased emotionality is frequently observed and is characteristic of adolescent depression when it is compared with the adult version. The highs seem higher and the lows seem lower as displayed by a depressed adolescent during the course of affective disorder. The *DSM-IV* does not include specific age-related material.

Assessment for major depressive disorder is one of the primary tasks of the adolescent clinician. It is important to have an organized approach to assessment. A comprehensive history aids the process; this can be achieved either through interview or written questionnaire and should include a detailed family history, genetic history, records of hospitalizations, and treatment response of family members to any psychotropic medications. A developmental history, completed by the parents, often fills in gaps. Histories of separations, losses, learning disabilities, and any related symptoms such as problems with eating or antisocial behavior should be included. Asking the adolescent to talk about his or her friends and school experience is also important. The mental status exam must access reality testing, and a suicidal assessment with the questions "Have you ever had ideas about ending your life? Do you presently have any ideas about that?" is important. If there is any concern, this part of the assessment should be expanded.

In a comprehensive examination, the adolescent should be seen alone and then with the family. Educative, evaluative family therapy that provides the family with education about affective disorders often gives the family the background to help them ask questions. Articles on antidepressants also are valuable in educating families. Developing a packet on affective disorders that can be handed out to the family during the assessment often introduces the family to this type of information.

The evaluation also should include questions about drug and alcohol use, arrests, and violent activity. Sexual activity should be evaluated in a confidential manner when parents are not present. After the clinician has conducted a comprehensive assessment, a number of different options are available. The adolescent can be admitted to the hospital if there is a serious risk of suicide. A course of antidepressant medication can be discussed with the family. When treating a depressed adolescent without suicidal risk, handing out the materials and arranging for another meeting to discuss treatment is a good strategy. A discussion of treatment options should include a description of the psychotherapies used in the treatment of affective disorders. Studies by Moreau et al. (1991) underscore the opportunity for brief focal psychotherapies in this age group, noting that studies have failed to demonstrate the superior efficacy of psychopharmacologic agents. One of the most frequently used treatment options is a three- to four-month psychotherapy that focuses initially on evaluating and then targeting depressive symptoms in the adolescent patient. There are also a large number of adolescents who are good candidates for fluoxetine or a tricyclic antidepressant. The selective serotonergic re-uptake inhibitors (SSRIs) are not presently FDA-recommended for the adolescent population, and the use of these medications poses a risk in the adolescent population (Ryan, 1990.) However, common clinical use has demonstrated their efficacy. Low doses of fluoxetine in 5-mg and 2.5-mg capsules can be specifically compounded, and the liquid form, although distasteful, can be used. The lower doses minimize the side effects of agitation and sleep disturbance associated with the larger doses.

Venkataraman, Naylor, and King (1992) suggest a strategy for treating adolescents with SSRIs beginning with low doses and increasing slowly to avoid adverse side effects. They report five cases of mania induced by the use of fluoxetine, but all patients were treated with more than 20 mg of the medication, some up to 60 mg. Low dose (2.5–20 mg/day) provides an alternative option.

SSRIs are now frequently used when there is a previously failed treatment with another antidepressant medication (often a tricyclic or monoamine oxidase inhibitor). Puig-Antich et al. (1984) as well as others report a disappointing lack of efficacy for tricyclic antidepressants in treating juvenile mood disorders, contributing to the hope that the SSRIs will be more successful (Ponton, 1993). Other clinical strategies for tricyclic failure include using higher doses of antidepressants in adolescents, with careful plasma monitoring because they may be metabolizing at a higher rate; and combined treatment approaches such as the use of two antidepressants of a different class, lithium carbonate, stimulants, thyroid hormone (T3) and antianxiety medications (Spencer, Wilens, and Biederman, 1995).

The four current SSRIs (fluoxetine, paroxetine, sertraline, and fluvoxamine) are structurally dissimilar and have differences in their side-effect profiles. Fluoxetine and paroxetine have been found to inhibit hepatic enzymes and thereby increase levels of tricyclic antidepressants. Sertraline is the least likely to interact with other medications (Spencer et al., 1995).

Tricyclic antidepressants, primarily imipramine and desipramine, have been used frequently in the adolescent population. Most of the tricyclic studies that have been conducted have looked at these particular agents in order to demonstrate efficacious treatment. Again, to date there have been only a limited number of double-blind trials, generally noting a 30% improvement with placebo versus 50% improvement with the medication (Boulos et al., 1991). Shaffer (1985) and Ryan (1990) note that it has been recommended that routine EKGs be carried out in any patient, whether child or adolescent, receiving 2.5 mg per kilogram or more of imipramine. Repeat EKGs should be obtained with dosage increases. A recent review article (Spencer et al.,

1995) has recommended a baseline EKG for all children or adolescents taking these medications, followed by serial EKGs throughout the treatment. Reports of sudden death in several cases of children treated with desipramine has favored this conservative approach (Riddle et al., 1991). Some of the studies (Saref et al., 1978) have indicated that plasma imipramine and desipramine combinations exceeding 155 nanogram/ml showed a significant clinical response, whereas in studies, only one-third of the patients with levels below this were improved, indicating that efficacy is related to blood levels and that there might be some sort of therapeutic window.

Strober and Carlson (1982) reported that 53% of adolescents with a unipolar depressive disorder responded well to antidepressants, but only 18% of those with a bipolar condition showed a positive response. When we are trying so hard to distinguish between adolescents with bipolar and unipolar disorders, it is important to remember that one-half of bipolar disorders present with depressive episodes.

Outcome studies indicate that 80% of all adolescents with depressive illness will recover within one year from treatment and that 90% will recover during a two-year period. The course of the illness if untreated is quite long. Two years is the average mean duration of the depressive illness (Kovacs et al., 1984). An examination of Kovacs and colleagues' outcome data is also revealing. They found that the mean duration of an episode of major depression at the time of diagnosis was 32 weeks, whereas those with dysthymic disorder had already been suffering for three years. The median time for recovery after diagnosis for dysthymia was three-and-a-half years, although the recovery rate with a major depressive disorder was much faster. Within five years from the time of diagnosis, they found that 69% of the dysthymic patients had had an episode of major depression and 72% of the patients with major depression had had a second episode. These studies were conducted with prepubertal children with depression, but they may have some applicability regarding adolescent recurrence.

BIPOLAR AFFECTIVE DISORDER

The diagnostic criteria for a manic episode as listed under bipolar disorders in the *DSM-IV* are 1) a distinct period of abnormally and persistently elevated expansive or irritable mood lasting at least one week, or of any duration if hospitalization is necessary; 2) during the period of mood disturbance at least three of the following symptoms must persist in a significant degree: inflated self-esteem or grandiosity; decreased need for sleep; increased talkativeness or pressure to keep talking; flight of ideas or the subjective experience that thoughts are racing; distractibility, including attention being drawn to irrelevant external stimuli; an increase in goal-directed activity, either socially, at work, at school, or sexually; and excessive involvement in pleasurable activities that have a high potential for painful consequences such as sexual indiscretions and unrestrained buying sprees; and 3) a mood disturbance severe enough to cause marked impairment in school functioning, social activities, relationships with others, or to necessitate hospitalization. This third criterion of sufficient mood disturbance separates manic episode from hypomanic episode. A hypomanic episode includes criteria 1 and 2 but does not include criterion 3. An additional diagnostic caveat for both manic and hypomanic episodes is that at no time during this period of disturbance can there have been the presence of delusions or hallucinations in the absence of prominent mood symptoms; this is obviously used to rule out other psychotic illnesses.

The treatment of bipolar affective disorders is currently centered around the medication lithium carbonate. Lithium carbonate is given in divided doses and is monitored by serum levels that are recommended to be between 0.7 and 1.2 mg per liter in blood serum drawn 12 hours after the last dose of lithium. It takes five to seven days to reach a steady state. Lithium carbonate is useful not only for manic depressive syndromes but also for aggressive behavior and hyperactivity in adolescents. Because there are fewer double-blind controlled studies in the child and adolescent population, an educational approach that alerts the family to risks and benefits is appropriate. The side effects are numerous and include transient hypothyroidism, hypothyroidism often accompanied by the development of goiter, possible renal damage manifested as a proteinuria, some adverse effects on learning, fine hand tremor in 30% of all patients, and the possibility that bone growth may be inhibited by the presence of the medication. Lithium also alters the hypothalamic pituitary axis, altering human growth hormone response to insulin-induced hypoglycemia. However, overall growth hormone output does not appear to be affected (Shaffer, 1985).

Geller and colleagues (1992) have recently tested adolescents dually diagnosed with bipolar and substance dependency disorders, and the preliminary results of the study indicate that lithium carbonate diminishes both symptom pictures.

Carbomazepine is a psychoactive drug that has been reported to be effective in controlling mania in adults and can be effective in treating lithium-resistant manic depressive illness (Shaffer, 1985). There is a strong indication for use of this medication in adolescents who have been lithium resistant, sometimes in combination with lithium. General use is to begin with a dose of 200 mg b.i.d. increasing to a full range dose between 1000 and 1600 mg b.i.d. It is very important to observe platelet and white blood cell counts closely because serious but infrequently reported side effects are aplastic anemia and agranulocytosis, of which leukopenia and decreased platelet count are one of the first signs. Valproic acid is also another alternative mood-stabilizing, antimanic agent with idiosyncratic reactions such as bone marrow and liver toxicity, which require careful monitoring.

At onset, bipolar illness frequently cannot be differentiated from early schizophrenia. Careful observation of the course of the illness is crucial.

Retrospective studies indicate that the course of bipolar illness often begins in the early 20s although there are many reported cases at an earlier age. The manic episodes typically begin with a rapid escalation of symptoms over a few days. The episodes usually last for a few days to a few months and end more abruptly than the depressive episodes. Estimates from the *DSM-IV* indicate that between 0.4% and 1.6% of the adult population has had bipolar disorder. Type I includes the prevalence of at least one manic episode. Type II (recurrent depressive episodes with hypomanic episodes) has a prevalence rate of 0.5% (American Psychiatric Association, 1994). It is now generally believed that these results may be low. In contrast to major depression, bipolar disorder is apparently equally common in men and in women. Treatment courses are variable but in about 30% of cases, there is a return to premorbid level of functioning between episodes. However, also in about 30% of cases, there is a chronic course of residual symptomatic impairment and this is more frequently associated with rapid cyclers and those with frequently recurrent episodes.

Werry et al. (1991, 1992) conducted a study of 59 adolescents diagnosed with the psychoses of schizophrenia or bipolar disorder and found that adolescents with bipolar disorder were more frequently misdiagnosed as schizophrenic, had a 50% homotypic family history, and had a better prognosis. At a mean of five years follow-up the bipolar patients were doing better than the schizophrenic patients. The indicators for best prognosis in the bipolar group were I.Q. and premorbid functioning.

CYCLOTHYMIA, SEASONAL AFFECTIVE DISORDER, AND DYSTHYMIA

The diagnosis of *cyclothymia* in children or adolescents requires the one-year presence of numerous hypomanic episodes (two years for adults), fulfilling all of the criteria for a manic episode except that of marked impairment. The treatment for this particular condition varies. Lithium carbonate has been used with some degree of success. The course is often without clear outset and follows a chronic course. Studies have reported a lifetime prevalence from 3% to 5% (American Psychiatric Association, 1994). The gender ratio is approximately even. Major depression and bipolar disorder are reported to be more frequent in first-degree relatives. Although *Seasonal* pattern specifier (which can be applied to Bipolar Type I, Bipolar Type II, or major depressive episodes or disorders) is rarely diagnosed in the adolescent population, it has been reported (Mghir and Vincent, 1991). This diagnosis requires a regular temporal relationship between the onset of a bipolar disorder or a recurrent major depression in a particular 60-day period of the year, usually between the beginning of October and the end of November, followed by full remissions. There must have been episodes of mood disturbance in two separate sequential years, or an observed pattern in a lifetime, making this difficult to diagnose with adolescents. Mghir and Vincent (1991) discuss treatment with phototherapy in their case study of a 16-year-old adolescent girl.

Dysthymia is also referred to as "depressive neurosis." The essential feature of this disorder is a chronic disturbance of mood consisting of depressed or irritable mood present for the majority of days during a two-year period for adults, and one year for children or adolescents. In addition, these periods of depressed mood are often associated with poor appetite or overeating, insomnia, or hypo-insomnia, low energy or fatigue, low self-esteem, poor concentration, difficulty making decisions, and feelings of hopelessness. In children and adolescents, social interactions with peers are frequently affected. Children with this condition often react negatively or shyly to praise and frequently respond to positive relationships with negative behavior. School performance may be affected. In children and adolescents, predisposing factors include the presence of attention deficit disorder, conduct disorder, mental retardation disorder, and some of the specific developmental disorders. Among adults, this disorder is more common in women. In children, it appears to be equal in both sexes and, again, one would expect the transition to occur in adolescence. A major depressive syndrome is characterized by one or more discrete major episodes that can be distinguished from the person's usual functioning, whereas dysthymia is characterized by a mild chronic depressive syndrome present for years. This disorder usually begins in childhood. Garrison et al. (1992) found that not living with both natural parents and being of lower socioeconomic status were both significant correlates of dysthymia in children and adolescents.

This condition is often evaluated and treated in a similar manner to the major depressive syndromes. Clinical experience demonstrates that psychotherapy is helpful with these individuals; the therapy is often focused on the depressive symptoms but also addresses decreasing isolation and promotes social interaction and changes in the family structure. Again, treatment with antidepressants is important to consider.

Suicide

Suicide is an important correlate of adolescent affective disorder. The Center for the Study of Suicide Prevention of the United States Public Health Service classifies suicidal behavior as follows: A *complete suicide* is defined as a willful self-inflicted life-threatening acts leading to death. The *suicide attempt* includes all willful self-inflicted life-threatening acts that do not end in death. *Suicidal ideation* is defined as all ideas or behaviors that suggest the possibility of a threat to the individual's life (Adam, 1985).

Nationwide, suicide is the most common form of death in the 18- to 24-year-old age group and the second leading cause in the 15- to 19-year-old age group, with the rate doubling between 1961 and 1975 in the adolescent age group (Hollinger, 1979), Suicidal ideation and behavior have been increasing in the adolescent population (Shaffer and Fischer, 1981). The age-specific mortality rate in 1978 was 0.81 per 100,000, which accounted for 2.4 deaths in the 10- to 14-year-olds. Among those aged 15 to 19 the mortality rate was 7.4 per 100,000 (Shaffer and Fischer, 1981).

Suicide attempts are one of the most common types of psychiatric emergencies faced by adolescent psychiatrists (Matteson, Sesse, and Hawkins, 1969). Shafi et al. (1985) noted a dramatic increase in the number of children with suicide attempts referred for psychiatric evaluation between 1970 and 1980. In 1973 there was a 530% increase in suicidal patients coming through the emergency services.

Completed suicide attempts, suicidal ideation, and emergency room visits related to suicide are increasing in young people, but these statistics still reflect underrepresentation of suicide in children and adolescents compared with the entire population, which is why Shaffer (1985) encourages exploration of protective as well as risk factors in this particular population. Adolescents have a higher rate of suicide than children, suicide attempts are more common in adolescent girls, and completed suicides are more common in adolescent boys. Adolescent boys in the United States most commonly kill themselves by firearms, hanging, or poisoning. Adolescent females most frequently employ poisoning. Suicide is generally more common in white adolescents than in nonwhites, so there are certain protective effects attributed to being nonwhite. Those who have made a suicide attempt in the past few months are at increased risk. Recent precipitating events include a disciplinary crisis, the suicide of a friend, and/or the diagnosis and presence of certain illnesses such as epilepsy, HIV, and others.

A major area of research in adolescent psychiatry focuses on whether there is psychiatric illness in the teens who complete or attempt suicide. Much of the current research is focused on teens who attempt suicide largely because they are more common and are, obviously, more accessible to study. Earlier diagnostic studies of teens who attempt suicide often examined only a small number and looked at only one or two psychiatric diagnoses. Most noteworthy among these was Crumley's (1979) study of 40 patients who attempted suicide; 24 were found to have a major depressive disorder and 22, borderline personality disorder. Adolescents who attempt or commit suicide have been found to have a wide variety of psychiatric diagnoses—affective disorder, conduct disorder, substance abuse, personality disorders, and attention deficit disorder (Levy and Deykin, 1989), but further evaluation is needed. In any study, all of the likely diagnoses have to be entertained.

Research on the treatment of the suicidal adolescent has been more limited. The initial evaluation of a patient presenting with suicidal ideation or following an attempt necessitates a careful assessment of suicide potential. Robbins and Alessi (1975) stressed the importance of interviewing the adolescent when inquiring about suicide and emphasized the adolescent's ability to accurately report symptoms. They also emphasized the importance of in-depth assessment of suicide attempts, stating that serious attempts are likely to be followed by others. An important juncture in treatment is the transition from the emergency room to outpatient setting at the time of the transfer. Thirty to sixty percent of those who attempt suicide fail to continue psychiatric treatment at that point. Emergency services have to be well integrated with outpatient facilities so that follow-up actually takes place.

Research also has focused on the value of limiting firearms in the United States. Because firearms are so frequently used in completed adolescent suicides, one should always inquire directly about the presence of firearms and recommend hospitalization strongly if safety cannot be maintained.

Theories of adolescent suicide are rarely addressed and are often one-dimensional. Adolescent suicide is a multifactorial problem, and more complex theories address it better. David Shaffer has attempted to do this by integrating some of the information from cohort studies, the increasing rate, an examination of the availability of firearms, exposure to suicide through cluster effect, and changes in the family structure, noting that all of these factors have some impact on the changing rate of suicide in the adolescent population (Shaffer, 1985).

Prevention

Prevention efforts are becoming increasingly important in the interfacing areas of adolescent psychiatric disorders and risk behaviors (DiClemente, Ponton, and Hansen, 1996). To date, many of the prevention strategies for juvenile mood disorders have targeted adolescent suicide and have included the development of community hotlines for adolescent suicide; creating special treatment services for populations at high risk using both the school system and the media to decrease the stigma of mental illness; improving the quality of assessment by mental health professionals; school-based programs that focus on increasing adolescents' self-esteem; and restricting access to firearms. Frequently, however, the all-important assessment components of these prevention programs have been lacking (Cohen, Spirito, and Brown, 1996).

Brent and colleagues (1993) have stressed the importance of developing psychoeducational programs for the families of affectively ill children and adolescents. A pilot of one such program has indicated an increase in parental knowledge about depression, including modification of false beliefs. Beardslee et al. (1993) did a comparison of a pilot that utilized both clinician- and lecture-based strategies and found that clinician-based strategies were more effective. Studies that include an assessment component and target prevention are key first steps in an area that is expected to grow in importance.

Summary

The topic of adolescent depression is as complex as the topic of adolescent suicide. Any worthwhile theory needs to explain adequately the complexity of these problems. Diagnostic criteria need to identify signs and symptoms specific to adolescents, and medications and other therapies should be prescribed accordingly when appropriate. Recent research advances in the areas of diagnostic criteria, scale development, epidemiology, neuroendocrinology, clinical medication trials, and suicide work together with clinical practice to improve understanding and provide more options for working with patients.

REFERENCES

Achenbach, T. M. & Edelbrock, C. S. (1978), The classification of child psychopathology: A review and analysis of empirical efforts. *Psychol. Bull.*, 85:1275–1301.

Adam, K. S. (1985), Symposium on self-destructive behavior. *Psychiat. Clin. N. Amer.*, 8:183–201.

Ambrosini, P. J., Metz, C., Bianchi, M. D., Rabinovich, H. & Undie, A. (1991), Concurrent validity and psychometric properties of the Beck Depression Inventory in outpatient adolescents. *J. Amer. Acad. Child Adoles. Psychiat.*, 30:5–7.

American Psychiatric Association (APA). (1980), *Diagnostic and Statistical Manual of Mental Disorders*, 3rd ed. Washington, DC: American Psychiatric Association.

———— (1987), *Diagnostic and Statistical Manual of Mental Disorders*, 3rd ed., rev. Washington, DC: American Psychiatric Association.

———— (1994), *Diagnostic and Statistical Manual of Mental Disorders*, 4th ed. Washington, DC: American Psychiatric Association.

Angold, A. (1988), Childhood and adolescent depression: Epidemiological and aetiological Aspects. *Brit. J. Psychiat.*, 1:601–17.

Beardslee, W. R., Salt, J. P., Porterfield, K., Rothberg, P. C., van de Velde, P., Swatling, S., Hoke, L., Moilanen, D. L. & Wheelock, I. (1993), Comparison of preventive interventions for families with parental affective disorder. *J. Amer. Acad. Child Adoles. Psychiat.*, 32:254–263.

Beck, A. T., Rush, A. J., Shaf, B. F. & Emery, G. (1979), *Cognitive Therapy of Depression*. New York: Guilford.

———— Ward, C. H., Mendelson, M., Mock, J. E. & Erbough, J. K. (1961), An inventory for measuring depression. *Arch. Gen. Psychiat.*, 4:561–571.

Boulos, C., Kitcher, S., Morton, P., Simeon, J., Ferguson, B. & Roberts, N. (1991), Response to desipramine treatment in adolescent major depression. *Psychopharm. Bull.*, 29:59–65.

Brent, D. A., Poling, K., McKain, B. & Baugher, M. (1993), A psychoeducational program for families of affectively ill children and adolescents. *J. Amer. Acad. Child Adoles. Psychiat.*, 32):770–774.

Carlson, G. A. (1983), Bipolar affective disorders in childhood and adolescence. In: *Affective Disorders in Childhood and Adolescence: An Update*, ed. D. P. Cantwell & G. A. Carlson. New York: Spectrum, pp. 187–226.

———— & Cantwell, D. P. (1980a) A survey of depressive symptoms, syndrome, and disorder in a child psychiatric population. *J. Child Psychol. Psychiat.*, 21:19–25.

———— & ———— (1980b), Unmasking masked depression in children and adolescents. *Amer. J. Psychiat.*, 137:445–449.

Cohen, Y., Spirito, A. & Brown, L. (1996), Adolescent suicide and suicidal behaviors. In: *Handbook of Adolescent Health Risk Behaviors*, ed. R. DiClemente, W. Hansen & L. E. Ponton. New York: Plenum Press, pp. 193–224.

Conners, C. K. (1973), Rating scales for use in drug studies with children. *Psychopharm. Bull.* (Special Issue, Pharmacology of Children).

Costello, A. J. & Angold, A. (1988), Scales to assess child and adolescent depression: checklists, screens and nets. *J. Amer. Acad. Child Adoles. Psychiat.*, 27:726–737.

———— & Edelbrock, C. (1983), Preliminary report on a diagnostic interview for children. Presented at a special meeting on diagnosis criteria. Washington, DC: National Institute of Mental Health.

Crumley, F. E. (1979), Adolescent suicide attempts. *J. Amer. Med. Assoc.* 241:2404–2407.

DiClemente, R. J., Ponton, L. E. & Hansen, W. B. (1996), New directions for adolescent risk prevention and health promotion research and interventions. In: *Handbook of Adolescent Health Risk Behavior*, ed. R. J. DiClemente, W. B. Hansen & L. E. Ponton. New York: Plenum Press, pp. 413–420.

Fergusson, D. M., Horwood, L. J. & Lynskey, M. T. (1993), Prevalence and comorbidity of DSM-III-R diagnoses in a birth cohort of 15 year-olds. *J. Amer. Acad. Child Adoles. Psychiat.*, 32:1127–1134.

Freud, S. (1917), Mourning and melancholia. *Standard Edition*, 14: 243–258. London: Hogarth Press, 1957.

Fristad, M. A., Weller, E. B. & Weller, R. A. (1991), The Mania Rating Scale: Can it be used in children? A preliminary report. *J. Amer. Acad. Child Adoles. Psychiat.*, 31:252–257.

Garrison, C. Z., Addy, C. L., Jackson, K. L., McKeown, R. E. & Waller, J. L. (1992), Major depressive disorder and dysthymia in young adolescents. *Amer. J. Epidem.*, 135:792–802.

Geller, B., Cooper, T. B., Watts, H. E., Cosby, C. M. & Fox, L. W. (1992) Early findings from a pharmaco-kinetically designed double-blind and placebo-controlled study of lithium for adolescents co-morbid with bipolar and substance dependency disorders. *Prog. Neuro-Psychopharm. Biol. Psychiat.*, 16:281–299.

Hamilton, M. (1960), A rating scale for depression. *J. Neurol. Neurosurg.*, 23:56–61.

Hollinger, P. C. (1979), Violent deaths among the young: Recent trends in suicide, homicide and accidents. *Amer. J. Psychiat.*, 136: 1144–1147.

Kashani, J. H. (1987), Depression, depressive symptoms, and depressed mood among a community sample of adolescents. *Amer. J. Psychiat.*, 44:931–4.

Kovacs, M. (1981), Rating scales to assess depression in school-aged children. *Acta Paedopsychiat.*, 46:305–315.

———— Feinbert, T. L., Crouse-Novak, M., Pavlavskis, S. I., Pollock, M. & Finkelstein, R. (1984), Depressive disorder in childhood: II. A longitudinal study of the risk for a subsequent major depression. *Arch. Gen. Psychiat.*, 41:643–649.

Levy, J. C. & Deykin, E. Y. (1989), Suicidality, depression and substance abuse in adolescence. *Amer. J. Psychiat.*, 146:1462–1467.

Matteson, A., Sesse, L. R. & Hawkins, J. W. (1969), Suicidal behavior as a child psychiatric emergency. *Arch. Gen. Psychiat.*, 20:100–109.

Merikangas, K. R. (1993), Genetic epidemiologic studies of affective disorders in childhood and adolescence. *Euro. Arch. Psychiat. Clin. Neurosci.*, 243:121–130.

Mghir, R. & Vincent, J. (1991), Seasonal Affective Disorder and its response. *J. Amer. Acad. Child Adoles. Psychiat.*, 30:440–442.

Moreau, D., Mufson, L., Weissman, M. W. & Klerman, G. L. (1991), Interpersonal psychotherapy for adolescent depression: Description of modification and preliminary application. *Amer. Acad. Child Adoles. Psychiat.*, 30:642–651.

Ponton, L. (1993), Adolescent affective disorders: Board review course for adolescent psychiatry. Unpublished manuscript.

———— & Philips, I. (1983), Recent development in the diagnosis of childhood depression. *West. J. Med.*, 138:410–411.

Poznanski, E. O., Cook, S. C. & Caroll, B. J. (1979), A depression rating scale for children. *Pediatrics*, 64:442–450.

Puig-Antich, J. (1982) Major depression and conduct disorder in pre-puberty. *J. Amer. Acad. Child Adoles. Psychiat.*, 21:118–128.

———— Goetz, R., Davies, M., Fein, M., Hanlon, C., Chambers, W. J., Tabrizi, M. A., Sachar, E. J. & Weitzman, E. D. (1984), Growth hormone secretion in pre-pubertal children with major depression: II. Sleep-related plasma concentration during a depressive episode. *Arch. Gen. Psychiat.*, 41:463–466.

———— Tabrizi, M. A., Davies, M., Goetz, R., Chambers, W. J. & Sachar, E. J. (1981), Pre-pubertal endogenous major depressives hypo-secrete growth hormone in response to insulin hypoglycemia. *J. Biol. Psychiat.*, 16:801–818.

———— & Weston, B. (1983), The diagnosis and treatment of major depressive disorder in childhood. *Ann. Rev. Med.*, 34:231–245.

Riddle, M. A., Nelson, J. C., Kleinman, C. S., Rasmussen, A., Leckman, J. F., King, R. A. & Cohen, D. J. (1991), Sudden death in children receiving Norpramin: A review of three reported cases and commentary. *J. Amer. Acad. Child Adoles. Psychiat.*, 30:104–108.

Robbins, D. R. & Alessi, N. E. (1975), Depressive symptoms and suicidal behavior in adolescents. *Amer. J. Psychiat.*, 142:588–592.

Roberts, R. E., Lewinsohn, P. M. & Seeley, J. R. (1991), Screening for adolescent depression: A comparison of depression scales. *J. Amer. Acad. Child Adoles. Psychiat.*, 30:58–66.

Rutter, M. (1985), The developmental psychopathology of depression: Issues and perspectives. In: *Depression in Childhood: Developmental Perspectives*, ed. M. Rutter, C. Izard & P. Read. New York: Guilford Press, pp. 18–36.

———— Tizard, J. & Whitmore, K. ed. (1970), *Education, Health and Behavior*. New York: Wiley.

Ryan, M. D., Puig-Antich, J., Ambrosini, P., Rabinovich, H., Robinson, D., Nelson, B., Iyengar, S. & Twomey, J. (1987), The clinical picture of major depression in children and adolescents. *Arch. Gen. Psychiat.*, 44:854–861.

Ryan, N. D. (1990), Heterocyclic antidepressants in children and adolescents. *J. Child Adoles. Psychopharmacol.*, 1:21–31.

Saref, K. R., Klein, D. F., Gittelman-Klein, D. F., Goatman, N. & Greenhill, P. (1978), EKG effects of imipramine treatment in children. *J. Amer. Acad. Child Adoles. Psychiat.*, 17:60–69.

Seligman, M. E. P. & Peterson, C. (1986), A learned helplessness perspective on childhood depression: Theory and research. In: *Depression in Childhood: Developmental Perspectives*, ed. M. Rutter, C. Izard & P. Read. New York: The Guilford Press, pp. 36–47.

Shaffer, D. (1985), Depression, mania and suicidal acts. In: *Child and Adolescent Psychiatry*, ed. M. Rutter & L. Hersov. Palo Alto, CA: Blackwell, pp. 698–719.

———— & Fischer, P. (1981), The epidemiology of suicide in children and young adolescents. *J. Amer. Acad. Child Adoles. Psychiat.*, 20:545–565.

Shafi. M., Carrigan, S., Whittinghill, J. R. & Derrick, A. (1985), Psychological autopsy of completed suicide in children and adolescents. *Amer. J. Psychiat.*, 142:1061–1064.

Spencer, T., Wilens, T. & Biederman, J. (1995), Psychotropic medication for children and adolescents. *Child Adoles. Psychiat. Clin. N. Amer.*, 4:97–121.

Strober, M. & Carlson, G. (1982), Bipolar illness in adolescents with major depression: Clinical, genetic and psychopharmacologic predictors in a three to four year prospective followup in investigation. *Arch. Gen. Psychiat.*, 39:549–555.

———— Morrell, W., Burroughs, J., Lampert, C., Danforth, H. & Freeman, R. (1988) A family study of bipolar I disorder in adolescence. *J. Affect. Disord.*, 15:255–268.

———— Morrell, W., Lampert, C. & Burroughs, J. (1990) Lithium carbonate in the prophylactic treatment of bipolar I disorder in adolescents: A naturalistic study. *Amer. J. Psychiat.*, 147:457–461.

Todd, R. D, Neuman, R., Geller, B., Fox, L. W. & Hickok, J. (1993), Genetic studies of affective disorders: Should we be starting with childhood onset probands? *J. Amer. Acad. Child Adoles. Psychiat.*, 32:1164–1171.

———— Reich, W. & Reich, T. (1994), Prevalence of affective disorder in the child and adolescent offspring of a single kindred: A pilot study. *J. Amer. Acad. Child Adoles. Psychiat.*, 33:198–208.

Tsung, M. T. (1978), Genetic counseling for psychiatric patients and their families. *Amer. J. Psychiat.*, 135:1465–1475.

Venkataraman, S., Naylor, M. & King, C. A. (1992), Mania associated with fluoxetine treatment in adolescents. *J. Amer. Acad. Child Adoles. Psychiat.*, 31:276–281.

Weinberg, W. A., Rutman, J., Sullivan, L., Pencek, E. D. & Dietz, S. G. (1973), Depression in children referred to an educational diagnostic center: Diagnosis and treatment. *J. Pediat.*, 83:1065–1072.

Weissman, M. W., Prusoff, B. A., Gammon, G. D., Merikangus, K. R., Leckman, J. F. & Kidd, K. K. (1984), Psychopathology in the children (ages 6–18) of depressed and normal patients. *J. Amer. Acad. Child Adoles. Psychiat.*, 23:73–84.

Werry, J. S. & McClellen, J. M. (1992), Predicting outcome in child and adolescent (early onset) schizophrenia and bipolar disorders. *J. Amer. Acad. Child Adoles. Psychiat.*, 31:147–150.

———— McClellen, J. M., Chard, L. (1991), Childhood and adolescent schizophrenic disorders: A clinical and outcome study. *J. Amer. Acad. Child Adoles. Psychiat.*, 30:457–465.

PART II

ASSESSMENT

10   HEARING THE S.O.S.: ASSESSING THE LETHALITY OF A YOUTH IN DISTRESS

BARONESS GHISLAINE D. GODENNE

Twenty years ago I gave my first presentation at a meeting of the American Society for Adolescent Psychiatry held in Dallas. The topic was "From Childhood to Adulthood: a Challenging Sailing" (Godenne, 1974). I will now pick up where I left off in 1972 and deal with how to hear the distress signal sent by an adolescent who is caught in a turbulent ocean, and having heard it, how to rescue the young sailor and help him or her reach a safe haven.

This reminds me of an experience I had while flying from New Zealand to Fiji island. We had just taken off from Auckland when the pilot asked all passengers if they would allow him to go off his course to find a boat that was sending an S.O.S. Previous attempts to locate the boat had been unsuccessful. We unanimously agreed to his request and were all asked to keep our eyes riveted on the ocean in order to spot the boat. The pilot flew over and over a radius of about 200 miles. Several times the pilot, after letting his landing gear out to slow the plane's speed, "dove" just above the water when he saw something that looked like a boat, only to find that it was a reflection of the sun on the waves. Finally one such dive was the right one, and we saw a yacht lying on a coral reef and at a little distance from it a man standing with a black box in his hands. It was the persistence and ingeniousness of the radio signaler that saved the man and his crew. Indeed, after sending S.O.S. for close to 48 hours, the batteries of his emergency signal box were almost out, and to spare what little power was left, he sent his S.O.S only when the plane was flying in his direction. "Mission accomplie!" exclaimed the pilot, who immediately radioed Auckland giving the exact longitude and latitude where the sinking vessel was spotted. Our flight resumed its course and arrived in Fiji four hours late. In the meantime a rescue helicopter went out to pluck the small crew out of the ocean and bring them to safe port.

This anecdote illustrates the point of my paper. The sailors whose ship was torn by a coral reef were ill prepared for the journey, as some teenagers are ill equipped for their journey into adulthood. The strength and unpredictability of the winds might so stress the young skipper that he or she abandons the fight against the elements and accepts the inevitable: disappearing into the ocean with a badly battered vessel. Fortunately, however, most young skippers send an S.O.S. when in serious difficulty. It is up to us to hear them and help rescue them. What accounts for the difference between these teenagers' reactions are many factors—like the particular stress experienced over a background of biological, sociological, and psychological factors.

Late Adolescence and Depression

Although depression seldom leads to suicide, which might be manipulative, vengeful, altruistic, or delusional, it seems appropriate to take a cursory look at depression in late adolescence.

Meeks (1988) suggests that adolescents feel alienated and depressed because they have to struggle with the push of independence versus dependence, the fluctuation of their friendships, and the fluctuation of their moods—all this at a time they have not as yet been able to see ambivalence as a way of life. Indeed, many college students suffer from depression. In the academic year 1992–93, 33% of students who felt enough distress to come to the counseling center at Johns Hopkins University checked "feeling depressed" on their personal inventory form, and 7% checked that they experienced suicidal thoughts. A few years earlier, when students seen at the counseling center and at psychiatric services were given, for insurance purposes *DSM-III-R* diagnoses, 45% were diagnosed as having adjustment disorders with depressive or mixed moods, 4% as being dysthymic, and 4% as having affective psychosis.

Why such a high incidence of depression on college campuses? Depression often follows the loss of an important libidinal object. The object can be external to the self or part of the self. The loss of a parent, sibling, close friend, even a favored pet usually brings with it a healthy period of mourning in which the youth's world is poor and empty. In some cases, however, the grief, which normally is short-lived and has its own resolution, turns into melancholia, and suicide then might become a serious option. This time it is the ego that is poor

212

and empty. Similarly the loss of a limb, of a body function, or of a body part is usually followed by a period of mourning and readaptation.

Narcissistic injuries, so frequent in this age group, often cause depressive reactions and lead to suicidal ideation in those youths who still rely mainly on others for their self-esteem. Broken romances that are experienced not only as the loss of a loved one but also as a severe narcissistic injury are among the main causes in youth suicide. The young person might kill himself or herself out of despair, rage, or vengeance.

Young adulthood is a life stage in which certain tasks have to be accomplished or certain issues resolved in order for the youth to become a healthy adult. Bocknek (1980) outlines how several authors conceptualize the tasks confronting this age group.

For Erikson,

the core issue of young adulthood is the conflict between intimacy and isolation. Intimacy covers a variety of experiences ranging from "physical combat" and "close affiliation" to orgasm and "intuition from recesses of the self." Isolation implies a readiness to see others as alien and dangerous. All too often the same person can be object of both intimacy and isolation. This is most likely to occur when the individual cannot differentiate between intense feelings, such as passion and combativeness [pp. 81–82].

Bocknek notes that Havighurst

evolved the concept of "developmental tasks," those things that constitute healthy and satisfactory growth in our society'. He identifies the "early adult" period as between the ages of 18 and 30. He sees it as made uniquely stressful by the varied and important task it contains. These include: 1) selecting a mate, 2) learning to live with a marriage partner, 3) starting a family, 4) rearing children, 5) managing a home, 6) getting started in a career, 7) taking on civic responsibility and, 8) finding a congenial social group [p. 85].

The "growth trends" identified by White and summarized by Bocknek (1980) are five in number: "1) stabilizing of ego identity,2) freeing of personal relationships, 3) deepening of interests, 4) humanizing of values, 5) expansion of caring" (p. 35).

213

Finally Bocknek writes that Wittenberg

> identifies five "metapsychologic characteristics" and three "socioeconomic factors" in young adults from their late teens to early 20s. The metapsychologic characteristics are: 1) A self-image crisis . . . 2) Brief sates of depersonalization . . . 3) End of role playing . . . 4) Awareness of time continuity . . . 5) Search for a partner . . . The socioeconomic factors are: 1) The economic bind, in which "young adults want to pay their own way" but . . . 2) Group formation, which is used to personify the young adult's ego-ideal . . . 3) Evolving *weltanschauung* or a philosophy of life . . . [pp. 87–88].

College students have a longer "young adult life" than those who join the workforce immediately after school. They consequently have more time to complete the tasks of this period, which might in part explain, as we will learn later, why their incidence of suicide is lower than that among their peers who are engaged in the workforce. But for college students, leaving home to go to college is often a stressful experience and necessitates a period of acculturation (Godenne, 1977, 1984).

Some college students, for instance, experience mild depression as they are separated for the first time from their parents, siblings, and high school friends. Some leave a boyfriend or girlfriend at home and are devastated when they receive a "Dear John" letter, their worst nightmare. In addition, those who on campus "fall in love" for the first time suffer the throes of despair when they experience the transitory quality of many college romances.

Moving away from home and gaining independence produces in some freshmen excessive anxiety and leads them to regress. Others look frantically for new experiences and abuse drugs and sex.

Most students are under a lot of parental and self-imposed pressure to perform. They are driven to succeed scholastically and socially. In addition, athletes have to live up to the expectation of their team and help bring it to victory.

College students fight their dependency needs while priding themselves on their ability to handle things alone. However, as their self-esteem is based mostly if not entirely on their outside achievements, a failure will shatter their ego. Whitaker and Slimak (1990) write that the macho student believes in "Death before Dishonor" (p. 84) as "machismo is a form of weakness peculiar to men who parody masculinity as a way to deny feelings of inadequacy"(p. 85).

Students who were big fish in small ponds while in high school suddenly find themselves little fish in large seas. For the first time they might doubt their ability to succeed and come to accept that they might no longer be at the top of their class.

Finally students who live side by side with a variety of peers of different cultures, religions, life goals, or sexual orientation might question once more, or for the first time, their true identity. This unexpected identity crisis might rock students' fragile foundations.

Freshmen who successfully weather their first year might experience a "sophomore slump" as the excitement of the starting college wears off and unresolved issues surface. Seniors and graduate students experience conflicts of their own. They have to face an imminent separation from college and their college friends, the necessity to adopt a career, and the urgency to form definite plans for the future.

African American students, Asian students, and Native American students not only have to deal with issues confronting the majority of students but, in addition, have to cope with the problems inherent in their minority status.

Adjustment disorders with depressive mood or with mixed depressed and anxious mood are thus not uncommon in college youth. Students are seen in counseling centers with complaints of feeling depressed, of changes in their sleep and eating patterns, of lack of concentration, of poor motivation and general anhedonia. Usually they respond well to short-term therapeutic interventions unless their present difficulties are experienced against a psychologically handicapped background. In the latter case, they might need not only long-term intervention but also pharmaceutical treatment, hospitalization, or both.

Suicide in Late Adolescence

Before discussing the empirical risk factors that play a role in the adolescents' comportment when facing stress, we should pause and look at suicide as a serious public health problem that has grown more severe in the last 10 years.

ADOLESCENT SUICIDE, A PUBLIC HEALTH PROBLEM

The rate of suicide in the 15- to 24-year-old population increased 40% between 1970 and 1980, and is still in ascendance, while the rate for the remainder of the population remained stable (Slimak, 1990, p. 18).

Former Surgeon General C. Everett Koop (1990) wrote:

U.S. suicide rates for persons between 15 and 24 more than doubled from 1950 to 1980, and suicide is now the second leading cause of death for this age group. One study of the economic impact of youth suicide and suicide attempts on our Nation placed the total costs for 1980 alone, at more than 3 billion dollars [p. ix].

Since 1980, the rate of suicides has progressively increased from 8.8/100,000 to 13.5/100,000. Among college students, however, the rate is about 10/100,000 (Schwartz, 1990). Although the incidence of suicide is relatively low for college students, it has been reported (Foreman, 1990) that 20% to 52% of students have contemplated suicide, of whom 10% had "very serious" suicidal thoughts and 4% to 15% had made suicidal attempts.

Why such a dramatic increase in adolescent suicides? The breakdown of the family through death or separation, the breakdown of organized religion, and the lack of employment opportunities for youth due to the post–World War II baby boom all might contribute to such an increase in our Western Hemisphere.

For Curran (1987), the tragic increase in youth suicide is due to the erosion of the stability of the nuclear family by divorce or separation; having two working parents; increased mobility; the lack of extended family; a decrease in the sense of community; the alienation of youth from a society they cannot influence; the increase in life stress; the general proliferation of the means and acceptability of avoidance methods of coping such as drugs and alcohol, sexual acting out, and suicide attempts; and the role of modeling. As the incidence of adolescents suicide grows, so does its familiarity. In addition, the suicide of a parent conveys in some way to his or her offspring that suicide is acceptable.

In a further attempt to explain the increase in suicidal behavior among contemporary youth, Curran (1987) writes: "Teenagers today are both blessed and cursed with an almost infinite variety of choices as to who, how, and what to be and do" (p. 9). Indeed, all of us who work with youth in their late teens or early 20s more and more frequently find them struggling with the issues of identity. They have, to quote Curran, "a heightened sense of marginality and confusion" and have difficulty tolerating "the seemingly endless period of waiting in a society they feel offers no guarantees and perhaps little support" (p. 9).

We know only too well that violence is perhaps the number one problem in our society, and the rate of suicide and homicide parallels the increase in violence. Violence engenders violence, and youth are trained to victimize and to be victimized.

EMPIRICAL RISK FACTORS CONTRIBUTING TO SUICIDE IN LATE ADOLESCENCE

Fortunately most of those in late adolescence bring their vessel to port without major problems. But this paper concerns itself with the few who are about to give up their effort to reach the adult harbor. They lack the energy, hope, vision, and inner strength to complete their difficult voyage.

Three group of risk factors are to be considered: the biological, the psychological, and the sociological. All three play a part in making the adolescent more susceptible to suicide when he or she is under great stress.

BIOLOGICAL

Suicide occurs with greater frequency in young people who suffer from certain psychiatric disorders such as unipolar or bipolar depression, schizophrenia, and panic disorders. It is also more frequently seen in those who suffer from chronic physical disease than in physically healthy individuals. Suicide thus might have biochemical and genetic roots. Stone (1992) writes:

> Schizoaffective males constitute a group at extreme risk and of extreme concern since they gave few warning signals to those who treat them. . . . the path to suicide is caused more by genetic/constitutional factors in the psychotic adolescent and more by family inflicted traumata in the borderline [p. 300].

PSYCHOLOGICAL

Under stress young people who show the following traits are more susceptible to suicide than their healthy counterpart: the borderline, emotionally unstable person; the withdrawn, schizoid individual; the highly dramatic, impulsive, reactive youth; the compulsive, perfectionistic adolescent; the antisocial youth; the substance abuser; and those attracted by life-threatening situations.

Stone (1992) believes that adolescents who have experienced an incestuous relationship are at higher risk of suicide, which they see as

TABLE 1
SUICIDE RATES AMONG YOUTH AND YOUNG ADULTS
ACCORDING TO ETHNICITY AND SEX, 1980*

	White		Black		Native American		Hispanic**		Japanese		Chinese	
Age Group	M	F	M	F	M	F	M	F	M	F	M	F
All Ages	19.4	6.2	11.6	2.6	24.2	4.6	17.8	4.0	11.1	5.0	7.9	8.0
15–24	21.9	5.0	12.6	2.7	49.0	7.0	19.0	4.4	14.1	4.5	8.0	4.7
25–34	27.0	8.0	23.1	4.8	41.2	9.1	25.1	6.1	16.7	7.8	8.6	5.7
35–44	24.3	9.9	16.1	4.3	31.4	6.2	21.0	6.3	9.8	8.2	10.8	13.9

*Age adjusted per 100,000 population
**1976–1980 cumulative data of five southwestern states
From: Group for the Advancement of Science. Reproduced by permission.

the only relief for their painful feelings. Indeed these youths live with a great deal of shame and fear that the incest might poison future sexual relationships. In addition they might receive death threats from the incestuous parent or alienate their families and thus lose their support if they divulge the information. Not infrequently, they suffer from guilt if the incestuous parent has been jailed on their account or from guilt toward the nonincestuous parent, whom they feel they have betrayed. Stone points out that the same is not true for adolescent victims of physical abuse as "it tends to induce instead, a sense of righteous indignation against the offending parent" (p. 301). The resulting aggression is thus diverted from the self and turned outward.

SOCIOLOGICAL

Among young people it is the single, depressed, unemployed white male in his 20s who belongs to the middle or upper class socioeconomically who has the highest incidence of suicide.

In a list of sociological factors that increase a person's risk of suicide, Foreman (1990) includes:

1. *Sex.* Males are at higher risk: two male suicides for each female suicide in the general population. In the college population males have five times as many suicide than females. Females, however, attempt suicide nine times more frequently than males.

2. *Age.* For males the suicidal rates increase with age, whereas for females it increases with age until the early 50s.

3. *Family status.* In depressed males from broken homes the risk to suicide is 10 times what it is in depressed males from intact homes. Depressed females from broken homes are five times as likely to commit suicide as depressed females from intact homes. Living alone increases the risk of suicide.

4. *Ethnic background.* Native Americans have the highest incidence of suicide in the United States—19/100,000 compared with 13/100,000 in whites and 9/100,000 in Asian Americans and 7/100,000 in African Americans (see Table 1).

Shaffer (1986) believes that African Americans have fewer suicides because they belong to a more affective social support system. They have, to quote Curran (1987), "less of a problem with relative status. They may derive a hidden benefit from 'we're all in this boat together'" (p. 21). Molock (1994) mentions that there is less suicidal ideation in African Americans, for whom suicidal behavior is most often an impulsive act rather than a planned event.

Asians comprise such a diverse group that it is difficult to generalize from findings concerning them. Although statistically it is reported that their suicide rate is lower than that of whites, in my experience Asians present a far greater risk of suicide in the face of failure. I am referring, of course, to Asian college students in the United States on student visas, recent immigrants, and even first-generation Asians still in the process of assimilation. Asians indeed have a different view of suicide. Hipple and Cimbolic (1979) mention the ritualistic suicide in the Japanese when there is an issue of honor. From an interpersonal perspective, Durkheim (1951) comments on the altruistic aspect of suicide such as that of the Kamikaze pilots of Japan. Uba (1994) mentions several other factors that play a role in suicide among Asians. These include stress caused by acculturation (Yu, 1989), the acceptability of suicide in the Asian culture (Nidorf, 1985), and the feeling shared by many Southeast Asians that their suicidal thoughts belong exclusively to them and should be no one else's business (Tung, 1985).

5. *Religious affiliation.* Religion probably plays a role in curbing the suicide rate, more by giving its followers a sense of community than though its teachings. To prove the point, Miller (1993) compares two mainly Catholic countries who have very different rates of suicide. "Roman Catholic Austria has almost the highest suicidal rate in Europe, Roman Catholic Ireland the lowest" (p. 364). Catholics and Jews, however, have a lower incidence of suicide than Protestants. In

the Moslem religion suicide is forbidden as it is for Catholics and Jews, who do not allow suicide victims to be buried in hallowed ground. Buddhists and Hindus view suicide in a different light because they believe in reincarnation. In a study on religiosity as it relates to suicidal ideation, Lester (1993) found that religiosity was not an important factor in the prediction of suicidability if one takes into account the neuroticism of the individual.

6. *Social class.* The white upper and middle social classes are overrepresented in the suicide statistics.

7. *Employment.* Retirees and unemployed have a higher rate of suicide, as do people in the helping profession.

8–11. *Health, personality factors, mental illness, and past suicidal behavior* complete Foreman's list. These factors are discussed elsewhere in this paper.

In addition, some authors report that the time of the year, the day of the week, and the time of the day influence the incidence of suicide in the college student population. September, January, and March have the highest rates of suicide rate as do Mondays and weekends. Most suicides of college students occur between 12 midnight and six a.m.

Suicide rates are higher when external restraints are weak and when individuals have to bear responsibility for their frustrations. For instance, in democracies the suicide rate is higher than in dictatorships, and during the German occupation of Western Europe, the suicide rate was very low, in part, I believe, because all energies were directed toward the struggle to survive. The climate of violence in society has repercussions on the incidence of suicide.

Jobes, in a 1995 workshop, offered a slightly different set of empirical risk factors, which he grouped as follows: 1) psychopathology, 2) behavioral characteristics, 3) family and parental characteristics, and 4) cognitive characteristics.

THEORIES SUGGESTED FOR UNDERSTANDING THE ACT OF SUICIDE

Here *suicide* encompasses suicide threats, suicidal gestures, suicide attempts, and completed suicide. However, authors who write about suicide may be referring to a variety of other lethal activities that can lead to death (Hipple and Cimbolic, 1979). Lester (1993) refers to completed suicide, attempted suicide, suicidal threats, and suicidal thoughts. Neuringer (1974) lists the following as suicide: intentional suicide, psychotic suicide, automatized suicide (e.g., the pill popper), chronic suicidal behavior (e.g., substance abuse), manipulative suicidal behavior (e.g., wrist cutting), accidental suicidal behavior (e.g., an attempt backfired), neglectful behavior (e.g., coronary disease), risky behavior (e.g., car racing), self-destructive behavior (e.g., heavy smoking), suicidal threats, suicidal thinking, and test suicide.

Schneidman (1986) discusses intended, subtended, (e.g., substance abuse), unintended, and contraintended (e.g., feigned) suicide. He offers 10 commonalities of suicide demonstrating the multidetermination of suicide:

> 1) The common purpose of suicide is to seek a solution. 2) The common goal of suicide is cessation of consciousness. 3) The common stimulus in suicide is intolerable psychological pain. 4) The common stressor in suicide is frustrated psychological needs. 5) The common emotion in suicide is hopelessness-helplessness. 6) The common internal attitude in suicide is ambivalence. 7) The common cognitive state in suicide is constriction. 8) The common action in suicide is egression. 9) The common interpersonal act in suicide is communication of intention. 10) The common constancy in suicide is with lifelong coping patterns [p. 4].

Throughout the years, many authorities in the mental health field have analyzed what might bring a person to end his or her life. The following are some of the more prominent theories.

Suicide results from extreme depression initiated by the loss of a significant love relationship and represents unconscious hostility directed toward the ambivalent love object.[1] When the significant love relationship is the self, as in narcissism, any failure might bring an individual to consider suicide owing to a sudden depletion of self-esteem built entirely on achievements instead than on inner qualities and attributes. Indeed, without an inner sense of self-worth, one is very vulnerable to failures that produce feelings of emptiness and nothingness. Owing to a form of "tunnel vision," the narcissistic student ignores his past achievements and, by concentrating exclusively on his

---

[1]Schneidman (1986) once called suicide "a murder in the 180 degree" (p. 7).

recent failure, believes that he or she is worthless and that the future holds no hope.

In discussing an interpersonal framework, Zubin (1990) mentions how Durkheim viewed the meaning of suicide: "The process leading to suicide is centered on a failure to accommodate oneself to the ecological niche one occupies, either because of too great acceptance or too little" (p. 7). Slimak (1990) reports that Durkheim described three types of suicide: 1) *altruistic,* "mandated by the society in which one lives" (p. 6) (e.g., the Japanese kamikaze pilot); 2) egoistic, when the individual feels rejected by society or feels unable to integrate with his or her social milieu; 3) anomic, "when a routine or established relationship between the individual and his or her society is suddenly broken" (p. 6). To avoid the painful state of anomie, a 15-year-old boy who was arrested for having stolen a bicycle hopes that the court will send him to the electric chair because then his name will appear in the newspaper.

Motto (1974) believes that the suicidal person looks for the relief of both physical pain and emotional pain but does not suicide out of a need to die. He established, according to Slimak (1990), "four basic patterns of suicide: depressive suicide, suicide for the relief of pain," of particular importance for college-student suicide), "symbolic suicide, and suicide resulting from organic disfunction" (p. 19).

Curran (1987) believes suicide to be a means of escaping confusion and stress, "eschewing mastery and growth in favor of nothingness" (p. xiii) and the suicidal behavior generally occurs within an "interpersonal context as a mean of communicating inner needs and as a mean of escape" (p. 66) "often not solely an effort to end one's life but rather to perhaps ameliorate it" (p. 67). Curran agrees with Jacobs (1971), who described the adolescent attempt as a four-stage process involving the following progression of experience:

> 1) A longstanding history of problems from childhood to the onset of adolescence; 2) A period of escalation of problems since the onset of adolescence and in excess of those normally associated with adolescence; 3) Progressive failure of available adaptive techniques for coping with old and increasingly new problems leading to a progressive social isolation from meaningful social relationships; 4) Chain reaction dissolution of remaining meaningful social relationships immediately prior to the suicide attempt [p. 52].

Broken homes, parental disturbance (through drinking), physical or sexual abuse by parents, modeling of behavior, poor physical health, and school problems are all additional factors that might bring an adolescent to attempt suicide.

Firestone and Seiden (1990) write that Novick sees suicide not as "an impulsive act but as the end point in a pathological regression" (p. 105).They advance the concept of *voice*, "a well-integrated pattern of negative thoughts that is a fundamental cause of an individual's maladaptive and self-destructive behavior" (p. 106). Suicidal patients have "an alien point of view, imposed originally from without" (p. 107). The voice is different from the conscience insofar as it does not represent a value system. Attack of the voice on the self leads ultimately to suicide, while suspicious, paranoid voices lead to homicide.

Firestone and Seidman (1990) note that Schneidman recognizes four psychological features that seem to be necessary for a lethal suicidal event to occur: "1) acute perturbation, 2) heightened inimicality and self hatred, 3) a sharp and almost sudden increase of constriction of intellectual focus, a tunneling of thought, and 4) the idea of cessation of pain" (p. 105). Pokorny (1974) reports that Schneidman proposed to divide suicide in three types: "a) Egotic: primarily psychological, intrapersonal, b) Dyadic: primary social, related to a significant other person, c) Ageneric: primarily related to the position of the individual in his society, in that he has 'fallen out' of his expected historical place" (p. 32).

METHODS OF SUICIDE

Substance ingestion is the method used most frequently in suicide attempts; tricyclics are responsible for 50% of near-lethal drug overdoses. Another common method is asphyxiation by covering one's face with plastic or by breathing carbon monoxide (e.g., from car exhaust or a gas stove). Hanging is also common, but occasionally death by hanging is accidental, a method of autoeroticism. For example, a student was found dead, hanging from a bedpost; while drunk, he had masturbated with a cord around his neck and accidentally fell to the floor. Firearms have become the main method of suicide by U.S. males. Table 2 shows the disproportionate number of suicides in which firearms were used in the United States compared with England and Wales.

TABLE 2
METHODS USED IN SUICIDE BY ADOLESCENTS
IN THE U.S. (1981) AND IN ENGLAND AND WALES (1983)

	10-14	15-19		20-24	
	U.S.	U.S.	E & W	U.S.	E & W
Firearms	52.9%	66.0%	5.9%	62.7%	9.4%
Hanging, strangling suffocation	31.0%	18.0%	29.4%	15.6%	27.7%
Poisoning by liquid & solids	12.8%	2.2%	23.5%	7.7%	22.7%
Poisoning by gas	0.6%	7.8%	5.9%	6.3%	18.8%
Other	1.7%	5.9%	35.3%*	7.8%	21.5%*

*Jumping from high places was common among the "other" methods in England and Wales.
From: Hawton, 1986. Adapted by permission.

EVALUATING THOSE AT RISK FOR SUICIDE

For those youth who are in the biopsychosociological high-risk group for suicide, stressful situations can trigger a suicidal reaction. Although suicide might be the end result of a depressive or psychotic illness of long duration, it might also be the outcome of a short-lived depressive reaction to an outside event. Although suicide threats and suicidal gestures can be manipulative, they should be attended to. Indeed, they are often cries for help, an S.O.S. sent by a youth desperately trying to convey an unmet need.

In some instances suicide might have delusional connotations, such as being a means to rejoin a loved one or an attempt to expiate one's crime or the crimes of the universe.

All students who state they feel depressed or appear depressed or act depressed are at risk for suicide, especially if they fit the biopsychosociological profile outlined earlier. The two main causes for suicide in college students are an argument or a disagreement with a significant other and academic problems. The significant other is usually a parent or a boyfriend or girlfriend. "For these adolescents the perceived rupture of a valued peer relationship . . . can be devastating, but only within the context of all that exists elsewhere in their lives and all that has transpired before" (Curran, 1987, p. 68). Academic problems not only bring them to doubt their competence but might also create in them a sense of guilt toward the parents who sacrifice themselves to send the student to college, or a feeling of shame for themselves, their family, their ethnic group.

Students who have been disciplined or who have been apprehended by the police for minor misdemeanors should be closely watched for suicide. For example, a young man shot himself in the mouth when the police came to his home to inquire about a "dirty phone call"; he did not die but he did disfigure his face. Another college student killed himself after he was taken to the police station for stealing candy from a convenience store; for two days, he became very depressed, but his roommates never suggested he visit the counseling center. Three mornings later, he looked "his old self" again and informed his dormmates that he had solved his problem and that they need not be concerned about him any longer. He hanged himself a few hours later. Another student tried to jump off a high building after a friend complained to the police about sexual harassment; fortunately, the police and fire departments were alerted to his precarious position on the roof, set up a net, and broke his fall.

Students who directly or indirectly make suicidal statements are at high risk. Robbins and colleagues (1959) studied 134 completed suicides and found that 41% had directly stated that they were planning to kill themselves, while 28% had made indirect statements to that effect.

Students who suffer from psychotic disorders, who have been discharged from a mental hospital within the past six months, who are chronically depressed or use drugs, who have a history of prior contact with the college counseling center or prior psychotherapy, who have a past suicidal history (past suicide attempt, suicide in the family, or suicide anniversary), and who are attracted to life-threatening situations are all in the high-risk category.

SUBSTANCE ABUSE AND SUICIDE

Abel and Zeidenberg (1985) believe that between 45% and 50% of suicide deaths in the 15- to 25-year-old age groups appear to be related to the use of alcohol and drugs. Rivinus (1990) mentions that Whitaker estimated that 70% of all college-student suicide attempts or completed suicides are related to substance use disorder.

Rivinus (1990) describes five general groups of suicidal gestures, attempts, or completed suicides related to substance abuse: 1) during intoxication, impulsive suicidal gesture; 2) during chemical withdrawal as the student might experience remorse over the events and the loss of control which occurred while intoxicated: "Many suicide attempts take place in the early morning, alone, after a humiliating or destructive act, occurring during intoxication" (p. 51); 3) while intoxicated, if the substance can no longer relieve the depression; 4) in students who are subacutely or chronically addicted to a psychoactive chemical; and 5) in students with dual diagnosis.

EVALUATION OF LETHALITY

Suicide may occur in students who are not clinically depressed but suffer from a transitional situational disturbance. Most frequently, however, they do show signs of depression, which can be of varying intensity ranging from dysthymic conditions to psychotic disorders and schizophrenic illness.

First and foremost, one should take a very careful history of the patient's depressive symptoms. One should attempt to elicit what precipitated them, when they first appeared, and if they are long-standing. Why does the student come *now* for help? In addition, one should ask about any previous episode of depression and how the current depression compares with the previous one. It is important to ask about prior suicidal ideation, gestures, or suicide attempts; Stone (1992) reports that 40% of youth who complete suicide made prior suicide attempts. It is also important to ask about depression or alcohol abuse in the family (including parents, grand parents, aunts and uncles, and siblings).

One should not shy away from asking if the student is thinking of harming himself or herself and if he or she 1) has any definite plans to kill himself or herself; 2) owns firearms or other weapons; 3) has access to a large quantity of drugs; 4) drinks heavily when depressed; or 5) lives in a high-rise apartment building.

One should inquire if the student has at least one close friend in town and find out if the student is associated with any group of peers or if he or she has a support system.

One should observe how the student relates to the therapist. Does the student communicate on a personal level? Does he or she allow eye contact? Can he or she smile in response to a humorous comment?

One should ask the student about his or her plans are for that same evening, for the following day. This is especially important with students who appear depressed but flatly deny any suicidal thoughts.

Indeed, students who have made up their mind to kill themselves in the next 24 hours will not admit to suicidal plans but will be totally incapable of answering what appears to be an innocuous question.

Finally one should find out through the student or through his or her friends if the student's behavior has changed recently. Try to learn if the student has become more withdrawn, has lost interest in his or her studies and hobbies, or has missed classes. Find out if the student has recently "put his or her house in order," that is, has written letters or given away belongings. Find out whether the student has been able to sleep recently or has been up all night. It is imperative to be vigilant about a student who suddenly, for no apparent reason, emerges from a deep depression and appears happy. A sudden "cure" probably means that the student has resolved his or her ambivalence about death and has decided to end it all.

Miller (1993) points out that if an adolescent has experienced the recent death of a loved one, it is important to find out whether under stress the adolescent thinks of the dead one and might have the fantasy of joining the deceased.

Psychological tests have been more or less useful in evaluating a person's degree of lethality, but for those of us who do not have easy access to testing, we must remember that nothing can take the place of good clinical judgment.

KEEPING THE SUICIDAL STUDENT FROM HURTING HIMSELF OR HERSELF

Once the student has admitted to suicidal preoccupations, one evaluates whether he or she should be hospitalized or whether his or her depression can be managed on an outpatient basis. Even though the student has come asking for help, he or she is still ambivalent about ending his or her life. It is believed that most people who kill themselves are ambivalent up to the last minute about ending their life.

If one feels "connected" to the student and if one feels that the student still has enough functioning ego, then having the student sign a contract not to kill himself or herself is often a useful maneuver. At least, it may help the student to live through the critical period of his or her depression while working through what led to it. A contract has to be time limited because asking a suicidal patient to contract never to kill himself or herself is asking the patient to give up forever what looks like his or her only solution. A reasonable contract should be limited to the next day, the next time the patient talks with us, or at the most, the next week.

When a student denies being suicidal but all indications make us doubt his denial, he or she should be immediately hospitalized. As he or she is serious about ending his or her life, the student cannot admit to suicidal preoccupations for fear that the last exit door will be locked for good. It is with this type of patient that the question about tomorrow is often very revealing.

"Very few people have thought through the idea of self-destruction so they are in a position to take their own lives based on logical and rational decision" (Hipple and Cimbolic, 1979, p. 3). "For many, death is not viewed as an absolute and total cessation of existence. Rather, death is conceptualized as a 'cessation of consciousness,' a respite from pain; or death will carry the person to a place where he or she may be free of the intense emotional pain being experienced" (Foreman, 1990, p. 131). Therefore, one might want to discuss in very down-to-earth terms with suicidal patients what will happen after their death. For instance, comment on the fact that although some people will grieve them for awhile, life will go on. We care for the living; there is nothing more we can do for the dead.

A useful question to ask a patient whom we suspect of wanting to kill himself or herself as a retaliation against someone who has deeply hurt him or her is, "Who will be hurt the most by your death?" The person named is probably the person toward whom, unconsciously, the suicide is directed, the person the patient wants to punish. Having gained that information one can then attempt to deal with the rage and redirect the anger to where it belongs.

Although suicidal threats or attempts are often manipulative, one should not neglect dealing with them. "Suicide attempters are often, paradoxically, attempting to solve a problem of living rather than hasten their death, to ameliorate rather than end their lives" (Curran, 1987, p. xii). Adolescent suicide attempts are nearly always to obtain assurance that people care, but unfortunately they are frequently seen by adults as manipulative (Curran, 1987). By ignoring suicide attempts, one simply reinforces the adolescent's need to attract attention. Despite their objections, students who make manipulative suicidal threats should be made to talk over and over again about the meaning of their threats. One should take them so seriously that the students come to realize that they don't have to show us, by killing themselves, that we should have believed in their threats.

Patients in treatment with us who become suicidal because of some transferential issues should be told that, although we are not omnipotent and thus cannot prevent them from committing suicide, we can help them to remain alive. Such a statement avoids a power struggle in which patients tell us, "You see, you can't stop me from killing myself. If I want to die, I'll kill myself despite your veto."

After a suicide attempt, it is important to evaluate the lethal intent of the action. One should look at where it took place, when, and in what circumstances. Students who overdose, for example, seldom intend to die and unconsciously attempt to arrange for their preservation.

Suicides often occur in clusters. Thus a suicidal student who is seen during an "epidemic" of suicide should be considered a great risk and treated accordingly. Suicides that are highly publicized on T.V. or the newspapers are often followed by a series of suicide attempts in youngsters who badly need attention.

In suicidal students who are substance abusers, both issues should be addressed simultaneously as alcohol abuse brings on a regression during which suicide is not uncommon. A note of caution is in order: when prescribing antidepressants, psychiatrists should refrain from giving out more than a few days' supplies. Tricyclic antidepressants have been responsible for a large number of suicide by ingestion. The difficulty in today's managed care system is that patients request large prescriptions in order not to have to pay out of pocket the $10 or $15 deductible on each prescription.

Although they believe that life is not worth living, some suicidal students don't want to take an active role in their demise but would welcome death taking them by chance. They cross streets without looking, they drive recklessly, and they engage in dangerous acts. For those students we can only hope that our efforts to relieve their depression will pay off before any fatal accident occurs.

In some counseling centers forms are devised that both the suicidal patient and the therapist fill in when a depressed and suicidal student is first seen at the counseling center and after the threat of suicide has subsided. This helps the therapist to remain focused on the suicidality of his or her patient.

THE PSYCHIATRIST'S ROLE
AFTER A SUCCESSFUL SUICIDE

As already mentioned, one suicide might lead to others, as they often take place in clusters. As soon as possible after a suicide, the therapist should meet with the family and friends of the deceased and with his or her close peers. One should not only commiserate on the premature death of a promising young adult but commiserate on what his or her death is doing to all those left behind. Every effort should be made not to "glorify the dead person" but instead help relatives, friends, and peers express their anger at such a hostile act. One should work at having them see suicide as ego dystonic. When a student who commits suicide was known professionally by the therapist, confidentiality has to be observed even after his or her death. At times like these, the therapist shares not only the grief but also some guilt, and he or she might have a tendency to lose sight of the confidentiality issue.

My hope in writing this paper is that we will always hear the S.O.S. sent by an adolescent in his or her journey on rough seas, that we will come to the adolescent's rescue, and that we will help the adolescent reach the adult harbor once he or she has learned to master strong winds.

REFERENCES

Abel, E. L & Zeidenberg, P. (1985), Age, alcohol and violent death: A postmortem study. *J. Studies on Alcohol*, 46:228–232.

Bocknek, G. (1980), *The Young Adult*. Monterey, CA: Brooks/Cole.

Curran, D. K. (1987), *Adolescent Suicidal Behavior*. New York: Hemisphere.

Durkheim, E. (1951), *Suicide*. Glencoe, IL: Free Press.

Firestone, R. W. & Seiden, R. H. (1990), Psychodynamics in adolescent Suicide. In: *College Student Suicide*, ed. L. C. Whitaker & R. E. Slimak. Binghamton, NY: Haworth Press, pp. 101–123.

Foreman, M. E. (1990), The counselor's assessment and intervention with the suicidal student. In: *College Student Suicide*, ed. L. C. Whitaker & R. E. Slimak. Binghamton, NY: Haworth Press, pp. 125–140.

Godenne, G. (1974), From childhood to adulthood: A challenging sailing. In: *Adolescent Psychiatry*, 3:118–127. New York: Basic Books.

———— (1977), Is being a college student a hazardous occupation? *Johns Hopkins University Magazine*, January:36–41.

———— (1984), College students. In: *Clinical Update in Adolescent Psychiatry*, ed. R. Marohn. New York: Nassau.

Group for the Advancement of Psychiatry (1989), *Suicide and Ethnicity in the United States*, GAP report #128. New York: Brunner/Mazel.

Hawton, K. (1986), Suicide in adolescents. In: *Suicide*, ed. A. Roy. Baltimore, MD: Williams & Wilkins, pp. 135–150.

Hipple, J. & Cimbolic, P. (1979), *The Counselor and Suicidal Crisis*. Chicago: C. Thomas.

Jacobs, J. (1971), *Adolescent Suicide*. New York: Wiley Interscience.

Koop, C. E. (1990), Foreword. In: *College Student Suicide*, ed. L. C. Whitaker & R. E. Slimak. Binghamton, NY: Haworth Press, pp. ix–x.

Lester, D. (1993), Is religiosity related to suicidal ideation after personality and mood are taken into account? *Person. & Individ. Differences*, 15:591–592.

Meeks, J. E. (1988), *High Times/Low Times*. Washington, DC: PTA Press.

Miller, D. (1993), Adolescent suicide etiology and treatment. In: *Adolescent Psychiatry*, 19:361–383. Chicago: University of Chicago Press.

Molock, S. (1994), Suicidal behavior among African American college students: A preliminary study. *J. Black Psychol.*, 20:234–251.

Motto, J. A. (1974), Refinement of variables in assessing suicidal risk. In: *Prediction of Suicide*, ed. A. T. Beck, H. L. P. Resnik & D. J. Lettieri. Bowie, MD: Charles Press, pp. 85–93.

Neuringer, C. (1974), *Psychological Assessment of Suicidal Risk*. Springfield, IL: C. Thomas.

Nidorf, J. (1985), Mental health and refugee youths: A model for diagnostic training. In: *Southeast Asian Mental Health*, ed. T. Owens. Washington, DC: US Dept. Health & Human Services, pp. 391–429.

Novick, J. (1984), Attempted suicide in adolescents: The suicide sequence. In: *Suicide in the Young*, ed. H. Sudak, A. Ford & N. Rushforth. Littleton, MA: Wright PSG.

Pokorny, A. D. (1974), A scheme for classifying suicidal behaviors. In: *The Prediction of Suicide*, ed. A. T. Beck, H. L. P. Resnik & D. J. Lettieri. Bowie, MD: Charles Press, pp. 29–44.

Rivinus, T. M. (1990), The deadly embrace: The suicidal impulse and substance abuse in the college student. In: *College Student Suicide*, ed. L. C. Whitaker & R. E. Slimak. Binghamton, NY: Haworth Press, pp. 45–77.

Robbins, E., Gassner, S., Keys, J., Wilkinson, R. Jr. & Murphy, G. (1959), The communication of suicidal intent: A study of 134 consecutive cases of successful (completed) suicide. *Amer. J. Psychiat.*, 8:74–89.

Schwartz, A. J. (1990), The epidemiology of suicide among students at colleges and universities in the United States. In: *College Student Suicide*, ed. L. C. Whitaker & R. E. Slimak. Binghamton, NY: Haworth Press, pp. 25–44.

Shaffer, D. (1986), Developmental factors in child and adolescent suicide. In: *Depression in Young People*, ed. M. Rutter, C. E, Izard & P. B. Read. New York: Guilford Press, pp. 383–396.

Schneidman, E. (1985), *Definition of Suicide*. New York: Wiley.

——— (1985), Some essentials of suicide and some implications for response. In: *Suicide*, ed. A. Roy. Baltimore, MD: Williams & Wilkins, pp.1–16.

Slimak, R. E. (1990), Suicide and the American college and university: A review of the literature. In: *College Student Suicide*, ed. L. C. Whitaker & R. E. Slimak. Binghamton, NY: Haworth Press, pp. 25–44.

Stone, M. H, (1992), Suicide in borderline and other adolescents. In: *Adolescent Psychiatry* 18:289–305. Chicago: University of Chicago Press.

Tung, T. M. (1985), Psychiatric care of Southeast Asians: How different is different? In: *Southeast Asian Mental Health*, ed. T. Wang. Washington, DC: US Dept. Health & Human Services, pp. 5–40.

Uba, L. (1994), *Asian Americans*. New York: Guilford Press.

Yu, E., Ching-Fu, C., Liu, W. & Fernandez, M. (1989), Suicide among Asian-American youth: In: *Report of the Secretary's Task Force on Youth Suicide*, ed. M, Feinlieb. Washington, DC: US Dept. Health & Human Services, pp. 157–176.

U.S. Center for Disease Control, Atlanta (1986), *Youth Suicide in the United States, 1970–1980*.

Whitaker, L. C. & Slimak, R. E., ed. (1990), *College Student Suicide.* Binghamton, NY: Haworth Press.

Zubin, J. (1974), Observations on nosological issues in the clarification of suicidal behavior, In: *Prediction of Suicide*, ed. A. T. Beck, H. L. P. Resnik & D. J. Lettieri. Bowie, MD: Charles Press, pp. 3–25.

11 USE OF STRUCTURED ASSESSMENT TOOLS IN CLINICAL PRACTICE

MARK D. WEIST AND MARY E. BAKER-SINCLAIR

Although the clinical interview remains the mainstay of diagnostic assessment of the adolescent, a variety of structured assessment tools are available to the clinician. The advent of more standardized diagnostic criteria and the importance of accurate diagnoses for treatment planning, not to mention the increased accountability of clinicians to outside parties, have made such structured instruments increasingly relevant to clinical practice. This paper will review instruments that are useful for the practicing psychiatrist to use in evaluating adolescent patients.

There are numerous assessment processes that can occur during the diagnostic process with adolescents. These processes include structured diagnostic interviews, direct observation, neurocognitive assessment, use of formal projective measures such as apperception tests, collection of checklists and rating scales from adults who know the youngster well and collection of self-report measures from the adolescent on his or her psychological functioning. Many of these measures are, however, impractical to use routinely in clinical practice. For example, structured diagnostic interviews such as the Schedule for Affective Disorders (K-SADS) (Ambrosini, 1986) are very time consuming, and therefore are typically used only in research projects. In addition, such aspects of neurocognitive assessment as intellectual testing are beyond the scope of most psychiatrists and are usually referred out to psychologists, as are projective measures. However, many measures are useful in clinical settings by psychiatrists or other mental health professionals who have a basic knowledge of how to use and interpret questionnaires.

In this paper, we focus on checklists and self-report measures that can be integrated pragmatically into the assessment efforts of practitioners. We review our conceptual schema in choosing domains for assessment, focusing on constructs that are most relevant in our work with adolescents from Baltimore. We provide a review of each construct, and then examples of specific measures that we use to assess them in our clinical practices. This is followed by brief discussion of the actual measures that we use in our clinical and research efforts, along with a process that we use to increase the "user friendliness" of these measures. Our goal is to provide our assessment strategy, and associated measures, as an example that should be generalizable to some degree to most clinicians who work with adolescents.

Conceptual Schema for Adolescent Assessment

It is important to operate with some conceptual basis in focusing on areas for assessment. The clinician's theoretical point of view will provide a framework that assists in selecting constructs most relevant to his or her practice. Ideally, the conceptual scheme should include not only general factors seen as important to adolescent adjustment, but also particular factors that are important for the clinician's adolescent population.

There is a myriad of constructs pertaining to adolescent psychological adjustment. In reviewing the literature for the preparation of this paper, we found over one hundred constructs applicable to adolescent adjustment that one might potentially want to evaluate. Attachment and attachment theory are two examples; the set of constructs subsumed under self-psychology are others. Not all constructs are equally useful in clinical practice. For example, it is useful to assess the construct of sensation seeking in older adolescents, but generally not useful to assess this construct in young children. In our work with children and adolescents in schools in Baltimore, a city with typical urban problems, constructs pertaining to urban life stress, violence exposure, and history of abuse and neglect are particularly relevant. These constructs are also relevant for many nonurban youth, since many suburban and rural youth are also exposed to violence, abuse, and neglect.

In our view, relevant constructs for adolescent assessment can essentially be classified into four major domains: 1. *stress factors* such as daily hassles, negative life events, traumatization, and problematic social and familial relations that often contribute to maladaptive functioning, 2. *protective factors*, or variables that either protect against the influence of stress factors, or directly or indirectly promote positive adjustment in adolescents, 3. *emotional/behavioral functioning*, including measures of internalizing (e.g., depression, anxiety), and externalizing (e.g., oppositionality, aggression) disorders, and 4. *social/educational functioning*, or the nature and quality of the adolescent's social relationships, school performance and extracurricular involvements. In our thinking, stress factors interact with protective factors to influence the adolescent's emotional and social adjustment. We recognize that given variables may be classified in more than one of these domains. For example, self-concept may be viewed both as a protective factor (e.g., adolescents with positive self-concepts may be less prone to depression) and as an aspect of emotional/behavioral functioning (e.g., feelings of worthlessness are a symptom of depression).

Desired Qualities in Assessment Measures

In these four assessment domains, the clinician should choose measures that are developmentally sensitive, that is, appropriate to adolescence (Yule, 1993) and culturally relevant, for example, created for or minimally used with urban youth (Ollendick and Hersen, 1993). Whenever possible, measures should be used that have an adequate normative base and strong psychometric properties. These properties include: 1. internal consistency, or the extent to which various scale items measure the same factor, 2. test-retest reliability, or the stability of scores over time, which should be expected to be higher for "trait" versus "state" measures, 3. interrater reliability, or agreement between different raters for checklists and rating scales, 4. content validity, or the degree to which the scale's items tap a representative sample of the domain to be measured, 5. construct validity, or the extent to which the scale measures the construct of interest, and 6. criterion-related validity, or how well scale scores relate to other relevant criteria such as diagnoses (Piacentini, 1993).

Too often, whether in clinical practice or in research efforts, convenience or easy accessibility are the basis for choice of measures rather than careful consideration of their adequacy (Ollendick and Hersen, 1993). Using measures that are not psychometrically sound increases the likelihood that decisions made during the clinical assessment process will be biased (Weist, Finney, and Ollendick, 1992). For example, many clinicians and even research investigators frequently create measures to assess a problem or phenomenon of interest that are not formally evaluated prior to their administration, and lead to the collection of invalid information. As an illustration, complicated measures requiring high school reading levels are created for use with children; when findings fail to meet expectations, the clinician or researcher often fails to realize that this is because the children could not understand the measure.

Assessment measures can also have a positive or negative effect of treatment outcomes. That is, use of the measure can directly or indirectly contribute to clinical outcomes (Hayes, Nelson, and Jarrett, 1987). Information discerned from measures can contribute to the development and implementation of an effective treatment plan, a positive effect. By contrast, excessively long or otherwise unpleasant measures can impair early rapport, or even contribute to the patient's dropping out from treatment. With adolescents, one must be particularly wary of the potential for such negative effects of structured instruments.

A frequent problem is the inappropriate translation of adult constructs for application with children, referred to as adultomorphism. For example, Weist and Ollendick (1991) traced a number of behaviors included in assertiveness training programs for children to studies training these same behaviors (e.g., requesting new behavior, refusing unreasonable requests) for adult psychiatric patients in the 1970s (Eisler, Miller and Hersen, 1973). This is not to say that assertiveness is an irrelevant construct for adolescents. Rather, we need to recognize that assertiveness by adults is different from assertiveness by adolescents, and we should ensure that the version we train in therapy is developmentally and culturally appropriate (Strain, Odom, and McConnell, 1985).

Clinicians should attempt to focus their treatment efforts on empirically validated treatment targets, or variables that have been shown to lead to clinical benefits for the adolescent population under study when they are improved. In prior work (Weist, Ollendick, and Finney, 1991), we have commented on problems that commonly occur in child and adolescent assessment and treatment efforts related to subjective selection of treatment targets, or goals. As such, clinicians should be cautious about training or promoting behaviors, such as assertiveness, that may be seemingly valid, but in actuality are ineffective for children or adolescents.

An example of an empirically validated treatment target is family cohesion and support. Numerous studies (e.g., Clark, 1983; Felner, Abu, Primavera, and Cauce, 1985) have documented the role of family cohesion and support in protecting youth against harmful influences, and in directly contributing to positive mental health and social/educational outcomes. Thus, treatment that aims at enhancement of family cohesion makes sense as a valid approach for most, though not all, clinical problems of adolescents.

In summary, the important point in selecting measures and thereafter focusing on particular treatment targets is for the practitioner to carefully consider whether these measures and targets are in fact important and meaningful to the individual adolescent with whom he or she is working.

Constructs and Measures for Assessment
of Urban Adolescents

In the following, we provide a brief review of constructs that we often assess with checklists or self-report measures in our work with adolescents. The discussion is focused around those areas in which we use such measures to augment the clinical interview. Obviously, one cannot assess all influences in a given measurement domain with the use of formal measures, as the clinical interview remains the most important and commonly used method of gathering information (Kleinmutz, 1984). For example, in the domain of *stress factors* we assess variables such as past and ongoing abuse and neglect through interview. We use checklists and self-report measures when we are interested in detailed probing of a given area, and when we are interested in normative comparisons that determine the relative intensity or quality of the variable under consideration as compared to other adolescents. Assessment of the adolescent's functioning in the domain of *social/educational functioning* is accomplished through interview, and at times direct observation in relevant settings such as school. Although checklists and self-report measures are available to assess functioning in this domain, these methods are less reliable and are not reviewed here.

STRESS FACTORS

NEGATIVE LIFE EVENTS/CIRCUMSTANCES

Numerous studies have documented that urban youth experience high levels of life stressors throughout their development, related to relatively increased exposure to abuse and neglect (Garbarino, 1976), problematic family environments, (West and Farrington, 1977), poverty and its associated impacts (Duncan, 1991), and exposure to domestic and community violence. This elevated life stress correlates with increased rates of emotional and behavioral problems (Farrington, 1987; Paster, 1985), involvement in drug dealing or abuse (Rhodes and Jason, 1988), teen pregnancy (Taylor, 1987), and school drop out (Rhodes and Jason, 1990). Effects of stress are felt to be both direct and indirect. For example, exposure to domestic conflict may directly stress an adolescent (e.g., physiological and emotional reactions to yelling and fighting), and also indirectly increase stress for her (e.g., missing school days to watch siblings).

Formal assessment of life stress is often indicated by our clinical observation—congruent with research findings—that highly stressed youth present relatively higher levels of internalizing disturbances such as depression, anxiety, and posttraumatic stress disorder. As such, documenting high stress indicates the need for expanded diagnostic assessment of these disturbances.

To assess life stress in adolescents, we use a self-report version of the Life Events Checklist (LEC) (Work et al., 1990) from the Rochester Child Resilience Project (RCRP), which taps stressful life events and *ongoing circumstances* experienced by inner-city youth and their families. Based on the RCRP's focus on youth exposed to severe, ongoing life stress, most of the items in the LEC pertain to chronic stressors (e.g., "our family had to move a lot") versus acutely stressful events (e.g., "a close family member died"). The LEC has an adequate normative base, is internally consistent, and its validity has been supported by correlations in expected directions with parent-, teacher-, and self-report measures of emotional/behavioral adjustment.

VIOLENCE EXPOSURE

Exposure to violence is a very serious problem for urban youth. Numerous studies underscore the severity of this problem. For example, Gladstein and Slater (1988), in a survey of adolescents receiving services in a Baltimore health clinic, found that 60% had witnessed severe aggression; shockingly, 24% of them had witnessed a homicide. In a study of African American adolescents from Chicago, Shakoor and Chalmers (1991) found that around 75% had witnessed someone being robbed, stabbed, shot, or killed. In reaction to such

240

violence exposure, urban youth show elevated levels of internalizing disorders including depression, anxiety and posttraumatic stress disorder (Hilton, 1992; Pynoos and Nader, 1988), externalizing behavioral difficulties (Prothrow-Stith, 1991), and cognitive and learning problems (Dyson, 1990; Shakoor and Chalmers, 1991).

Assessment of the impact of violence exposure on youth is in its infancy, with few measures existing that have established psychometric properties. One measure that does have supportive psychometric data is a self-report measure, the Survey of Community Violence (Richters and Saltzman, 1990), which contains 51 items that pertain to violence that is heard about, witnessed, or experienced. Research on the measure has provided support for its interrater reliability in that parent and child reports of violence exposure converged. Validity has been demonstrated by finding a significant relationship between violence exposure and level of distress in children.

We also use a brief measure of violence exposure and victimization derived from self-report measures by Bell et al., (1988), and Gladstein and Slater (1988). The Exposure to Violence Screening Measure (EVSM) (Weist et al., 1996) includes nine types of violence; for example robbery with a weapon, sexual assault, stabbings, and shootings. For each type of violence, the adolescent indicates whether he or she has witnessed it in the past, knows of a victim who is a friend or family member, or has been victimized by it. Analyses indicate that the measure has adequate psychometric properties including internal consistency and construct validity (Weist et al., 1996).

PROTECTIVE FACTORS

In contrast to stress factors that increase the likelihood of maladaptive outcomes, protective factors serve to reduce the probability of illness or maladaption.[1] Below are some of these factors, with associated measures, that we have found particularly useful in our clinical efforts with adolescents.

FAMILY ENVIRONMENT

As mentioned above, family variables have been shown to exert protective functions for urban adolescents, and adolescents in general.

---

[1]For a more detailed and technical discussion of protective and related factors see Pellegrini (1990).

For example, family cohesion, that is, closeness and supportiveness, has been found to protect boys against the development of discipline problems under high stress (Weist et al., 1995), and to promote academic achievement in urban youth (Clark, 1983). Other studies have documented that family cohesion provides general protective benefits to youth under stress (Garmezy, 1987; Luthar, 1991).

There are numerous measures of family functioning. One measure that we have found useful is the FACES III (Olson, Porter, and Lavee, 1985), a self-report measure for adolescents that contains 20 items that assess perceived family functioning and 20 items that assess ideal functioning in two major domains: cohesion (e.g., emotional closeness, supportiveness), and adaptability (e.g., leadership, family roles or rules). The discrepancy between perceived and ideal functioning scores provides a measure of family satisfaction. The FACES III has excellent test reliability, internal consistency, and validity and is designed for use with youth down to age 12.

To assess perceived family supportiveness we use a measure that was designed for use with urban teenagers by Wills, Vaccaro, and McNamara (1992). The measure contains seven items that assess perceptions of emotional support (e.g., "I can share my feelings with my parent"), and eight items that assess perceptions of instrumental support (e.g., "I can ask my parent for help with my school work") provided by the primary parental figure. The measure was developed with a large sample of urban adolescents; thus normative data are available for this population.

LOCUS OF CONTROL

The degree to which a person believes that he or she has control over life events and consequences is known as locus of control. Studies have documented that youths who have a sufficient locus of control present lower levels of emotional and behavioral problems than those who feel little personal control over their lives (Martin and Pritchard, 1991; Nunn and Parish, 1992). Even more striking is the consistent finding of other studies (e.g., Luthar, 1991) that internal locus of control helps to protect urban adolescents from the effects of life stress.

To assess locus of control, the Children's Nowicki Strickland Internal-External Locus of Control Scale (CNS-IE) (Nowicki and Strickland, 1973) is useful. The CNS-IE contains 40 items that are answered yes or no, and assesses perceptions of personal control over events and consequences for youth in grades 3 through 12. The measure has adequate internal consistency for adolescents, but somewhat low test-retest reliability (Reynolds, 1993). However, its relevance and validity for urban adolescents has been supported by our own research (Weist et al., 1995).

SELF-CONCEPT

As mentioned, positive self-concept may be considered either as a protective factor or a measure of psychological health, while poor self-concept may be seen as reflecting emotional disturbance. Our preference is to categorize self-regard as a protective factor, but admit that it could appropriately be placed in the domain of *emotional/ behavioral functioning*. Studies have supported the importance of positive self-concept for emotional and social functioning in children of mentally ill parents (Murphy and Moriarity, 1976), and in urban youth (Felner et al., 1985).

There are a number of very good measures of self-concept for adolescents. The Offer Self-Image Questionnaire for Adolescents (Offer, Ostrov, and Howard, 1984) is a 130-item self-report measure that provides standard scores on a number of subscales including body and self image, family relations, impulse control, psychopathology, and superior adjustment. Psychometric qualities including internal consistency, reliability, and validity of the measure have been reported to be strong. The time involved to administer this instrument limits its usefulness in clinical situations.

A somewhat less time-consuming but still fairly comprehensive measure of self-concept is the Self-Perception Profile for Adolescents (Harter, 1988), which assesses self-perceptions of functioning in domains that include academic competence, behavioral conduct, friendships, global self-worth, and social acceptance. Psychometric properties of this measure have been reported to be adequate.

When time constraints prevent detailed assessment of self-concept, the Rosenberg Self-Esteem Scale (Rosenberg, 1965), may be used. This is a very brief measure, using only 10 items, that has demonstrated reliability and internal consistency. Even though this measure is now over 30 years old, it remains relevant for use with adolescents.

EMOTIONAL AND BEHAVIORAL FUNCTIONING

Depression, anxiety, and behavioral problems reflect core disorders of adolescence, and we and others have documented their increased occurrence among urban youth in relation to higher levels of poverty, life stress and violence exposure (Weist et al., 1995). These constructs are certainly central to the assessment and treatment of adolescents with emotional and behavioral disorders. As such, psychiatrists who work with adolescents should be familiar with instruments for the assessment of these constructs. Structured instruments can be very useful in determining a baseline level of impairment and symptom severity, and for monitoring change over time. In the era of managed care, where reporting of patient status is often mandated by third party payors, the results of standardized assessments can provide a shorthand for communication of assessment findings and treatment response. They have the additional advantage of preserving some degree of confidentiality, as an aggregate score of depression can be reported for a group of individuals before and following intervention, with the anonymity of individual respondents preserved.

DEPRESSION

We most commonly use the Reynolds Adolescent Depression Scale (RADS) (Reynolds, 1987) related to its outstanding normative and psychometric qualities. This 30-item self-report measure for youths aged 13 through 19 contains norms for more than 11,000 teenagers from various sections of the U.S., and has strong internal consistency, test-retest reliability, and validity that is construct and criterion related (Reynolds, 1993). The relevance of the measure for urban youth has been supported by its ongoing use in our clinical and research efforts.

For early adolescents (e.g., youths aged 11 and 12) and for older adolescents with suspected developmental delays, we prefer to use the Children's Depression Inventory (CDI) (Kovacs, 1981), which contains 27 items, and is designed for youth aged 8 through 17. The CDI has been reported to have good internal consistency and validity, and adequate test-retest reliability, and is widely used in research investigations with children and adolescents.

ANXIETY AND FEAR

To measure anxiety specifically, we use the Revised Children's Manifest Anxiety Scale (RCMAS) (Reynolds and Richmond, 1978), which is a measure of self-reported anxiety in children and adolescents aged 6 through 19 years. The RCMAS contains 27 items measuring anxiety symptoms and 8 items that comprise a lie scale, reflecting the youth's tendency to provide false responses. The measure is reported to have adequate internal consistency, and validity that is content and construct related (Goldman, Stein, and Guerry, 1983).

To measure fear in youth presenting other anxiety symptoms, we have found the Fear Survey Schedule for Children-Revised (FSSC-R) (Ollendick, 1983) to be useful. This 80 item self-report measure of specific fears in youths aged 6 to 18 has acceptable internal consistency and test-retest reliability over a short time interval.

BEHAVIORAL PROBLEMS

Perhaps the most useful self-report measure we use with adolescents is the Youth Self-Report (YSR) (Achenbach, 1991), that contains 112 items which assess aspects of emotional and behavioral functioning in youths aged 11 through 18. The YSR has an extensive normative base, and yields T scores (with a mean of 50 and standard deviation of 10) on social competence, internalizing, externalizing, and total behavior problem scales and subscales including depression/anxiety, attention problems, thought problems, and delinquent behavior. Clinical cutoffs are provided; as a general rule, T scores exceeding 67 are considered clinically significant. We use a computerized scoring program for the YSR that takes around five minutes to use, and yields a printout for the adolescent with T scores across the various subscales. Psychometric qualities for the YSR are outstanding; it can give an overall sense of degree of disturbance, and can also point to specific clinical syndromes, such as depression, or conduct disorder, although it is not designed to generate specific diagnoses. By reviewing the responses to specific questions, the clinician can inquire further about them and obtain additional information useful in making a diagnosis.

Two checklists tap similar behavioral domains as the YSR. The Child Behavior Checklist (CBCL) (Achenbach and Edelbrock, 1983) is a parent-report measure of internalizing and externalizing behavior problems in youths aged 4 through 16. The Teacher Report Form (TRF) (Achenbach and Edelbrock, 1986) is similar to the CBCL in format and content, except that behaviors most relevant to the school setting are assessed. Both the CBCL and TRF have strong psychometric qualities, computerized scoring programs like the YSR, and a means for clinicians to obtain perceptions of the adolescent's functioning from significant adults.

Improving the "User Friendliness" of Assessment Measures

We have found—in our own practices, and in our observations of trainees—that the use of checklists and self-report measures generally do not occur unless these measures and background information about them are easily accessible. Busy practices do not allow for the extra time needed for finding the right measures, learning about them, and trying to figure out how to score and interpret them. To increase the probability that staff and trainees will use such measures in their clinical work, we have created a simple system for organizing and using the measures.

The system involves creating files for each assessment measure, with the files maintained in a central location that is easily accessible to the clinical staff in our program. In each file, we place copies of the measure, and any background articles that we can locate. At the front

TABLE 1
EXAMPLE OF SUMMARY SHEET FOR ADOLESCENT MEASURES

Children's Depression Inventory	
Ages:	8–17
Scoring:	27 items; child chooses one of three responses for each item. Each item is scored 0, 1 or 2, with higher scores indicating higher levels of the symptom. Cutoff for presence of some level of depression = 13
Normative Background:	Extensive normative base; used in numerous research studies with children and adolescents
Internal Consistency:	Good (.70–.89)
Reliability:	Test-retest is adequate (.74–.77 after 3 weeks)
Validity:	Criterion-related established with social skills, dysphoric mood, anxiety, and stress. Construct validity supported by convergent parental reports
Strengths:	Able to discriminate between depressed and nondepressed youth, sensitive to treatment effects. Good measure for youth with poor reading abilities (can be completed with assistance from the therapist)
Limitations:	More of a screening measure that comprehensive measure of depressive symptoms
From:	Kovacs, M. (1981)
Publisher:	The Psychological Corporation Order Services Center P.O. Box 839954 San Antonio, TX 78283–3954 1-800-228-0752

of the file, we include a summary sheet that includes the name of the measure, scoring information, normative data, psychometric qualities, comments on strengths and limitations, a reference, and a phone number and address of the publisher. This summary sheet, usually just one page, can then be used by clinicians for multiple purposes from quickly learning about the measure and how to score it to reporting on the measure in presentations and written articles. We have found that this system saves considerable time, and also increases the probability that clinical assessment efforts by our staff will be augmented by use of checklists and self-report measures. In Table 1, a sample summary sheet is provided.

Concluding Comment

We have presented our personalized strategy of assessing adolescents, along with measures that we have found useful. We have reported on constructs that we most commonly assess in our clinical efforts; there are many other constructs important to adolescent adjustment (e.g., anger, attentional disturbance, hopelessness, social skills) that we have not reviewed. Undoubtedly, since we work in a program serving almost exclusively inner-city youth from lower socioeconomic backgrounds, some of the constructs that we assess with their associated measures (e.g., violence exposure) may be less relevant for clinicians working in other settings. Most of the measures presented in this paper, however, reflect core constructs, and are generally applicable to adolescents. We hope we have presented an assessment approach, and corresponding checklists and self-report measures, that will provide some guidelines for beginning level trainees and perhaps add something to the clinical armamentaria of seasoned professionals.

REFERENCES

Achenbach, T. M. (1991), *Manual for the Youth Self-Report and 1991 Profile.* Burlington: University of Vermont Department of Psychiatry.

_____ & Edelbrock, C. S. (1983), *Manual for the Child Behavior Checklist and Revised Child Behavior Profile.* Burlington, VT: Author.

247

————— & Edelbrock, C. S. (1986), *Manual for the Teacher Version of the Child Behavior Checklist and Revised Child Behavior Profile.* Burlington, VT: Author.

Ambrosini, P. J. (1986), *Schedule for Affective Disorders and Schizophrenia for School Age Children.* Unpublished manuscript.

Bell, C. C., Taylor-Crawford, K., Jenkins, E. J. & Chalmers, D. (1988), Need for victimization screening in a black psychiatric population. *J. Natl. Med. Assn.*, 80:41–48.

Clark, R. M. (1983), *Family Life and School Achievement.* Chicago: University of Chicago Press.

Duncan, G. (1991), The economic environment of childhood. In: *Children in poverty,* ed. A. C. Huston. New York: Cambridge University Press. pp. 23–50.

Dyson, J. L. (1990), The effect of family violence on children's academic performance and behavior. *J. Natl. Med. Assn.*, 82:17–22.

Isler, R. M., Miller, P. M. & Hersen, M. (1973), Components of assertive behavior. *J. Clin. Psychol.*, 24:295– 299.

Farrington, D. P. (1987), Epidemiology. In: *Handbook of juvenile delinquency,* ed. H. Quay. New York: Wiley.

Felner, R., Abu, M., Primavera, J. & Cauce, A. (1985), Adaptation and vulnerability in high risk adolescents: An examination of environmental mediators. *Amer. J. Comm. Psychol.*, 13:365–380.

Garbarino, J. (1976), A preliminary study of some ecological correlates of child abuse: The impact of socioeconomic stress on mothers. *Child Devel.*, 47:178–185.

Garmezy, N. (1987), Stress, competence, and development: Continuities in the study of schizophrenic adults, children vulnerable to psychopathology, and the search for stress- resistant children. *Amer. J. Orthopsychiat.*, 57:159–174.

Gladstein, J. & Slater, E. J. (1988), Inner city teenagers' exposure to violence: A prevalence study. *Maryland Med. J.*, 37:951–954.

Goldman, J., Stein, C. & Guerry, S. (1983), *Psychological Methods of Child Assessment.* New York: Brunner/Mazel.

Harter, S. (1988), *Manual for the Self-Perception Profile for Adolescents.* Denver, CO: University of Denver.

Hayes, S. C., Nelson, R. O. & Jarrett, R. B. (1987), The treatment utility of assessment: A functional approach to evaluating assessment quality. *Amer. Psychol.*, 42:963–974.

Hilton, N. Z. (1992), Battered women's concerns about their children witnessing wife assault. *J. Interpers. Violence,* 7:77–86.

Kleinmutz, B. (1984), The scientific study of clinical judgement in psychology and medicine. *Clin. Psychol. Rev.,* 4:111–126.

Kovacs, M. (1981), Rating scales to assess depression in school- aged children. *Acta Paedopsychiatrica,* 46:305–315.

Luthar, S. S. (1991), Vulnerability and resilience: A study of high-risk adolescents. *Child Devel.,* 62:600–616.

Martin, M. J. & Pritchard, M. E. (1991), Factors associated with alcohol use in later adolescents. *J. Studies on Alcohol,* 52:5–9.

Murphy, L. B. & Moriarity, A. (1976), *Vulnerability, Coping and Growth.* New Haven, CT: Yale University Press.

Nowicki, S. & Strickland, B. R. (1973), A locus of control scale for children. *J. Consult. Clin. Psychol.,* 40:148–154.

Nunn, G. D. & Parish, T. S. (1992), The psychosocial characteristics of at-risk high school students. *Adolescence,* 27:435–440.

Offer, D., Ostrov, E. & Howard, K. I. (1984), *Patterns of Adolescent Self-image.* San Francisco: Jossey-Bass.

Ollendick, T. H. (1983), Reliability and validity of the Revised Fear Survey Schedule for Children. *Behaviour Research and Therapy,* 21:685–692.

Ollendick, T. H. & Hersen, M. (1993), Child and adolescent behavioral assessment. In: *Handbook of Child and Adolescent Assessment,* ed. T. H. Ollendick & M. Hersen. Needham Heights, MA: Allyn & Bacon.

Olson, D., Portner, J. & Lavee, Y. (1985), *FACES III Manual.* St. Paul, MN: Family Social Science.

Paster, V. S. (1985), Adapting psychotherapy for the depressed, unacculturated, acting-out, black male adolescent. *Psychother.,* 22:408–417.

Piacentini, J. (1993), Checklists and rating scales. In: *Handbook of Child and Adolescent Assessment,* ed. T. H. Ollendick & M. Hersen. Needham Heights, MA: Allyn and Bacon.

Pellegrini, D. S. (1990), Psychosocial risk and protective factors in childhood. *J. Devel. Behav. Pediat.,* 11:201–209.

Prothrow-Stith, D. (1991), *Deadly Consequences.* New York: Harper-Collins.

Pynoos, R. S. & Nader, K. (1988), Psychological first aid and treatment approach to children exposed to community violence: Research implications. *J. Traumatic Stress*, 1:445–473.

Reynolds, C. R. & Richmond, B. O. (1978), "What I think and feel": A revised measure of children's manifest anxiety. *J. Abn. Child Psychol.*, 6:271–280.

Reynolds, W. M. (1987), *Reynolds Adolescent Depression Scale Professional Manual*. New York: Psychological Assessment Resources.

———— (1993), Self-report methodology. In: *Handbook of Child and Adolescent Assessment*, ed. T. H. Ollendick & M. Hersen. Needham Heights, MA: Allyn and Bacon.

Rhodes, J. E. & Jason, L. A. (1988), *Preventing Substance Abuse Among Children and Adolescents*. New York: Pergamon Press.

———— & ———— (1990), A social stress model of substance abuse. *J. Consult. Clin. Psychol.*, 58:395–401.

Richters, J. E. & Saltzman, W. (1990), *Survey of Children's Exposure to Community Violence*. Bethesda, MD: National Institute of Mental Health.

Rosenberg, M. (1965), *Society and Adolescent Self-image*. Princeton, NJ: Princeton University Press.

Shakoor, B. & Chalmers, D. (1991), Co-victimization of African-American children who witness violence and the theoretical implications of its effect on their cognitive, emotional, and behavioral development. *J. Natl. Med. Assn.*, 83:233–238.

Strain, P. S., Odom, S. L. & McConnell, S. (1985), Promoting social reciprocity of exceptional children: Identification, target behavior selection and intervention. *Remedial & Special Ed.*, 5:21–28.

Taylor, R. L. (1987), Black youth in crisis. *Humboldt J. Social Rel.*, 14:106–133.

Weist, M. D., Finney, J. W. & Ollendick, T. H. (1992), Cognitive biases in child behavior therapy. *The Behavior Therapist*, 15:249–252.

———— Freedman, A. H., Paskewitz, D. A., Proescher, E. J. & Flaherty, L. T. (1995), Urban youth under stress: Empirical identification of protective factors. *J. Youth & Adoles.*, 24:705–721.

———— Myers, C. P., Warner, B. S., Dorsey, N. & Varghese, S. (1996, June), A brief screening measure for violence exposure in urban youth. Presented to the Maryland Psychiatric Research Center, University of Maryland School of Medicine, Baltimore.

———— & Ollendick, T. H. (1991), Toward empirically valid target selection with children: The case of assertiveness. *Behav. Mod.*, 15:213–227.

———— & Finney, J. W. (1991), Toward the empirical validation of treatment targets in children. *Clin. Psychol. Rev.*, 11:515–538.

West, D. J. & Farrington, D. P. (1977), *The Delinquent Way of Life*. London: Heinemann.

Wills, T. A., Vaccaro, D & McNamara, P., (1992), The role of life events, family support, and competence in adolescent substance use: A test of vulnerability and protective factors. *Amer. J. Commun. Psychol.*, 20:349–374.

Work, W. C., Cowen, E. L., Parker, G. W. & Wyman, P. A. (1990), Test correlates of stress affected and stress resilient outcomes among urban children. *J. Primary Prevention*, 11:3–17.

Yule, W. (1993), Developmental considerations in child assessment. In: *Handbook of Child and Adolescent Assessment*, ed. T. H. Ollendick & M. Hersen. Needham Heights, MA: Allyn and Bacon.

12   ON THE USES AND MISUSES OF PSYCHOEDUCATIONAL EVALUATIONS

JONATHAN COHEN

Learning problems are among the most common experiences that complicate and interfere with growth and development in and outside of the classroom. Some learning problems are due to psychological difficulties, but most are due to a complex mix of psychodynamic conflicts, constitutional vulnerabilities, and cognitive weaknesses, as well as how the youngster has consciously and unconsciously (mis)understood the learning problem (Cohen, 1983). Many educators and mental health professionals are keenly aware of the potential complex constellations of factors that may be undermining achievement and/or learning. As a result, psychoeducational diagnostic testing[1] is often recommended as a part of the initial clinical evaluative process.

At its best, a psychoeducational diagnostic evaluation helpfully clarifies the youngster's strengths and weaknesses in a way that leads to recommendations that will address intrapsychic, interpersonal, and educational difficulties and facilitate learning and development. In fact, a diagnostic evaluation can change a child's life as well as others' perceptions of the youngster in profound and healing ways. The diagnostic report that emerges from the evaluative process can enhance teachers' understanding and help educators to teach more effectively and develop short-term and long-term strategies that help the child to effectively address educational, cognitive, and, sometimes, emotional

---

[1] In this essay, *psychoeducational diagnostic testing* refers to the wide array of test batteries, educational, psychological, and neuropsychological, administered to children who present with learning difficulties. When I comment on the particular practices of a certain school of testing, I specify this and do not use the term *psychoeducational*.

difficulties. Testing can powerfully enable parents to be more understanding and empathic. Testing can help parents to recognize and understand why a certain therapeutic intervention is worth considering. Testing can potentially increase the child's understanding of him- or herself in a way that has profoundly positive educational and psychosocial consequences. Testing can sometimes help mental health professionals in an integrative, differential diagnostic understanding of the youngsters. In short, testing can further integrative understanding and work, a basic therapeutic and educational goal; but, too often, diagnostic evaluations do not accomplish all of these goals.

There are many ways in which psychoeducational tests are inadvertently misused. For example, diagnosticians commonly use tests for the wrong purposes, invest more meaning than they should in test results, or treat results as absolute (Sattler, 1990; Eyde, Robertson, and Krug, 1993). In this essay I will assume that the tester does understand what tests to use and how to score and interpret the test findings properly. This essay focuses on why professionals, parents, and the youngster himself often do not learn all they can and need to before, during, and after testing. As I will detail below, this lack of learning profoundly undermines the usefulness of this potentially powerful diagnostic and therapeutic intervention.

It is difficult to know how many children and adolescents are diagnostically evaluated in public and independent schools today. I do not believe that there are epidemiologic data available about how many tests are given in the public or private sectors. It has been estimated that between 100 and 200 million students are given psychological and "intelligence" tests every year (Hanson, 1993). My impression as a consultant to many parents and independent schools is that testing is common and can be costly. Depending of the type of evaluation and where it is done, the cost of evaluations ranges from $300 or $400 at state and/or federally funded clinics that have sliding fee schedules to $1200 to $2500 in the private sector. The economics of psychoeducational testing is important not only because of the significant expense for parents, but also because fee management inadvertently contributes to the misuse of test findings.

This essay is a clinical exposition based on two decades of observing and participating in the diagnostic evaluation of childhood and adolescent learning problems in a variety of settings: public and private psychiatric hospitals, community clinics, independent and public schools, in the private practice sector as a diagnostician and consultant to parents, and as a teacher in a university where graduate students are taught how to perform these evaluations. The impetus for this essay emerged primarily from my work in recent years as a consultant to parents, schools, and mental health professionals in which I have seen countless instances of parents, children, and teachers who have not had an opportunity to learn from diagnostic evaluations and benefit from the findings. I will describe what factors before, during, and after the diagnostic evaluation of learning and psychosocial problems inadvertently limit the usefulness of testing. Next, I will suggest how to enhance the usefulness of diagnostic testing. Some of these suggestions are not new: they constitute good clinical work practiced in many settings. However, a variety of factors limit the wider use of certain aspects of good practice.

Before Testing

There are specific practices and a pervasive attitude that inadvertently limit the usefulness of diagnostic testing before, during, and after the actual evaluation. Before, some educators and many diagnosticians begin to communicate an attitude about testing that colors the whole experience in an inadvertently unhelpful manner. What is the role and responsibility of the psychoeducational diagnostician? How this question is answered by the tester and, to some extent, by the parents, school, and/or the referring mental health professional importantly determines what occurs in the testing process. Is it the tester's job to find the problem, to fix the problem, to educate parents about the benefits and limitations of testing and about the short-term and/or long-term implications of the test findings, or to make sure that the parents, the school, and the child understand all of the findings? The answer to some of these questions are clear: At least part of the tester's job is to discover what is the problem, but it is not the tester's responsibility to fix the problem. Virtually all testers would agree that their job includes making recommendations to further the growth and development of the youngster. However, what the tester looks for and how he or she attempts to be helpful is complicated and, in practice, varies greatly.

Most psychoeducational testers have been taught to believe that testing is an *event*: It is a diagnostic intervention in which the tester discovers what the current situation is and reports the findings to the parents, remedial, and/or mental health professionals, and sometimes, the youngster. This model is akin to visiting a neurologist: to find out what is wrong and to be told. This is the "x-ray technician" model. Sometimes this model is taken to the extreme: A summary of test scores is sent to the parents with a phone call or very brief meeting to "explain" the results. More commonly, the tester will meet with the parents or talk briefly on the phone before the testing and then meet with them once after the testing to provide "feedback." This approach to testing is not helpful.

The x-ray technician model is not helpful because understanding the parents' questions and the nature of a child's learning difficulties and strengths is always a long-term process in a number of ways. The relatively short time typically spent before and after the actual testing limits everyone's capacity to use what parents, teachers, and child already know before the testing and what the tester has learned from the testing. Psychoeducational testing is typically inexact: What we learn is rarely definitive but instead points to patterns and tendencies that always need to be compared and contrasted with reports from parents, teachers, and, often, the child. A youngster's learning abilities and disabilities and the match between the child and educational demands is always changing. These factors need to be understood and addressed over time for the testing results to be assimilated, used, and helpful. For example, the implications of a particular dyslexic and organizational disability at age 7 has very different educational and emotional meanings than it does for an 11- or 17-year-old.

The x-ray technician model is one that primarily focuses on "the problem" and not on the youngster's strengths. To be most helpful, we need to understand the child's strengths as well as weaknesses in order to develop strategies to build self-esteem and foster a more realistic, integrated image of self. Testing provides unique opportunities to learn about a youngster's strengths. Although most testers are aware of the long-term importance of understanding and underscoring a child's strengths, they do not emphasize these in practice. The discussion of how to use strengths is often a minimal aspect of "feedback" and the test report itself; the "news" of testing is often what is the nature of the "problem." A more extended dialogue about the youngster's strengths as well as weaknesses not only makes it easier to understand and assimilate information about the weaknesses, but to think concretely about how to build on strengths. Depending on a number of factors, mental health professionals may or may not want to be directly involved with developing behavioral interventions to build on strengths. Nonetheless, this is always potentially valuable information that testing can reveal. As the tester is virtually always asked, "Depending on the test findings, what will help?" it is the diagnostician's responsibility to understand and use the youngster's strengths to further growth.

The x-ray technician model discourages a collaborative effort between the parents and tester and between the school and tester. Testers usually want to understand what questions the parents have, and they provide the test findings to the parents and make themselves available for further questions and discussion. Parents do not have a chance to think about what all of their questions are before the testing, and parents and child usually do not understand all the implications of the test findings after just one feedback session. I believe that it is the tester's responsibility to work collaboratively with parents and child before and after the testing to make it maximally useful.

The idea that the psychoeducational testing is a part of an ongoing process and that the tester has a responsibility to work in collaboration with the parents (and optimally, with the school) leads to another aspect of how diagnosticians do or do not address parental questions and expectations before the testing actually begins. The more parents and, if at all possible, the child, have a chance to become aware of all of their questions before the diagnostic evaluation, the more useful the testing can be. Sometimes parents are not given much of a chance to think about all that they know and do not know about their child. The more the tester understands all that the parents do know about their child and want to know the better able the tester is to understand the child and address the parents' concerns and questions.

When the tester, parents, and mental health professional do not have an opportunity to understand the breadth and depth of what parents and the youngster know and want to know before the testing, it undermines learning in several important ways. The parents' and child's knowledge and areas of confusion will critically direct the tester in his inquiry. If we do not explicitly communicate that the initial consultation and the process of diagnostic testing are necessarily collaborative, we reinforce the common fantasy and wish that the tester will provide "all the answers." To some extent, the psychoeducational diagnostician—like any specialist to whom the patient is referred in the early stages of treatment—is consciously and/or unconsciously viewed as the individual who will "help us to find out the nature of the problem and fix it." As mental health professionals and all parents who have had their children tested know, testing cannot answer all questions. Not addressing this fantasy before the testing can lead to disappointment and resentment by the parents and the youngster after the testing. This disappointment can contribute to patients' not being able to use the test findings that have emerged from the process. The consulting and/or referring mental professional is in a unique role to anticipate and address these expectations and potentially complicating practices.

In essence, the referring mental health professional and the tester have a responsibly both to educate parents about the uses and limitations of psychoeducational testing and to learn about parental concerns and expectations before the testing begins. When parents understand that testing is part of a long-term collaborative process, focusing on strengths as well as weaknesses, the stage has been set for maximally useful testing.

There are many reasons why testing may not be maximally useful, including how testing is taught in graduate school and the rarely discussed economics of testing. In learning to administer and understand testing, the graduate student's experience is like learning to drive a car. However, doing testing is more like driving a car with two stick shifts, each of which has seven gears. The student needs to learn about an overwhelming number of factors that must be kept in mind simultaneously. The student, faculty, and supervisors focus on the actual process of testing, the "basics." What is least emphasized is what happens before and after the actual testing. Emphasis on the actual test administration, scoring, and interpretation also contributes to the "x-ray technician" state of mind. Although experienced testers are often attuned to how to use the time therapeutically before and after testing, economic and other factors contribute to testers' not being as helpful as they could be.

Economic factors influence in powerful and typically covert ways what is and is not done during psychoeducational testing. In the public school system, parents are not charged for these testing services; any child who is having trouble learning is entitled to a free and "comprehensive" diagnostic evaluation. Although any parent can request that a psychoeducational evaluation be done for his or her child, more commonly testing is recommended when a child is identified by a teacher as showing learning or behavioral problems. In either case, the process of how psychoeducational assessment is managed is dictated by federal and state regulations (Strickland and Turnbull, 1990). This process leads to the development of the Individual Educational Plans (IEP). In theory, parents play an integral role in the process of psychoeducational testing in the public schools and, in fact, are legally empowered to authorize whether testing is done or not. Parents should determine that the testing has addressed their concerns about their child's difficulties and affirm their support for the recommended plan to address the problem. Often, this does not occur.

The lack of funds for psychologists to do the actual testing limits how much time they can spend in collaborative work with parents, teachers, and other professionals before and after the testing itself. It also limits the amount of time that testers feel they can spend with any one child and family. The testers are often under tremendous pressure to evaluate a growing backlog of youngsters in the public school system. Understandably, the psychologists may believe that if they spend too much time with any one family, other children in need will not receive any attention—a tragic outcome, because the children who are evaluated often do not benefit from the process as much as they could and need to.

In the independent school sector, educators typically identify a child as showing learning or behavioral problems. At a certain point, educators recommend that parents seek a psychoeducational evaluation for their child to help clarify the nature of the problem. Actual testing is rarely done in independent schools but instead is completed in the private sector. There are two ways that fees for testing tend to be managed by private practitioners, a flat fee and an hourly fee. Most testers in the private sector set a flat fee for the whole process. How the "whole process" is defined varies. It sometimes involves one meeting with the parents before testing to understand what are the parents' questions and to learn about the child's history; the actual testing (which varies tremendously in content and time); and one (or, occasionally, two) meetings to describe and discuss the test findings, the "feedback" meeting.

Testers estimate how long the testing process takes and set their fee based on market rates. The problem with this approach is that there is a financial incentive for the tester not to meet more than planned, before, during, and after the testing. The more time they spend, the less they make. On the other hand, testers are concerned that if they charge an hourly rate, parents will be concerned that there is an incentive to spend too much time before, during, and after the testing. In any case, fees are a force that consciously or unconsciously can affect how much time the tester spends with parents before the actual testing begins to learn about their concerns and questions. It can also be a powerful force that affects how much time the tester spends with the youngster during the actual testing and with members of the family during the feedback process.

There is a simple and critically important solution to this problem: Parents need to be educated that testing is a *process*—not only does it take time to clarify and identify the questions that parents and the youngster have, but also if we do not understand what the range of our questions are and what test findings mean educationally, socially, and psychologically, we lessen the usefulness of the diagnostic testing intervention.

During Testing

What is actually done during psychoeducational diagnostic testing? The tester attempts to learn about one or more aspects of functioning by asking the child to answer questions and perform on a variety of tasks. In theory, how the child performs in this testing situation is related to how he or she functions in other learning situations.

In fact, what psychoeducational testers focus on and how much they correlate their findings with the child's learning experience in school varies tremendously. Some testers focus on educational functioning, some on cognitive functioning, some on neuropsychological functioning, some on psychological functioning, and many on some combination of these domains. Other testers virtually never talk with parents, teachers, and school administrators to learn about the detailed nature of the match between the child and the classroom where he or she is learning and or having trouble learning. These testers believe that the child's performance on the tests administered has merit in its own right and can and will be used profitably by parents and teachers. At the other end of this spectrum, there are diagnosticians who believe it is more useful to look closely at the match between the child and his or her learning environment or what has been called the nature of the "instructional environment" (Choate, et al., 1992). To a great extent, this method of evaluating a learning problem is a reaction to serious concerns that traditional psychoeducational assessment does not provide reliable and specific information to help educators to effectively teach students with learning problems.

Many testers find their own balance between utilizing more traditional psychometric tests (e.g., the Wechsler intelligence tests) and understanding what is the nature of the match between the child and his learning environment. Most often, this means that the tester talks with the child's teachers about their perceptions, concerns, and questions about the student. Increasingly, testers administer in-depth educational tests to recreate learning situations that directly echo what occurs in the classroom. In this way, they believe that they come closer to the child's educational experience in the classroom, and in fact they do. Unfortunately, many of these testers do not evaluate other important aspects of the child's functioning (e.g., psychodynamic processes), and the tester's report risks resembling one of the proverbial sightless reports of one or two parts of the elephant.

The tendency of many testers to focus on one or two domains of the child's experience and not to attempt to integrate these findings into the interactive process of the child with his actual learning environment tends to undermine the usefulness of testing. It is rare for one diagnostician to have expertise in all of the many domains that complicate learning and psychosocial development—educational, cognitive, neuropsychological, and psychological. There is some, but not enough, debate within the testing world about the relative merits of various types of test batteries. Some argue that if a child is having difficulty learning to read or write, it is always useful to have an evaluation that focuses on the child's educational abilities and weaknesses, and that it is not necessary to evaluate the nuances of psychodynamic functioning. Sometimes it may not be necessary for a tester to evaluate more than one aspect of the child's functioning. For example, when a 6-year-old is having trouble learning to read and there is no indication of psychological problems at school or home, it may not be necessary to assess emotional functioning in any detail. However, psychological reactions to school difficulties that endure longer than six to nine months always accompany psychogenic reactions that affect psychological functioning (Cohen, 1984). In time, these reactions color the "nooks and crannies" of the mind and become ongoing aspects of self-experience with the development of particular defenses and symptoms. Hence, it is important to understand how cognitive and psychological factors are interacting in the later childhood years.

Too often psychological testing reports are too narrowly focused. Consequently, parents, educators, and occasionally the child learn a great deal about certain aspects of the child's functioning but do not "see" and come to understand the whole child. Two common examples are psychological/emotional issues being left out and detailed educational evaluation and recommendations being given short shrift.

There are many evaluations that tell us a great deal about the youngster's cognitive or educational capacities but nothing about how the child's or adolescent's psychodynamics influence learning. Emotional and motivational issues become as important as, and often more important than, the specific learning disability itself as the child gets older. This complex constellation of psychological factors should be integrated into an understanding of the child's learning experience.

Many other evaluations describe the psychodynamic and/or cognitive functioning of the child in exquisite detail but tell us very little about the educational experience and capacity of the youngster. Although many children who present to mental health professionals with "learning problems" are simply showing a symptomatic expression of an underlying psychogenic problem, it is much more common that when a learning problem is the presenting problem, there are indeed significant cognitive/educational problems that need to be understood in conjunction with the youngster's psychodynamics. There are several ways in which many evaluations are lacking educationally. Too many evaluations simply do an inadequate job attempting to assess the complex array of skills that youngsters utilize in the classroom. The tests that are used often have little relevance to what the child or adolescent is actually struggling with in school. Another critical aspect of educational functioning has to do with the questions of the match between the learner and the learning environment.

We have learned that many difficulties in childhood are not simply the child's problem, but rather a function of a mismatch between the youngster and the environment. This is not a new idea in psychiatry, psychology, or special education, but it is often forgotten and not commonly integrated into many psychoeducational evaluations done today. Testers often evaluate the child with little knowledge about what his or her classroom environment is really like, and the actual tasks presented in the testing situation are far different from the tasks the child confronts in the classroom.

After Testing

After the testing has been completed, the results are often presented in a manner that does not facilitate understanding and helpful application. This is perhaps the single most serious way that psycho-educational testing is misused. When the actual testing is completed, the diagnostician usually meets with parents once. A test report for parents and, if authorized, for educators, is prepared. Testers rarely meet with children to discuss the diagnostic findings, but they usually meet with adolescents to provide feedback.

This method of informing parents and the youngster about the findings is in accord with the x-ray technician model: The findings are conceptualized as being relatively straightforward, and it is thought that the patient can assimilate this information in one (or occasionally two) meetings in conjunction with the actual test report. This is not so. Three factors contribute importantly to the inability of parents, the child, and teachers to understand and use test findings presented in one or two sessions and/or in the test report: 1) the overwhelming amount of factual information presented; 2) emotional reactions to test findings; and 3) the fact that using the information needs to occur in a gradual, collaborative manner to be helpful.

Psychoeducational testing reveals a tremendous amount of information about the youngster. In my experience, it is simply unrealistic to expect that anyone will be able to assimilate and use this information in one or two meetings. This is true even for professionals who are versed in the categories that organize the tester's presentation of the findings: cognitive, linguistic, visual, perceptual, memory, and neuropsychological functions. Parents are overwhelmed with information in the 5- to 14-page reports issuing from the psychoeducational testing process. Parents and the adolescent also need to learn a new language and new ways of thinking about learning, learning problems, and mental functioning. This is a difficult task even when testers translate findings into plain English.

Parents' and children's emotional reactions to test findings are often powerful and complicate the understanding of test findings. For example, a mother said to me, "When I first received the feedback from the tester, I didn't really hear a word. . . . I brought my sister because I knew I wouldn't really be able to comprehend." This is often a way to manage or react to anticipatory anxiety—to be overwhelmed and/or to deny. It also easy to understand why the child or adolescent may experience significant anxiety about hearing testing findings from a psychodynamic perspective. Along with the time needed simply to understand the findings, it takes time to know how to use the findings.

In addition to children, adolescents, and adults alike not being able to understand fully the content of test findings in one or two meetings (and by reading the reports), there is an another reason why using this information must happen gradually. Unlike a medical test that results in a specific treatment recommendation, psychoeducational evaluations typically yield complex findings with specific and general implications that change as the child develops and faces new academic and psychosocial tasks year after year.

At its best, a psychoeducational evaluation reveals much information about strengths, weaknesses, and coping/defensive strategies. These findings facilitate a dialogue between the youngster and those working with him or her about their experience and performance. This dialogue can help the youngster develop a more realistic sense of self. Test findings can also provide rich therapeutic opportunities to discuss adaptive and maladaptive defensive styles, interests, wishes, fears, and experiences. A major reason why this is not done is that the results are not presented in a manner that facilitates either understanding and curiosity about how parents, professionals, and the youngster agree and disagree with the findings or an extensive discussion about how the test findings can be used.

Three ways to enhance the effectiveness and comprehension of psychoeducational testing are 1) rejecting the x-ray technician model and instead entering the process as a diagnostic inquiry that will also be a short-term psychotherapeutic intervention; 2) engaging in intensive, collaborative, and educational work with parents to understand what they know and want to learn as well as to educate them about what may emerge from the testing process; and 3) ensuring that the child, parents, and professionals understand the information in a way that fosters application and learning.

Several factors contribute to testers' not taking responsibility to assure that the child, parents, and professionals understand the test findings. When practitioners are first taught to perform psychoeducational tests in graduate school, little attention is paid to helping make the findings understood and used helpfully. Nor is there training in how economic/fee-related matters affect what is and is not done before, during, and after the testing.

Five specific practices can dramatically increase the likelihood that test findings will be understood and used to further understanding and learning, and to change the life of the youngster: 1) a letter to the child; 2) parents' writing a summary of the test findings; 3) meetings with the teacher at school; 4) writing reports clearly; and 5) the six-month follow-up.

Seldom do children and adolescents understand what has been learned in a psychoeducational evaluation. In the public school system, the team of testers rarely meets with the child to provide feedback. In the independent school sector, where testing is often done by private practitioners or in clinics, the child is sometimes seen once for feedback. Most practitioners would say that children under five will not be able understand any of the details of test findings, but even young children yearn to understand their experience and fatefully attribute meanings (realistic or not) to their successes, frustrations, and failures. In fact, even young children's understanding of their strengths and weaknesses can be dramatically enhanced when test findings are provided in a way that they can understand. One of the most powerful ways to do this is to talk with the child and to write him or her a letter of the findings that serves as the child's "test report." When a one-page (or for older children, sometimes a two-page) letter is written to the youngster at a developmentally and psychologically appropriate level, that child then has something from which he or she not only can learn, but which he or she can go review—alone and in discussions with parents—about the experience. The children and adolescents who have received such letters have had their understanding of the test findings dramatically enhanced.[2]

It can be extraordinarily useful to ask parents to write a summary of the test findings. When we write a summary of what we understand, we always realize what is clear and not clear in our mind. After the tester has met with parents once to provide feedback about the test findings and given them a copy of the test report, it is highly useful to recommend that they write a summary of what was told them verbally and in the test report. It is often surprising to parents how much they still do not understand, and this process makes it easier for them to talk about what is and is not comprehensible about test findings. Although most parents are initially surprised to be invited to write such a summary, they are typically invested in doing everything that they can to further their understanding and capacity to help. Parents' being clear about test findings allows them to be empathic with their child and helpful advocates for him or her.

Test reports should be written clearly and understandably. Many test reports are poorly written and filled with "psychobabble." Test reports given to parents should be written so that any intelligent adult can

---

[2]I am grateful to Dr. Richard Echler, who introduced this idea to me.

understand them. Often, a report is written both for professionals (e.g., a psychotherapist, a teacher, a remedial expert) and for parents, and although professionals understand the concepts and vocabulary in the report, the parents often do not.

Understanding the youngster's strengths, weaknesses, and cognitive styles is just the first step in the psychoeducational evaluative process. To be helpful, we have to use the findings that have emerged in the diagnostic process. Too many test reports are read once, understood little, and put in a drawer. To be most useful, the tester and the parents—and when possible, the youngster—need to talk with educators and other professionals who are involved (e.g., mental health professionals and remedial experts) to discuss collaboratively two critical questions: How do these findings compare and contrast with your experience of the youngster? How can we use these findings to promote learning and growth? When these questions are addressed collaboratively, they can lead to the group of adults—and eventually the youngster—working together in powerful ways (Cohen, 1993). One specific implication of this is that it is routinely useful for the tester to meet with the youngster's teachers at school. It is typical that testers let parents, the child, and other professionals know that they are available to be helpful in the months and years after the testing is completed, but it is rare that this invitation is heeded. On the other hand, it is always helpful for parents and the child to review what was learned, what psychological and/or educational plans were made to remediate weaknesses and enhance strengths, and to what extent these goals have begun to be realized. When the tester meets with parents six to nine months after the testing has been completed, it typically provides therapeutic opportunities to build on the initial test findings.

Conclusion

I have described how most children and adolescents who are having significant learning problems are referred for psychoeducational diagnostic test evaluations. The assessment of a youngster's strengths and weaknesses can invaluably aid the child, parents, educators, and mental health professionals to facilitate understanding, learning, and development. However, diagnostic testing is often unhelpful and inadvertently misused. Aspects of current practice before, during, and after the testing have been described that undermine its potential usefulness.

Before the testing, psychoeducational diagnosticians' adopting an "x-ray technician" model of professional behavior lessens the likelihood that they will learn all that they can and need to from parents, other professionals, and the youngster, prior to the actual testing. Testing needs to be viewed as a short-term psychotherapeutic endeavor—as well as a diagnostic inquiry—to ensure that the tester will learn what he or she needs to learn before the testing, and that the youngster and parents will have an opportunity to understand and use the test findings. During the testing, it is invaluable for the tester to understand the youngster comprehensively (i.e., to assess cognitive, educational, neuropsychological, and psychodynamic functioning) and to learn about strengths as well as weaknesses. After the testing, it is shocking how often the youngster, parents, and professionals do not understand what the testing discovered. Even when there is some understanding of the test findings, it is quite common that the tester does not help others to use the findings to make educational, social, or intrapsychic interventions to facilitate change. A series of specific suggestions have been made that can enhance the likelihood that testing will be better understood and used: a letter to the youngster; a summary of the test findings written by the parents; an actual meeting at the school; clearly written and intelligible reports; and a six- to nine-month follow-up meeting with the tester.

Mental health professionals are in a powerful position to ensure that psychoeducational tests will be understood and used to further therapeutic and educational goals. Experienced mental health professionals know that it is often relatively easy to understand the nature of someone else's difficulties, but more difficult, and more important, to use our understanding to facilitate change. Too often, in diagnostic testing situations, the diagnostician understands the youngster without helping him or her to use the information to change, learn, and further the developmental process. Diagnostic testing is a powerful tool that can facilitate integrative learning about oneself. The major pitfall of this powerful tool is that the findings are too often not understood by parents and the youngster. When mental health professionals recommend psychological testing, I believe that it is their responsibility to ensure that this diagnostic intervention and the findings that emerge from it are understood and employed to facilitate therapeutic change. I have here described an attitude and a number of practices that further the therapeutic utilization of psychoeducational diagnostic evaluations.

REFERENCES

Choate, J., Enright, B., Miller, L., Potect, J. & Rakes, T. (1992), *Curriculum Based Assessment and Programming,* 2nd ed. Needham, MA: Allyn & Bacon.

Cohen, J. (1983), Learning disabilities and the college student: Identification and diagnosis. *Adolescent Psychiatry,* 11:177–198. Chicago: University of Chicago Press.

———— (1984), Learning disabilities and adolescence: Developmental considerations. *Adolescent Psychiatry,* 12:177–196. Chicago: University of Chicago Press.

———— (1993), Attentional disorders in adolescence: Integrating psychoanalytic and neuropsychological diagnostic and developmental considerations. *Adolescent Psychiatry,* 19:301–342. Chicago: University of Chicago Press.

Eyde, L. D., Robertson, G.J. & Krug, S.E. (1993), *Responsible Test Use..* Washington, DC: American Psychological Association Press.

Hanson, F. A. (1993), *Testing, Testing..* Berkeley: University of California Press.

Sattler, J. (1990), *Assessment of Children,* 3rd ed. San Diego, CA: Sattler.

Strickland, B. R. & Turnbull, A. P. (1990), *Developing and Implementing Individualized Educational Programs,* 3rd ed. Columbus, OH: Merrill

PART III

ISSUES IN PSYCHOTHERAPY

13 ADOLESCENT ANALYZABILITY RECONSIDERED

MICHAEL G. KALOGERAKIS

It is more than 40 years since Anna Freud stated that in her opinion adolescents were not analyzable. Since that time psychoanalysts who work with adolescents have differed on the question, most agreeing that classical analysis, as developed for adult patients, is neither appropriate nor possible, at least until late adolescence. Still, the issue remains controversial and has left many questions unanswered.

Many writers on psychodynamic approaches to the treatment of adolescents have muddied the waters by seemingly dealing with classical analysis and psychoanalytically oriented psychotherapy as interchangeable constructs. Others, while emphasizing that they were not using classical technique, have failed to clarify precisely how basic analytic technique should be modified in work with adolescents. What parameters are appropriate, at what points in the therapy, and the rationale for their use are seldom clearly delineated. This lack of clarity has led to considerable confusion over which might be the appropriate therapeutic intervention in a given case, at the same time delaying the development of a comprehensive and reliable psychodynamic treatment model for adolescents. indications and contraindications, constraining factors, alternative treatments and appropriate mixes, adaptations of the basic technique and the role of the therapist/analyst—all essential components of the individual treatment plan that must be drawn up after the requisite diagnostic evaluation—have received little of the needed attention.

This paper is a first step toward a systematic delineation of the developmental, psychopathological, familial, reality and other factors that must be considered in deciding on the elements of an optimum treatment plan when the choice is between classical psychoanalysis and psychoanalytically oriented psychotherapy. The concomitant use of pharmacotherapy, although often appropriate, will not be considered in this paper.

Since Anna Freud's time, there have been important contributions to psychoanalytic theory that have come from developmental research with infants and from attachment theory. Other significant ideas that have relevance for adolescent work have come from the self psychology school originated by Kohut. Note will be taken of some of these findings and ideas, where they are particularly relevant to the psychodynamic treatment of adolescents.

A symposium on "Indications and Contraindications for the Psychoanalysis of the Adolescent" held at the spring meeting of the American Psychoanalytic Association in 1971 (Sklansky, 1972) was the first and, to my knowledge, remains to this day the only comprehensive attempt to address the issue of adolescent analyzability. Different schools of thought would define psychoanalysis and therefore analyzability in different terms. However, the common denominator, which will serve as the basis for this discussion, is the notion that there are aspects of the childhood experience which exist as memories beyond awareness ("unrecognized meanings and structures") that play a significant role in current psychopathology. The individual's capacity to recognize these memories and/or the forces that they unleashed, which is highly variable, defines that person's analyzability. At the meeting referred to, there was general agreement that few adolescent patients are analyzable and that, where analysis is attempted, a variety of techniques involving parameters far beyond those used in the classical analysis of adults must be employed.

The major themes that emerged in the discussion concerned the fluidity and volatility of the adolescent's psychological state, the adolescent's orientation to the present and amnesia for the past, the tendency to relate to the analyst as a real object and the related inability to develop a regressive transference neurosis that, in the classical Freudian tradition, is what must be analyzed for a successful treatment outcome. It was further noted that adolescent narcissism, a normal developmental phenomenon, precludes analysis until it is renounced in late adolescence.

Others have pointed to the marked tendency for periodic regression in adolescents under stress. This tendency constitutes a specific contraindication to fostering regression in analysis, because the adolescent ego is struggling to move developmentally in the opposite direction, toward integration and stability. The analyst is confronted with the difficult dilemma of giving up a critical element of technique in the interest of promoting current growth and development, or adhering to the technique in the face of a worsening symptom picture with the hope that, in the long run, the patient's needs will be better served.

I shall try, in the remarks that follow, to address two questions: First, when is psychoanalytically based individual psychotherapy the treatment of choice for the adolescent (as opposed, for example, to biological approaches, cognitive therapy, or family therapy? Second, when, if ever, is adult-style classical analysis indicated?

Before proceeding to a more general discussion of these questions, it is essential to review the relevant aspects of normal adolescent development and adolescent psychopathology.

The Developmental Perspective

Adolescent development proceeds along five major lines: biological, emotional, cognitive, moral and social.

BIOLOGICAL

Adolescents, by their midteens, have usually achieved adult levels in the biological sense, including hormonally. Thus, the adolescent who has attained full growth, generally by 16 years of age, does not differ significantly from the adult. The fact that an adolescent may not have achieved full physical development, does not per se constitute an impediment to adult-type psychoanalysis. The obstacles lie elsewhere.

EMOTIONAL

Normal adolescents are not likely to achieve emotional maturity until they are well past their teens. Their struggle for individuation, for independence and autonomy; their efforts to establish mastery over impulses and normal adolescent narcissism and omnipotence; and their quest for identity are among the major issues with which they must deal. Are these analyzable? Not really, because we analyze what is pathological or inappropriate to the stage of development, not what is normative. We may support a youth going through these struggles, challenge what is maladaptive, and provide some insight and encouragement. For the most part, however, these conflicts must be allowed to run their course. Any interference is likely to he disruptive, with unpredictable and undesired consequences.

COGNITIVE

Although Piaget's studies (Piaget and Inhelder, 1958) have shown that formal operations (abstract thinking} are achieved by 14 years of age, subsequent work has cast doubt on the universality and completeness of this developmental milestone. Empirically, those who work with adolescents know that there are areas of cognition that continue to develop throughout the teens and beyond. A good example is perspective: intelligence and the capacity for abstraction do not give the adolescent the ability to stand back and see himself or herself with the objectivity that can come only with distance. The observing ego remains rudimentary in vital areas. At a later age, such lack of perspective can be considered pathological and analyzable. Not so during the teenage years when it is the normal state and presents a potential barrier to a rigorous application of psychoanalytic method.

MORAL

Kohlberg's (1976) explorations of moral development have led him to postulate three developmental stages, paralleling the Piagetian stages of concrete operational thinking and formal operational thought: the preconventional, which is focussed on the individual and is egocentric; the conventional, characterized by a societal focus; and the postconventional, in which values are universal, transcending any particular culture.

We know that an individual's value system figures prominently in adult psychoanalysis, notably with respect to getting and giving. Egocentricity, selfishness, altruism, generosity, concern for others, and so on are vital aspects of our work with adults. Commonly, the adolescent retains a good measure of preconventional thought (normal adolescent narcissism), which, at a later age, would represent a breakdown of healthy values. The establishment of a mature value system is closely linked to a developing sense of responsibility and accountability. These remain in an early stage of development during adolescence. The harbingers of a coherent and internally consistent value system may well be in evidence, and good measurements of responsibility and accountability are already being used. However, the

274

demands adults place on adolescents tend to be limited because of their age. (A troubling legal development, which has already been sanctioned by the U.S. Supreme Court, is to ignore such developmental markers and, increasingly, to treat younger and younger adolescents as fully responsible for the commission of violent crimes).

SOCIAL

Social development proceeds apace throughout adolescence. It is, in fact, one of the defining characteristics of adolescence. "Good" friends and "best" friends are an important part of the teenage years and are regular features in any form of psychotherapy with adolescents. In part, this social development is a direct continuation of the peer relationships established during the latency years. What is new is the sharp increase in heterosexual interest and a deepening in the emotional involvement. The sexual awakening adds a powerful new dimension to peer relations, affecting them profoundly for the remainder of the adolescent period and beyond.

Sexual activity is commonly initiated during the second decade of life, very often clumsily and with little preparation. Conflict surrounding sexuality is virtually universal, but may not be readily acknowledged by adolescents. Oedipal components in such conflict are often obvious, as Blos (1967) has pointed out, and compound the difficulties of adjustment.

In addition to the adolescent's inevitable oedipal struggle and the often uncontainable pressure of sexual urges, there are the added hurdles of learning new skills. Making conversation, broaching the subject of sex, performing adequately—all can be terrifying challenges. Yet, once these are negotiated, sexual activity can become surprisingly conflict free. The adolescent may achieve passion as well as orgasm. Noticeably lacking, however, and probably not achievable until late adolescence, as Erikson (1950) has shown, is intimacy: a psychological experience characterized by deep feelings of love, genuine give and take, and some measure of commitment.

It is noteworthy that many sexually active adolescents in therapy seldom mention their sexual behavior spontaneously. For some, this is evidence that the area is too highly charged to deal with openly. For others, it.would appear that sexual relationships are compartmentalized in such a way as to protect emotions the youth is incapable of managing. Because the capacity for responsible, shared intimacy is scarcely tested, it is impossible to predict with any certainty what the future sexual adjustment of the youth is likely to be.

Adolescent Psychopathology

Virtually all forms of psychopathology seen in adults may be seen in adolescents, some more commonly than others. Much adult psychopathology has its onset during the adolescent years, where it may be observed *in statu nascendi*. Schizophrenia, psychoneuroses, and personality disorders are common examples.

Some of the psychopathology of adolescence is characteristic of that stage of development (e.g., maladaptive behaviors such as truancy and running away, gang activity, academic failure, promiscuity and teenage pregnancy). We know these activities frequently to be symptoms of internalized conflict, the elucidation of which is a prime psychoanalytic goal. Aichhorn (1936) first made this point 70 years ago while working with delinquents in Vienna, thereby initiating the psychoanalytic exploration of adolescence. Since that time, scarcely any form of adolescent psychopathology, neurobiological syndromes such as attention deficit hyperactivity disorder (ADHD) and learning disorders included, has escaped psychoanalytic exploration. The syndromes most likely to benefit from psychoanalytic treatment are the psychoneuroses, which, in *DSM-IV* (American Psychiatric Association, 1994) are primarily subsumed under anxiety disorders and mood disorders, and personality disorders, to the extent that these may be identifiable at an early age. (In *DSM-IV*, 18 is the earliest age at which a personality disorder is presumably identifiable; however, many adolescent psychiatrists feel that personality structure and its pathology are often laid down some years earlier).

Here it is important to recall that diagnostic labels rarely provide an adequate clinical description of a disturbed adolescent. In part, this is a result of their having been designed to describe what is amiss with the individual, not with his or her world. Adolescents, who live at home, attend school, interact with peers, and are otherwise engaged with their environment, may suffer because of dysfunction in any of these areas, or, as is often the case, in several at the same time. A psychodynamic formulation that does not address all these aspects of a youth's life is incomplete.

Adolescents who come into treatment will invariably present with difficulties in the three major areas of psychic activity: reality, the

276

interpersonal sphere, and the intrapsychic sphere. In my work with adolescents, I have found it absolutely essential to distinguish among these three areas, and to think about them, individually and collectively, as a prerequisite to devising an appropriate treatment plan. Often, the possible role of some form of psychoanalytic intervention is based on a careful elucidation of these areas.

REALITY

Adolescents who enter treatment almost always have some reality problems (i.e., problems in which they are the victims of circumstances beyond their control). These may include physical illness such as diabetes or skeletal anomalies, handicapping conditions such as ADHD or a learning disorder, a psychotic mother or sadistic father, or an incompetent teacher. Although adolescents invariably suffer consequences from these realities, they are not always certain about their perceptions or clear about their responsibility, especially where it concerns their parents' beliefs and behavior. Like younger children, they may blame themselves for what may in fact be parental psychopathology.

Traditionally, the approach has been to inquire into the adolescent's adjustment to such realities, as if this were all one could do. However, hearing out the youth's grievances, expressing empathy, helping to clarify perplexing questions, providing consensual validation of accurate perceptions of others, advising him or her on how to handle a particular problem and offering support are all necessary and appropriate actions for the therapist. The youth is appreciative, gains respect for the therapist who has not automatically assumed that any problem with the adult world must be the young person's fault, develops a measure of trust, and becomes more amenable to the self-inquiry that will be needed as the therapy moves on to the more complicated interpersonal and intrapsychic issues.

THE INTERPERSONAL SPHERE

Some of what transpires interpersonally may stem from the kinds of reality problems referred to above. Here, however, it is the interaction between the parties that is of concern. Attempts to deal with this interaction by working exclusively with the adolescent are often doomed to failure. Anna Freud originally pointed to the need to see parents when working with younger children, but this was primarily for the purpose of sharing information. Since her time, there has been a major shift to a family approach in child psychiatry. More recently, mother–infant studies have underscored the degree to which parents need counselling and other support. Shapiro and Esman (1992) have emphasized that this is just as true when the identified patient is an adolescent.

In my work with adolescents, I have used a number of techniques that involve contact with parents. At times, I have seen the adolescent together with his or her parents for a session or two, or for an extended period running into months. Generally, this has been in addition to continuing individual therapy.

The goals of such a family focus will depend on the reason for introducing this modality, among which frequently are significant problems of communication, parental overcontrol, misunderstanding of the teenager's behavior, mutual hostility and destructiveness, or a combination of these. The goals may range from providing some simple guidelines and engaging the parents in the therapeutic process, to helping the parents to understand their child's ideas and behavior, to identifying serious parental pathology. The therapist may need to serve as interpreter and advocate for the adolescent, even while evincing empathy for the parents as they confront their difficulties. It is usually desirable to maintain the individual therapy of the adolescent both for continuity's sake and so that he or she will not feel that something has been taken away. This also makes it possible for the adolescent to take up in individual sessions any issues that have emerged in the family therapy.

Often, such family intervention serves to clear away obstacles that stand in the way of the adolescent's dealing with his or her intrapsychic conflicts. When, in the therapist's mind, this is clearly a goal, the work with the family may have to be kept to a minimum, and the parents may have to be referred to another therapist for additional treatment.

THE INTRAPSYCHIC SPHERE

It is here that analytic principles can be truly applied. As in adult analysis, the goal is to identify unconscious conflict by means of interpretation of symptoms, fantasies, and dreams. Transference

278

reactions will occur and may be carefully interpreted, generally when negative, and then at an ego-psychological level (i.e., in terms of their defensive importance). As mentioned earlier, a regressive transference neurosis is not likely, and should not be encouraged. Despite this, free association can be appropriate and useful, although few adolescents seem able to make use of this method. The majority of adolescents are more responsive to a give-and-take approach; thus, the therapist is generally required to be more active than when working with adults. Experienced therapists are apt to permit more of their own personality to enter the therapeutic interaction with adolescents. Use of this is, however, conditional on ongoing, careful attention to countertransference reactions, distinguishing these from appropriate emotional responses to the adolescent patient. Perhaps more so than in work with adults or younger children, a therapist's responses to an adolescent patient are likely to be interwoven with the vicissitudes of his or her own corresponding period of development. The associated importance of a personal (didactic) analysis as preparation for such work cannot be overemphasized.

Much of the therapeutic work I find myself doing with adolescents involves tracing the origins of their symptoms and conflicts, and making their self-defeating and self-destructive behavior comprehensible. For some of our colleagues, this is the essence of cognitive therapy, with its emphasis on cause and effect and irrational assumptions. For others, this is precisely what analytic work is all about, that is, reviving lost meanings and connections. By whatever name, such work is insight producing, and the hope is that such insight will permit the youth to change. Needless to say, this is often an elusive goal, even with adults. With adolescents, the limitations on the use of the analytic method increase the chances that the understanding gained will be largely intellectual, and have little emotional impact. As a result, treatment goals may have to be modest, restricted, say, to symptom relief, or fostering an improved social adjustment. Behavior modification techniques may be instituted, although the changes achieved by the adolescent may be partial, cosmetic, and short lived. They may nonetheless have a beneficial impact and make a difference in the youth's life.

By and large, once the adolescent's reality and interpersonal aspects are dealt with in therapy, I find that the remaining work tends to focus on the elucidation of the personalities and behavior of the parents or other caretakers, especially as they relate to the impact on the adolescent from his or her earliest years and through each stage of development. Much of this involves inference, all the more so because of the aforementioned adolescent amnesia for early childhood. Direct contact with the parents can provide significant insights, which, taken together with the adolescent's memories (and distortions), provide a working model of what has actually transpired in the relationship that is psychologically significant. Specific traumatic events are likely to be less significant than the ongoing, day-today parent-child communications, as the infant research to which I have already alluded has shown.

In this regard, my own clinical experience is consistent with the seminal research of Zeanah and colleagues (1989). These authors' observations led them to underscore the importance of context in development and to propose a continuous construction model of development to replace the fixation-regression model of classical psychoanalytic theory. The findings of Zeanah and colleagues have led them to observe that the origins of psychopathology are not necessarily tied to specific critical or sensitive periods of development (e.g., the oral or anal-retentive). In fact, their findings place greatest importance on the subtle interactions between parent and child, which they see as determining the vulnerabilities and invulnerabilities that will accompany the child through his or her growth and development. The internal representations of these vulnerabilities and invulnerabilities are what subsequently emerge in transferences, including those observed in psychodynamic psychotherapy. The specific components of the parent–child interaction that emerge as important, according to Peterfreund (1983), are "emotional availability, dependability, empathic attunement, sensitivity to developmental needs and provision of comfort and security". These are also the prerequisites of the therapeutic relationship, which is seen as an essential vehicle for change of the relationship pathology.

Zeanah and colleagues remind us that it is still not clear whether insight-producing therapy permits actual change in the disordered personality and psychopathology that derive from the internal representations, of whether it merely provides understanding of the patterns of vulnerability and invulnerability. This leads the authors to underscore the importance of using a variety of types of therapy as a means of maximizing the chances of change.

Case Vignette

To illustrate much of the foregoing, I shall describe the case of Paul, who was 16 when first seen by me and remained in treatment for the next 11 years, with a couple of interruptions when he was away at college and during his post-college period.

Paul came into treatment after running into academic and interpersonal problems in boarding school and making what appeared to be a suicide attempt. He had a history of academic underachievement despite high intelligence, and troubled social relationships.

Relevant family history included a highly successful, mercilessly demanding and emotionally remote father who had little patience with "psychological gobbledygook," as he would call it, and a more empathic, overinvolved, and overanxious mother, who was, however, quite controlling. His younger siblings had relatively untroubled childhoods and did well in school.

It was apparent from the outset that the psychopathology included a strong biological component, the specifics of which were not clear. (Later, it developed that the problem involved attention deficit disorder, which was confirmed by psychological testing.) In addition, the youth was depressed, angry, grandiose, and, with the exception of one male friend, socially quite isolated. He was vociferous in his criticism of his parents, in particular his father, whom he experienced as a tyrant lacking in any compassion. Characterologically, the boy had become a liar, was very manipulative, and was not in very good touch with reality about his adjustment. Nonetheless, there was a distinctly likeable quality about him, he was capable of genuine warmth, and, with his intellectual strengths, he seemed to me to offer some hope for resolution.

Therapy was truly multifaceted. His parents, very child centered and used to success, were despondent and very much at their wits' end. The father had finally recognized that all was not well with his son and was ready to seek professional help. The mother feared that he might hurt himself and was guilt ridden. They desperately needed to know what the problem was and what could be done. They were seen by me several times, and telephone communication was made available. They needed support, an opportunity to air their concerns, a clear and honest statement about their son's prognosis (I indicated it was guarded), and reassurance that they had placed their son in competent hands.

More than anything else, Paul needed a rational, empathic listener. Though there was much to confront him about—his lying, his manipulations, his grandiose fantasies in the face of repeated failure, his excessive rage at his parents—it had to wait until a solid therapeutic alliance could be established. Gradually, as he came to trust me and saw that I was not merely his parents' hireling, as he recognized the role of ADHD in his academic and interpersonal difficulties and felt relieved that he was, in fact, not just stupid and lazy, he could admit that he had lied, even to me; he could tolerate confrontation, though I had to go gently at first; and he could begin to look within, at his terrible feelings of inadequacy and impotence, at his despair that he would ever make it in life. Most of this, which finally permitted serious analytic exploration, came later in his treatment, when he was past adolescence and well into his adult years. I was able to help him understand why he had, in the context of his home and biological legacy, resorted to lying, manipulation, and embarrassing self-inflation, therapeutic work which was initiated while he was still an adolescent.

Despite taking a year off from college when he was 19, failing at a variety of small jobs, and subsequently flunking out of law school, he finally found a niche for himself in a job involving managerial responsibility, which he performed competently. In the social sphere, he established a relationship with a woman ten years his senior who was herself rather unstable emotionally. The relationship survived for two to three years, although the unmistakable oedipal elements could not be interpreted, despite his having attained full adult status. At 28, Paul remained quite sensitive to criticism, and although proud of having finally proved to his parents that he was not a total loser, continued to resist deep (id) interpretations and to dismiss them as "pop psychology."

As should be apparent from this description, Paul's problems had at least three major sources. First, an inborn biological deficit, which manifested itself as attention deficit disorder, made him different from his brother and sister and handicapped him academically in that, superior intelligence notwithstanding, he could not keep up with his peers. It also stood in the way of normal socialization throughout his childhood. Second, parents who were ill suited, by virtue of their own personality organization and psychopathology, to provide an environment that was sufficiently nurturing for a child with specialized needs. Third, dysfunctional ego development which compounded the problems significantly, interfering with his efforts to build self-esteem, and further impacting on his social relationships.

It is also clear that if I had failed to deal with the ADHD and his parents as external realities over which he had little control, any therapeutic efforts would have been unproductive. Handling these issues first during the initial phase of therapy—as it turns out, while he was still an adolescent—made it possible to move him increasingly toward more serious self-inquiry during his adult years.

Discussion

Psychoanalysis is a technique of psychiatric intervention that presumes that unconscious forces are at least partially responsible for the psychopathology in evidence, and that bringing these forces into awareness is an essential step in the relief or elimination of that psychopathology. As it has evolved, the method has relied heavily on the interpretation of transference phenomena. The point has been made that, although psychoanalysis was conceived originally as a treatment for adult psychoneuroses, its use has been extended, with modifications, to other forms of psychopathology and other age groups. I have attempted in this paper to review its applicability to adolescents. In summing up, let me now address the three basic questions:

1. What are the indications for the use of psychoanalytic techniques (whether classical psychoanalysis or psychoanalytically oriented psychotherapy) in adolescents?
2. What are the contraindications?
3. What modifications of the basic technique are appropriate when working with this age group?

INDICATIONS

As with adults, whenever there is evidence that the clinical picture is in any way related to damage inflicted in earlier childhood, for which the patient may be amnesic as the result of forgetting or repression; whenever it is clear that the patient's symptom or behavior is in part determined by internal forces beyond his or her awareness; the therapist's resort to analytic technique is indicated. Any technique that fails to elucidate such dynamics cannot hope to arrive at a definitive resolution of the pathology. No other form of psychiatric treatment pretends to expose unconscious conflict, and no other therapy makes use of transference and countertransference and has working through as its modus operandi. As previously described, the psychopathologies that most clearly apply during adolescence are the psychoneuroses and personality disorders.

In the official nomenclature (*DSM-IV*), this would include all anxiety disorders (e.g., obsessive-compulsive disorder, generalized anxiety disorder, posttraumatic stress disorder, panic disorder), and all personality disorders (e.g., narcissistic, dependent, obsessive compulsive, borderline, antisocial). Selectively, the technique may also be of value, as one of a number of therapies being employed, with conduct disorders, the psychoses, adjustment disorders, problems of drug abuse, and other pathologies.

CONTRAINDICATIONS

To the extent that the adolescent's problems concern the here and now, real objects, and matters he or she personally can do nothing about, an analytic approach is inappropriate and would be counterproductive. All psychotherapies presume that the patient is in a position to change his or her life. Analysis presumes that the change needed is internal (intrapsychic), and that if this is accomplished, the other desired changes will follow naturally.

In the case presented, the therapist had to be a real object, thus precluding the neutrality and abstinence that would be conducive to the development of transference. I frequently had to bolster the patient's faltering ego and support his struggle for autonomy, maneuvers that countered rather than fostered regression and dependency.

Because dependency is still in some measure appropriate to the adolescent condition, it is not subject to interpretation with a youth as it would be in an adult patient. Similarly, feelings of inadequacy, so common a theme with adult patients, are partly associated with the emotional, cognitive, and social immaturity that are part and parcel of adolescence. Egocentric concerns (narcissism) are also developmentally normal and therefore not subject to analysis, which would interfere with the growth process. As mentioned earlier, the problems of career and intimacy, invariably central to adult maladjustment, do not become issues for the adolescent until late in the teens. Finally, because adolescents have only partial control over their lives (parents, teachers, and others dictate most of their activities), the essential analytic condition of full personal responsibility and accountability is not present.

Modification of Analytic Technique

Whatever one's theoretical orientation, no properly trained psychiatrist (this biological era notwithstanding) can have any doubt that psychoanalytic or psychodynamic theory is one of the pillars of our understanding of mental processes and mental illness. It is the "psycho" part of the biopsychosocial approach that defines contemporary psychological medicine. For the psychoanalyst, it is an ever-present consideration, informing all treatment decisions.

Freud long ago alerted us to the dangers of "wild" psychoanalysis. In the conduct of any classical psychoanalysis, the skilled analyst knows when to apply a given technical maneuver, when to modify it, and when not to use it. Most of the necessary modifications to traditional technique have been touched on in the foregoing discussion. What follows is a review of these principles, which adds some specifics to the technical adjustments that I believe are advisable.

To begin with, the frequency can be limited to two to three times a week. The patient should not be on the couch but seated and facing the therapist. Although, as nearly as possible, the agenda should be the patient's, the therapist may on occasion decide that some unfinished business needs to be readdressed. Free association can be encouraged but not demanded. In general, the therapist must remain fairly active. I believe it is a mistake to allow long silences without breaking in and trying to interpret their meaning. Offering advice where it is clearly indicated is often appropriate.

Although all of the technical maneuvers used in classical analysis may find some application at one time or another, clarification and confrontation are likely to prove more useful than interpretation. Interpretation of fantasies and dreams may, however, prove valuable and should be based, as always, on the patient's readiness. The point has already been made that ego interpretations based on manifest content are more likely to be productive than deeper interpretations stemming from latent content that may come up in the patient's associations. Transference reactions and resistances are appropriate material for analysis but, as with every other maneuver, must be considered in the context of what is uppermost in the adolescent's concerns. The therapist must in fact constantly be considering what the patient needs most from therapy at the particular moment.

Countertransference reactions to adolescent challenges and acting out are of course common and call for sensitive handling.

As is apparent, this necessarily abbreviated list of modifications involves considerable departure from classical technique. At the same time, the essence of what psychoanalysis is all about is preserved. Perhaps more than anything else, it lies in the manner of listening, in the empathy that the therapist brings to the treatment, and in the belief in an unconscious and in its power over psychic life. What this approach adds is a measure of flexibility and ecumenism that I believe are necessary to successful work with adolescents.

Over the years of working with adolescents, I have been struck by two themes that seem to me most frequently to define adolescent concerns: These themes are competence and control. In this respect, I find myself in agreement with Basch (1988) and others in the self psychology tradition, who assert that the search for competence is the overarching motivational system driving behavior throughout life. For Basch, this subsumes curiosity, mastery, effectance, and even sex and aggression. It is the means by which self-esteem is established. It is a prerequisite to maintaining control over one's life, which is the second core concern. Repeatedly, in my clinical work, I have seen that when the quest for competence is impeded, self-esteem suffers, and depression is the result. When normal control over one's life is lost, anxiety is the consequence. Such control is achieved gradually and painstakingly through learning and is measured by one's degree of mastery over one's environment. It applies to every aspect of life and is the central driving force of our existence. It is present from infancy and infuses not only all developmental tasks, but day-to-day living at all stages of development.

Beyond their importance in normal development, issues of competence and control are relevant concerns in all psychoneuroses and personality disorders. They are therefore, I believe, the central concerns of all psychoanalytic treatment. The degree to which they can be adequately addressed or definitively resolved differs with the age of the patient and is the primary difference distinguishing analytic work with adolescents from that with adults.

Finally, I return to the original question regarding the place of traditional psychoanalysis in work with adolescents. It should be clear from the foregoing that I believe that the cases in which a clinician might choose classical psychoanalysis rather than psychoanalytically oriented psychotherapy for an adolescent below the age of 17 should be few indeed. They would most likely involve instances that combine the following:

1. A specific indication for deep, intensive psychotherapy aimed at resolving intrapsychic conflicts, usually to be found in one of the anxiety, depressive, or personality disorders.
2. A relative absence of significant intergenerational conflict, which when present, requires a family approach.
3. Good ego strength on the part of the adolescent, and a willingness to commit to the rigors of an appointment schedule of three to five times a week over a period of years.
4. Full support for such an approach from the family, both emotionally and financially. In today's climate, this is likely only in highly motivated parents, often those who have themselves undergone traditional psychoanalytic treatment.

This leaves unanswered the question of whether definitive change (e.g., in the structure of a neurosis) is possible during early to mid-adolescence. If it is not, as I believe, then such adolescent analysis must necessarily be viewed as mere preparation for later, more thorough work during adulthood.

REFERENCES

Aichhorn, A. (1936), *Wayward Youth.* New York: Putnam's Sons.
American Psychiatric Association (1994), *Diagnostic and Statistical Manual of Mental Disorders.* Washington, DC: American Pschiatric Association.
Basch, M. F. (1988), *Understanding Psychotherapy: The Science Behind the Art.* New York: Basic Books.
Blos, P. (1967), The second individuation process of adolescence. *The Psychoanalytic Study of the Child,* 22:162–186. New York: International Universities Press
Erikson, E. (1950), *Childhood and Society.* New York: Norton.
Kohlberg, L. (1976), Moral stages and moralization: The cognitive-developmental approach. In: ed. T. Lickona, ed., *Moral Development and Behavior: Theory, Research and Social Issues.* New York: Holt, Rinehart & Winston, pp. 31–53.
Peterfreund, E. (1983), *The Process of Psychoanalytic Therapy.* Hillsdale, NJ: Lawrence Erlbaum Associates.

Piaget, J. & Inhelder, B. (1958), *The Growth of Logical Thinking from Childhood to Adolescence*. London: Routledge and Kegan Paul.

Shapiro, T. & Esman, A. (1992), Psychoanalysis and child and adolescent psychiatry. *J. Amer. Acad. Child & Adoles. Psychol.*, 31:6–13.

Sklansky, M. A. (1972), Indications and contraindications for the psychoanalysis of the adolescent. *J. Amer. Psychoan. Assoc.* 20:134–144.

Zeanah, C., Anders, T. F., Seifer, R. & Stern, D. N. (1989), Implications of research on infant development for psychodynamic theory and practice. *J. Amer. Acad. Child and Adoles. Psychol.*, 28:657–668.

14   FAILURES IN EVERYDAY PSYCHOTHERAPY

RICHARD C. MAROHN*

What is expected of someone who would speak about therapy failures? That he bare his soul? That he catalog failures in some rational way? That he blame some theory or teacher? Or blame patients' limitations? Or their unsuitability for a particular form of treatment?

Somehow I could never accept a patient's being "unsuitable." It has always seemed to me that my job was to make the treatment work, unless, of course, the patient needed a kind of expertise that I simply didn't have. This was my goal when in 1969 we confronted our first hospitalized delinquent adolescent (Offer, Marohn, and Ostrow, 1976; Marohn et al., 1980) and remains my intention today when I ponder whether what I am doing is psychoanalysis or psychotherapy. In fact, it seems to me that the distinction between psychoanalysis or psychotherapy is rapidly disappearing. {For example, the concept of *enactment*, as used in the current literature, suggests that the therapist's personality inevitably has impact on the patient; parameters now have become necessary and therapeutic interventions to the successful analysis of the transference; and newly formulated perspectives of intersubjectivity and social constructivism shift our attention once again to the therapeutic relationship. Of course, this is not news to many clinicians, but I remind you that Greenberg and Mitchell (1983) have written an important volume on just this controversy within psychoanalysis.

The Notion of Failure in Psychotherapy

There is some mention of failure in the psychotherapy literature but usually in empirical studies, such as how families in therapy reunite to

*An earlier version of this paper was presented at the Annual Meeting of the American Society for Adolescent Psychiatry, March, 1984, Scottsdale, Arizona.

expel the therapist and abruptly terminate the treatment (Young, 1991) or how subjects in therapy fail because of their inability "to become involved in a therapeutic relationship and to work productively within the framework proffered by the therapist" as because of "countertransference reactions that seriously interfered with successful confrontation and resolution of the . . . negative transference" (Strupp, 1980)

This certainly sounds like a psychoanalytic perspective, but most references to failure in the psychoanalytic literature are to developmental failures. The word itself is in neither the index of Freud's writings nor the index of Kohut's writings. (Detrick, 1991).

Whether in psychotherapy or psychoanalysis, whether from an empirical or an intrapsychic perspective, one can speak objectively about failure—the treatment ends abruptly or without success or cure according to some predefined criteria. Then, there is a more subjective definition—as seen from the patient's perspective or from the psychotherapist's. {I recently had the opportunity to discuss this matter with two other experts, my daughter and son-in-law, neither one a mental health professional. Both are "experts" because they have both been psychotherapy consumers, and I well remember my teen-age daughter searching for one to two years until she connected with a psychotherapist, her fourth. When I asked them what accounts for failure in psychotherapy, they answered in unison "the relationship" and the "personality" of the therapist. Although there was a time in my professional life when I would not have accepted such naive wisdom, I am convinced that the relationship *is* fundamental, in other words, how successfully this therapist can function as this patient's selfobject. I do not mean that the therapist is a "nice guy" or a pleasant person, but that the therapist struggles to be "with" the patient and has the strength, flexibility, and depth of personality, as well as affective and cognitive skills, to tune in to an understanding of this person's unique experience.

Two recent professional experiences emphasized this issue for me. A patient described how she had been diagnosed as a "borderline personality," and her therapist proceeded to discuss her family. Instead of helping the patient explore her experiences with parents and siblings, however, the psychiatrist said that she "knew" what the patient's parents were like, because they were "the parents of a borderline." At a recent conference, several presenters decried the gratification of patient needs inherent in a "deficit" model of development and treatment and warned that, unless therapists refrained from trying to cure their patients with "love," the negative transference, deriving as it does from an aggressive drive (death instinct), would never emerge. One patient lay on the couch for 30 minutes looking at her analyst, begging him to say something affectionate, but he said nothing. After 30 minutes of silence, she became enraged, thus uncovering the underlying destructiveness! I do not question this analyst's good intentions, but I do wonder whether the patient wasn't responding to an unnecessary narcissistic injury.

I could present here testimonies or complaints from my patients about the success or failure of their treatment with me, but those statements are valuable only if they can be understood, formulated, and conceptualized in ways that would help you and me to learn more. Similarly, there is no point in cataloging here those patients, particularly adolescents, who simply quit after a short time unless I can present some reliable grasp about what happened and unless that could lead to some fruitful learning. So my purpose here is to describe clinical information that can be understood and will help explain the "failure."

Presenting such material involves self-revelation, which plays a crucial role in both successful and failed psychotherapy. Although the relationship between therapist and patient is asymmetrical, patients know a lot about their therapists, and therapists reveal a great deal— simply by what they discuss and don't, how they speak and breathe, how they sit, their familiarity with certain topics, and on and on. This idea is not new, but the self-revelation that is often our focus is the therapist's telling the patient something about himself or his life. I think that self-revelation results from the development of a **psychotherapeutic self**, whereby one is no longer concerned about the rules of taking gifts or not but recognizes the powerful impact of one's personhood on the patient's experience and will easily and naturally share something about oneself because it will either facilitate the empathic bond or move the treatment forward. On many occasions, however, such sharing is simply being human, which must be, above all, the therapist's first attribute. Thus, we hear about discussing countertransference experiences (Boyer, 1994), or of the shared intrapsychic experience from the intersubjective perspective, (Stolorow and Atwood, 1992), or how both patient and therapist construct their relationship with each other (Hoffman, 1993).

Clinical Illustrations

Given this background, I would like to discuss two instances that I as an adolescent psychotherapist experienced as failures: in the first, my theoretical orientation prevented me from understanding how the patient was experiencing the therapy; in the second, I did not anticipate a suicide early in treatment.

THE CASE OF KERRY

Kerry was 15 years old when I first met her at a girls' residential facility 27 years ago. Two years before I met her, when she was in sixth grade, she had come to the attention of both the public schools and the Juvenile Court because of academic underachievement, running away, and sexual delinquency. She was referred to the treatment center and had been living there about a year when I was asked to see her in consultation because she had become depressed and had ingested some nail polish remover. She was apparently distressed over the impending loss of her house mother, who was being transferred elsewhere. This loss resonated with earlier losses: her father's death in an auto accident, which she witnessed when she was about three, and her subsequent placement for about a year in an orphanage until her mother could get herself back together, remarry, and establish a new home for Kerry and her sister.

I began seeing Kerry in weekly psychotherapy sessions. She was often silent and said that she was seeing me only because others wanted her to. She told me a little more about herself only when, after several frustrating sessions, I attacked her wall of silence. I suppose that I was correct in addressing her defensive withdrawal, but I was clumsy. I interpreted that she did not want to become attached to me because she feared she would lose me too. In essence, I was interpreting her narcissism as a resistance to object relating. Her angry reply was, "Are you going to see me for 50 years?" She expressed her fear of my dying, as her biological father had, and wanted to terminate therapy.

I began to understand that she could not explicitly acknowledge that she did want to see me in therapy; but, with her impending release from the group home after six months of psychotherapy, we both recognized that she was continuing with the sessions by choice, and she acknowledged that therapy was important to her. Once, when I related to her a phone conversation I had had with her adoptive father about her progress and had told him that I was unsure about whether she needed long-term or short-term therapy, she angrily told me to "make up your mind." I replied, "Long-term," and she then told me more about her desolation, how she used to run away from home because she felt lonely. She was explicit about wanting my attention; for example, what did I think of her new hairstyle? She also became more serious about her boyfriend and planned to "get a ring for Christmas." She alternately called me the "great psychiatrist" who had helped her and then she would criticize my tie. She described her boyfriend as a good dresser, brought him to meet me, and was radiant. In sessions, we talked about the parallels between the two relationships, and she recognized not only how much she wanted me to approve of her, but also that she wanted me to adore her.

After she left the group home, her office psychotherapy lasted about one year until her mother and stepfather discontinued it because of the cost and their belief that she was not motivated to change. Kerry called me to tell me this and said that it "didn't matter" to her, but five months later, troubled by intensified sexual activity with her boyfriend, she asked to return to treatment. It distressed her that she was angry so often and did not enjoy sex.

She seemed more committed to our sessions than before, asked me many questions about my work, and said that she now liked talking to me. Before too long, her participation in therapy became sporadic; she was pregnant. She missed one appointment because she had secretly planned a criminal abortion and expected that I would try to stop her. We arranged for a therapeutic abortion, after which she became depressed and could not talk about the procedure and the loss, topics I felt we had to try to address. She began using marijuana, amphetamines, and LSD more frequently, continued to miss appointments, and ran away from home. Even though I tried diligently to interpret her acting out and secretly believed that she was acting out unspoken transference issues, as she had in getting pregnant, nothing worked. I felt powerless—I could only sit and wait. She finally called and said that she wanted to quit therapy because it was a "waste of time and money." I heard no more from her directly although I learned a month later, from her mother, who called me, that Kerry, hoping to find someone to love and blaming her mother for the abortion, had written a note speaking of despair and suicide. She had also been abandoned by her boyfriend. I encouraged the mother to try to get her back into therapy, but no one contacted me again. I considered my work with her a failure.

About 20 years after first meeting Kerry, I learned that her adoptive father had died, and I sent her a sympathy note. She wrote back, "It seems like an eternity since I last saw you, although I have not forgotten those sessions." She recounted how, in the intervening years, she had married, had a son three years later, was divorced three years after that, started college within a year, and graduated *summa cum laude*. She was entering her final year at a prestigious professional school. She thanked me for my expression of sympathy and asked to see me to discuss something. When we met, Kerry told me of her doubts about whether her nine-year-old son should visit his father, who had just been imprisoned on a drug conviction. She thought it would be a good idea to have him continue to see his father, her ex-husband, especially because her son's male psychotherapist had recently left the city. She also wondered about his starting with another therapist.

I was pleased, though a little surprised, that she recognized the importance of therapy for her son—surprised until she began to reflect on her own experiences. Kerry talked about her problems with loss and reminisced about her own therapy with me, her inability to talk and express herself, and how worthless she had felt. She said she remembered therapy quite well and had enjoyed it, but used to wonder why I "bothered" with her—after all, she was "just a piece of shit." That I had continued to see her and to try to help her, especially with the abortion, was very significant to her. She said that she "stored up a lot of this" but could use it only "later." As a result, she said, she would always feel free to contact me in the future if she felt the need.

Today, I can see better how my functions as a selfobject, both mirroring and idealized, helped Kerry find herself. At the time, I tried desperately to apply a drive and conflict model, tried to break through her narcissistic defenses and help her work through how previous losses had prevented her engaging with me because she feared another loss. I failed to appreciate that she *was* engaged with me. I well remember my frustration that she just wouldn't see it the way I did! This was resistance, but I failed to deal effectively with it because she got pregnant, used drugs more, ran away, and quit treatment. Now I attribute these failures to how one listens to a patient and how one's theoretical orientation facilitates or hinders one's empathic ability. I considered this therapy a failure and can now point to my "errors." Had I not tried to convince her that I was an important object but quietly accepted my role as selfobject, she might have stayed around. I am sure that she felt misunderstood, but all I could see at the time was that my efforts weren't working. One could attribute my approach to inexperience; I was just a few years out of residency, had just begun my personal analysis, and lacked the tact and finesse of an experienced therapist. To my amazement, the patient says she had a different experience, that what she found helpful was precisely what I did unintentionally, that is, mirror her while I struggled to help her. Obviously, that I cared enough to help her get the abortion was important, and, at some level, she must have identified with my respect for her, that she was not a "piece of shit."

THE CASE OF ROGER

Roger, an 18-year-old from a Chicago suburb, contacted me several years ago and was seen a few days later. His 60-year-old father, in psychotherapy with a psychoanalytically oriented psychiatrist for many years, had called me late the year before because he believed that Roger was not doing well in his freshman year in college in another state and had encouraged him to come home and get involved in psychotherapy in Chicago. The father's psychiatrist had suggested me as a resource, and I agreed to see his son for an evaluation. I had no further contact, however, until Roger called me several months later.

Roger said that he wanted to see me for reasons different from his father's. The father had told me he was concerned about Roger's poor grades and alcohol abuse, but Roger was evasive and would not tell me why his father was so concerned about these problems, nor how his father had found out about his problems with alcohol. Roger said that he was currently enrolled in a local college but had lost his job at a fast food restaurant about a month before because he worked too slowly and was forgetful. This bothered him because he felt less competent than his lower-class and poorly educated coworkers. More recently, he had felt depressed and suicidal. He had no definite plan, nor had he felt a *strong* urge to kill himself. In our first session, he told me that his mother had died of cancer seven years before (when he was 11), and he cried. He was surprised that her death still affected him so strongly. He said that he was doing well at the local college and drinking less.

My initial impression was that he was experiencing unresolved grief over the death of his mother, was depressed, and might have significant problems with alcohol and substance abuse.

I saw Roger again three days later. He was puzzled by what therapy is and how it would help him, especially because he would prefer to avoid painful discussions of his mother's death. He seemed blocked about memories of her. A 10-year-old sister died about two years before he was born, because of a brain tumor, and he believed that this death had strongly affected his parents and his older sister, 15 years older than he and three years older than the deceased sibling. I wondered to myself if he might have been experienced as a replacement child.

He noted that his family's investment in their religion declined after his mother's death, but that, while in college out of state, he had become more aware of his religious heritage. He could remember no childhood symptoms but did remember getting into fistfights from age five onward. He had had a fight during the previous Thanksgiving vacation break with his physician-cousin in the presence of his father, when his cousin kept accusing him of being an alcoholic. This episode apparently prompted his father to suggest that he come home and get into psychotherapy, and this was what he had avoided telling me initially. I felt reassured that Roger would eventually tell me what troubled him.

Roger denied that he used drugs to any significance, but I felt that we needed to assess his use of alcohol more thoroughly. He had been sexually active in foreplay and had had sexual intercourse twice. Often he felt shy and inadequate with girls. I told him that I would be recommending that he get involved in psychotherapy, with me or with another therapist of his choice, and that we would discuss that and other issues more thoroughly in the next session. Roger told me that the previous session with me had increased his feelings of depression, and he seemed reluctant to leave the office.

I saw him again one week later, and he acknowledged that he had thought of himself as a "replacement" for his deceased sister. One year after his sister's death (and one year before his birth), his mother overdosed, although this incident was never discussed in the family. He recognized this tendency to avoid painful issues. I recommended psychotherapy, discussed with him the process, the frequency, and the use of the couch, indicated that I would like to work with him. He said that he would like to think it over.

He called me for an appointment and came in one week later. He said that he had decided to come in once a week and wanted to try lying down on the couch because it would enable him to talk more freely with me. We agreed on Thursday afternoon sessions. He described how he had been drinking at a fraternity party at another local college the night before, that he felt lonely there and out of place and that he was shy, like his father, had no friends, and had had some transient suicidal thoughts. I wondered to myself if a part of him had died with his mother.

In the next week, he called me twice and seemed to be grieving, sporadically. I saw him the following Thursday. Sometimes, he would cry with no images, and sometimes, he felt aggrieved with memories of his mother. At times, he felt choked up and found it hard to breathe; he was talking a lot with friends about his mother. He asked for more frequent sessions, and we agreed on twice-a-week sessions, Mondays and Thursdays.

I was out of town the next Friday and Saturday for a meeting which did not affect his schedule. Ironically, the meeting was a work group of psychiatrists preparing a monograph on adolescent suicide; I was, at that time, hearing of the latest research in the field—risk factors, the assessment process, and the like.

On the next Monday, he said that he was no longer feeling so moved by the loss of his mother and even wondered if he had been forcing it. As he was about to leave the session, he said that he would no longer need to come in twice a week and wanted to cut back to once a week. I refused to do this and said that we would need to discuss this further on Thursday. He seemed to acquiesce to my request. Roger called me that evening, however, to say that he was intent on cutting back to once a week, and that he was canceling the next two sessions (Thursday and Monday) and would see me on Thursday of the next week. I disagreed with him and told him that we needed to continue, at least to talk over his ideas about cutting back. To emphasize this, I told him that, as we had agreed, I would be charging for these two appointments and that I hoped that he would keep them with me. In retrospect, I sense that I made this threat because I felt desperate.

Roger's father called me the next evening, Tuesday, about 11:30 PM to say that Roger had killed himself by jumping off the roof of the parking garage next to my office building about 3 PM that afternoon. He died a few hours later at a local hospital. I was in such disbelief that I had to confirm this with a nursing supervisor on duty. Father asked, "What did he talk about with you Monday?" I told him, and then he added that Roger had been doing better and had been pleased with an A in a course. Father was obviously distraught but said that he felt supported by his female companion who had now moved in with him. A mental health professional, she told him that often suicide cannot be predicted. Father was concerned because he had been out of town over the weekend, "when you were out of town." I was surprised to hear that he knew I had been gone for the meeting and assumed that Roger had tried to call me but left no message. I described how Roger had wanted to cut back on sessions and that I had refused but that he had called back and insisted. Father said that he knew about this. I told Father that I would call him in the morning. I wanted to be sure that he was in touch with his own psychiatrist to help him during this terrible experience. I also wondered whether Roger had come to my office that Tuesday afternoon, when I was with other patients, but I had no way of knowing.

I spoke to Father again the next morning. He and I both expressed shock and surprise at Roger's suicide. Father said that Roger had been laughing while talking on the phone Sunday night with another student, a girl with whom he often spoke. Father then read me the note Roger had left him. It said that Roger loved him, that he hated to give Father another loss after Sister and Mother, but that he could not go on, that suicide was "inevitable"—that ever since Mother died, he had been depressed and that there was no alternative. He thanked Father for trying to help him by getting him into therapy. He said that he was going to jump off the building where Father had come looking for him; he listed my office address. I was confused about what this meant, and Father explained that after Roger's Monday session with me, he could not start his car in the adjacent parking garage because he had left the headlights on, and so he called his father for a battery jump. By the time Father arrived at the garage, Roger had gotten a jump from a security guard and gone home. Father was aware of our phone conversation about canceling and had encouraged Roger to keep the appointments, especially if he was going to have to pay for them. Father said he would be seeing his psychiatrist with whom I spoke and who told me that he was aware of the suicide and was also surprised, especially because Roger seemed to be "object related." I mentioned the site of the suicide, next to my office, and he wondered about a "psychotic transference."

A few months later, Roger's sister called me from the city where she lives. She asked for my thoughts about Roger's suicide. She described how she had helped her father sort out Roger's belongings and that she had been surprised by the "depth" of the high school essays they found. No one ever suspected that he had been suicidal, although she had strongly urged him not to return to the out-of-state school for the second semester and to get into treatment. She was matter of fact with me on the phone and seemed satisfied with what I had said in reviewing the treatment. She obviously felt some guilt about not being able to prevent the suicide. I said that she should call me whenever she wished. She said that her father was continuing in treatment and that his friend was a source of great help to him.

I was shocked and seriously moved and saddened by this suicide, the first I had had in 24 years of practice. I thought it ironic that I was participating in ongoing workshop discussions about adolescent suicide. I tried to master the experience partly by reviewing what we had been discussing and by planning to share this experience with my colleagues at our next meeting. Roger had discussed with me his suicidal ideation, but I did not think he was at risk; there was no plan, no lethality, no strong urges. There is, however, a family history of a suicide attempt, a family history of depression, a death he experienced and another in the family before his birth. Other important factors are that he was male, that he used alcohol, and that he was impulsive. His history did not substantiate a career of impulsivity, but his behavior with me in suddenly deciding to decrease the frequency of the sessions was impulsive. Certainly, I am aware that some depressed persons feel better when they have decided on suicide and have a plan, but I did not judge that relevant here because Roger had said that he would keep his Thursday appointment the following week. I fully expected to see him again.

Jumping from the garage adjacent to my office is relevant and strongly suggests a transference response, but I don't know what more to infer from this. Roger wrote his father a very explicit note, maybe hoping that the father would stop him, but his father was at work. He may have come by the office to see me. He may have been enraged with me. Yet I saw no evidence of the "psychotic transference" and felt that we were developing an alliance in the six sessions we had had over the course of a month. Was it a mistake to let him use the couch? He seemed to have no difficulty moving from the couch to the outside world, and I saw no evidence of a strong or irreversible regression. I thought that he was grieving and that this was begun partly because I had correctly interpreted to him his unresolved reactions to his mother's death. I felt that I was in empathic contact with him. Retrospectively, I wonder about my leaving the one-week gap between sessions when he had called me twice, but I had no open times in my schedule and did not feel that he had to be seen on an emergency basis. I don't know whether my absence over part of the weekend was an issue; it did not interfere with any scheduled session, but obviously both his father and he were aware of my being gone.

So I continue to feel bad that Roger killed himself—guilty and defensive—but I still don't know if I could have prevented it. I never considered hospitalization to be necessary, and I did not prescribe an antidepressant because he had no vegetative signs. Yet the risk factors were there: a family history of suicide attempt and of depression, male, impulsive, depressed, a loss, and alcohol usage. In reviewing and rewriting this paper, I noticed that I had mentioned these risk factors earlier, but I decided to leave them in because they demonstrate how I am still going over the data. My colleagues have been gentle with me, but one suggested hospitalization and another a family diagnostic with the father present. How well or how poorly was I listening? What about the risk factors my colleagues and I were discussing? I sensed that my relationship with Roger had not yet got moving. After all, isn't the nature of the relationship the best protection against a suicide?

It is obvious that I continue to be troubled by this suicide, to a great extent because I couldn't or didn't do the right thing. This is a matter of personal and professional pride. This manifestation of transformed personal grandiosity is important to the healthy functioning of a psychotherapist—it is professional self-esteem, confidence in oneself. We must wonder, though, if, at times, such pride can interfere with one's therapeutic work or interfere with introspection about such an event.

Discussion

As I review these two treatment reports, I see similarities in how I understand them and why I consider them failures. All involve in one way or another my preoccupation with my own professional competence and skill. In each instance, narcissistic concerns interfered with my ability to listen to my patients.

Kerry was a difficult adolescent to treat because at the same time as she communicated a desperate need for contact and attention, she also rejected it, fought it, and tested it. The feeling of omnipotence that had moved me to seek medicine as a career and had prompted me to try to "save" others was severely tested here. During my psychiatric training, I began to learn that good intentions were not enough, that sound clinical theory would help, and so, I tried to apply theory, at times vigorously, to try to keep Kerry from "acting out." Yet my redirected diligence prevented me from relaxing and letting the mirror transference unfold. Such transferences had only then begun to be defined by Kohut, but I could have done more by "doing less"— simply by listening to her and not demanding of her the allegiance no adolescent can give. I could have done more had I not needed to protect myself from her neediness by insisting that she verbalize it. On the other hand, I did act like a committed "doctor," and that seems to have accomplished something.

Roger's suicide continues to puzzle and plague me. I wonder whether my belief in the power of the "relationship" caused me to ignore the risk factors that he presented. I wonder whether something prevented me from listening to him, from recognizing the devastation he had experienced when his mother died, and perhaps from recognizing that initially I had abandoned Roger by leaving too much to his own choosing, by not structuring the relationship more firmly, and by not being more available to him. Roger left his father a note, but he sent me a strong message as well.

Tensions between one's role as psychotherapist and one's personality may interfere with listening. Hoffman (1993) sees such tension as not simply inevitable, but as essential to the therapeutic process and to a positive outcome and cure. He notes the dialectic between the therapist's discipline and his expressive participation, between therapeutic authority and personal authenticity, and between the asymmetry and the mutuality of the psychotherapeutic encounter. Hoffman notes that the patient needs the psychoanalyst (or psychotherapist) to survive in his role, discipline, authority, and asymmetry, while simultaneously, at the deepest level, the patient is nourished by the psychoanalyst's (psychotherapist's) personality, participation, authenticity, and mutuality. This is the patient's dialectic, because both are necessary to a successful outcome. This perspective is not unlike Kohut's (1984) emphasis on the importance of both the understanding phase, with empathic contact, and the explanatory phase, with interpretation and reconstruction.

I suggest that there is another perspective to the therapist's struggle, similar to the dialectic of role and personality—how certain transformations of primitive narcissism are involved in the therapeutic process. The therapist's empathic ability, therapeutic ambition, confidence, ideal paradigm, wisdom, creativity, and sense of humor all participate. I suspect that in our model therapist these are all operating harmoniously and without conflict. Yet, depending on the therapist's unique organization, one may occupy central stage to the detriment of another. I suspect further that such an imbalance can lead to therapeutic failure.

If I am preoccupied with pursuing my therapeutic model and fulfilling my theoretical ideals, I might fail to be empathically in tune with my patient. If I am unable to respond creatively and with humor to an irreverent adolescent like Kerry because I feel my therapeutic ambitions thwarted and confidence threatened, I am unable to listen to her and follow her needs. In other words, it helps the patient that I try to be right, that I strive to be perfect, but that can also interfere seriously with my listening to my patient. On the other hand, if I listen but have no way of organizing the data, I may fail my patient as well. Here, I could become infatuated with the power of attunement and neglect the wisdom of others' models. As you may have guessed, I still wonder if I failed to recognize that Roger was at severe risk, or that he was telling me that this was all too much, that he had to curtail the intensity of what he felt. As you can see, the dialectic continues—and perhaps it continues and continues, as long as one struggles to become a psychotherapist—until one achieves wisdom!

Conclusion

What is failure in psychotherapy is open to many definitions. In this presentation, I have tried to view failure from the therapist's perspective and review clinical material that is sufficiently detailed to stimulate inference and formulation. I have tried to consider how the therapist's various narcissistic preoccupations can disrupt his clinical skill. The issue is not that one has pride in one's work or that one tries to learn and grow, but rather that intense immersion in theory or technique can sometimes interfere with listening. Only by reviewing and studying our failures can we as professionals justify our patients' trust. Only by recognizing that our work involves struggle can we learn to trust ourselves.

REFERENCES

Boyer, L. B. (1994), Countertransference. *J. Psychother. Prac. & Res.*, 3:120–137.

Detrick, D. W. (1991), Index to the complete works of Heinz Kohut. In: *The Search for the Self, Vol. 4*, ed. P. Orenstein. Madison, CT: International Universities Press, pp. 741–848.

Greenberg, J. R. & Mitchell, S. A. (1983), *Object Relations in Psychoanalytic Theory*. Cambridge, MA: Harvard University Press.

Hoffman, I. (1993), Dialectical thinking and therapeutic action in the psychoanalytic process. Presented at Chicago Psychoanalytic Society, March 23.

Kohut, H. (1966), Forms and transformation of narcissism. *J. Amer. Pschoanal. Assn.*, 14:243–272.

——— (19840, *How Does Analysis Cure?* ed. A. Goldberg & P. Stepansky. Chicago: University of Chicago Press.

Marohn, R. C., Dalle-Molle, D., McCarter, E. & Linn, D. (1980), *Juvenile Delinquents*. New York: Brunner/Mazel.

Offer, D., Marohn, R. C. & Ostrov, E. (1979), *The Psychological World of the Juvenile Delinquent*. New York: Basic Books.

Strupp, H. H. (1980), Success and failure in time-limited psychotherapy: Further evidence. *Arch. Gen. Psychiat.*, 37:947–954.

Stolorow, R. D. & Atwood, G. E. (1992), *Contexts of Being*. Hillsdale, NJ: The Analytic Press.

Young, D. W. (1991), Family factors in failure of psychotherapy. *Amer. J. Psychother.*, 45:499–510.

15 SELF PSYCHOLOGY PERSPECTIVES ON ADOLESCENTS*

GUSTAVO LAGE**

In this paper, I have chosen to discuss several different topics related to Self-Psychology about which I have, over many years of practice, developed some strong views. As I developed my own concepts I realized that I was thinking differently from my beloved teachers, a very disturbing thought because they had provided the foundations on which I could build and create. Although these are people that I admire, I would like to demonstrate that we have to look at adolescents differently from the way that we have all tended to look at them. Throughout our psychiatric literature we talk about "we mature adults" and "those immature adolescents". That suggests some hostility toward them. I am not questioning the validity of those writings in expanding our understanding of adolescents, but if we examine them more closely, we can learn even more. Further on in this paper I speculate on some of the reasons for the gap that we create between adolescents and ourselves.

The Continuing Life of the Oedipus Complex

I would like to begin by exploring some basic theories of adolescent development, a further expansion of them by Peter Blos, and my suggestions for an extension of that theory. Blos (1977) wrote that psychoanalytic theory "postulates that the Oedipus complex was resolved, for better or for worse, at the end of early childhood, and reappears, essentially unchanged, at puberty. . . . " He goes on to say

*This chapter is a revised version of Dr. Lage's Schonfeld Award Address, March 1994.

**I would like to thank Philip Katz, past president of ASAP for his assistance in editing this paper.

that "during adolescence, however, a continuation, not only a recapitulation of the oedipal conflict, becomes apparent" (p. 7) I think that this is a very important contribution, and I would like to take it a step further. The Oedipus complex continues not only from childhood into adolescence but on into and throughout adulthood. The process of development never ends, it is never completed, in any of its various lines, but moves ever onwards. The Oedipus complex, which first appears at age 4 continues, becoming more visible at puberty, during the adolescent years, during parenthood, and again when we become grandparents. It is very important to see it as an ongoing developmental process.

In my clinical practice, I have seen adolescent developmental struggles continue into adulthood—young, mature, middle, and senior adulthood. It is essential to see that we therapists, continue to struggle with the problems of our own adolescence. If we cannot accept our own adolescence, then we are not able to treat adolescents appropriately. In my view, the recognition of the continuation of adolescent conflicts into adulthood is a very important step in the development of our abilities to treat adolescents.

The Depreciation of Adolescents

There is a tendency in our society and in our profession to separate off the adolescents from the adults, to create a we–they division. This tendency has been evident in our literature for a long time. "I see no hope for the future of our people if they are dependent upon the frivolous youth of today, for certainly all youth are reckless beyond words. . . . When I was a boy, we were taught to be discreet and respectful of our elders, but the present youth are exceedingly wise and impatient of restraint." This quotation, although almost modern in sound, was written by the ancient Greek poet Hesiod and dates approximately from the eighth century B.C. (cited in Pumpian-Mindlin, 1965, pp. 2–3).

Aristotle, 400 years later, but 2300 years ago, commented:

> The young are . . . prone to desire and ready to carry any desire they may have formed into action. Of bodily desire it is the sexual to which they are the most disposed to give way, and in regard to sexual desire they exercise no self-restraint. They are changeful, too, and fickle in their desires, which are as transitory as they are vehement. . . . they are passionate, irascible, and apt to be carried away by their impulses. . . . they have high aspirations; for they have never yet been humiliated by

the experience of life. . . . if the young commit a fault, it is always on the side of excess and exaggeration. . . . they regard themselves as omniscient and are positive in their assertions; this is, in fact, the reason of their carrying everything too far [p. 18].

These reactions to adolescent behavior are manifested in our contemporary life in statements like, "Hire adolescents while they still know everything," and "It is amazing how much my parents learned when I was between the ages of 17 and 21." There seems to be a strong need to depreciate our youth, not only by adults, but even by psychiatrists and psychoanalysts, who many times in their theoretical formulations have shown subtle notes of depreciation of adolescents.

Blos (1977) described the adolescent tasks as being: achieving ego continuity, proceeding through the second individuation, forming a sexual identity, and the working through of residual trauma. He sees them as developmentally specific tasks at the end of adolescence. This implies that the passage into adulthood signals the end of the immaturity and confusions of adolescence, and the arrival of stability, good judgment and clarity of vision. It implies a "holier than thou" attitude toward the adolescents. Why do we need to dig a gulf between adolescence and adulthood?

Pumpian-Mindlin describes omnipotentiality as consisting primarily of the feeling and conviction on the part of the youth that he can do anything in the world, solve any problem in the world if given the opportunity, and if it is not given, he will create it. There is no occupation which is inaccessible, no task which is too much for him. As his perspective of the world broadens, as his horizon widens, he begins to question everything which his elders have come to accept. Nothing is impossible, nothing can be taken for granted. He can indulge in wild flights of the imagination, soaring speculations, incredible adventures. He knows no limits in fantasy, and accepts grudgingly any limits in reality. Yet, at the same time, he finds it difficult to do one thing and follow it through to completion, because to do so would mean to commit himself to one thing primarily, and this he is not yet prepared to do.

I have made many commitments in my lifetime, not all of which I followed through, and I have many more to make. The exaggeration in the description of adolescent behavior by Pumpian-Mindlin does imply a bias—that adolescents are egocentric, omnipotent, omniscient, and megalomanic. Such behavior by adolescents is frequently observed, but is not the rule. I would suggest that even though the clinical manifestations of omnipotence are present in teenagers, they are there as well when we are dealing with mature adults. And I would further suggest that narcissistic developmental tasks continue throughout our lives, and that the struggles with such narcissistic issues as grandiosity don't end in adolescence.

The Continuation Throughout Adulthood of Adolescent Developmental Tasks

Settlage (1972) wrote:

This process of measuring oneself and one's culture and modifying one's ideals and aspirations requires relinquishments which may engender a sense of loss, feelings of depression, and a kind of mourning. In relation to the self, one may have to give up a long held wish for perfection. Such a relinquishment during adolescence is comparable to a similar relinquishment which occurs during a successful analysis, frequently as a part of termination. In both instances, the acceptance of one's personal limitations, along with the reality that time is finite for everyone, causes a painful sense of loss. But this acceptance also has its rewards, since, after the sense of loss is worked through, the individual finds that he sets more reasonable goals which can be more readily met, and he enjoys a new-found sense of achievement and self-esteem. In relation to culture and society, one may have to give up some cherished ideals and learn to live with uncertainty, ambiguity, and only partially attainable goals. In this connection, I offer the recently made statement of a well-known public servant: "Throughout our history we believed that effort was its own reward. Partly because so much has been achieved here in America, we have tended to suppose that every problem must have a solution and that good intentions should somehow guarantee good results. Utopia was seen not as a dream, but as a logical destination if we only travelled the right road. Our generation is the first to find that the road is endless, that in travelling it we will find not utopia but ourselves. The realization of our essential loneliness accounts for so much of the frustration and rage of our time." (Henry Kissinger, 1972) [pp. 90–91].

Settlage says that at the end of adolescence there is a relinquishment of ego ideals and an acceptance of attainable goals in their place. I do not think we ever relinquish our ego ideals for attainable goals. I believe that the modification of our ego ideals is a never-ending process, a struggle within ourselves, throughout our life cycle, and that the ego ideals continue all through our lives as realistic and unrealistic sustaining thoughts. They are the origins of our imagination and creativity.

The modification of our ego ideals is a part of the process of maturation from archaic selfobjects to more mature selfobjects. When we enter therapy it is with the hope of finding an omniscient and omnipotent therapist who will fulfill our infantile wishes. During the course of therapy we realize that our infantile wishes will continue to exist throughout our lives, necessitating constant modifications, as we struggle with the limitations of our relationships.

There is considerable ambivalence amongst our theoreticians about this relinquishment of magical beliefs for attainable goals. Sigmund Freud (1930) wrote:

> The fateful question for the human species seems to me to be whether and to what extent their cultural development will succeed in mastering the disturbance of their communal life by the human instinct of aggression and self-destruction. It may be that in this respect precisely the present time deserves a special interest. Men have gained control over the forces of nature to such an extent that with their help they would have no difficulty in exterminating one another to the last man. They know this, and hence comes a large part of their current unrest, their unhappiness and their mood of anxiety. And now it is to be expected that the other of the two "Heavenly Powers," eternal Eros, will make an effort to assert himself in the struggle with his equally immortal adversary. But who can foresee with what success and with what result? [p. 145].

Freud talks about the need to be realistic but ends with wishes for a magical solution.

My grandson recently played the role of a munchkin in *The Wizard of Oz*, a play in which, if one does the right thing and follows the yellow brick road, one will find the Wizard, an omnipotent being. In reality, he is not a wizard. He plays the role of a therapist, who helps others to find what they need within themselves, whether it is a heart, a brain, or courage. The play ends with the idea that reality does not prevail, you just click your heels, and you find your way home. The return to magical beliefs resumes. This particular phenomenon, that at times of stress we need to believe in the omnipotent powers of others in order not to feel deflated, is ongoing throughout our lives.

So, my criticism of these theories—of Blos's theory that there are specific tasks to be accomplished by the end of adolescence, which when accomplished transforms one into an adult; of Pumpian-Mindlin's picture of adolescence, highlighted by an omnipotence that practically disappears in adulthood; and of Settlage's theory that at the end of adolescence there is a transformation of grandiosity to attainable goals—is that I see all those phenomena continuing to a significant degree right through adulthood rather than demarcating the end of adolescence.

Treatment Difficulties Due to the Therapist's Own Adolescent Conflicts

I do believe, though, that many adults, and many therapists, have difficulties with adolescents because of their own conflicts about these developmental processes. They haven't coped with and worked through their problems with their own parents, and this handicaps them, sometimes paralyzes them, when it comes to dealing with their patients, and often, their own adolescent children. They are still dancing to the background music of their own adolescent years, instead of hearing the adolescent's background music.

We have seen that there is much subtle and often overt hostility on the part of the adult world toward its adolescents, even on the part of adolescent therapists. This raises the following questions:

1. Are adults afraid of the reactivation of their own Oedipal conflicts?
2. Are adults afraid of the return of their own repressed omnipotent beliefs?
3. Are adults concerned that in the process of separation-individuation the adolescents will abandon them?
4. Are adults afraid that the adolescents, the next generation, will be different from them?

I suggest that for adults the worst fears arise when they see fragmentations occurring in adolescents, for they are then reminded of their own vulnerability, and the fears of their own fragmentation. These fears make it difficult for the therapist to immerse himself or herself in an adolescent patient's experience. Schwaber (1983) stated her belief that the major contribution of Kohut in regard to the therapeutic process can be illustrated by our need to change our position— from separateness from the patient to becoming immersed through introspection in what the patient's experience is like.

310

In the preceding quotations of Blos, Pumpian-Mindlin, and Settlage, adolescence is formulated from a position of the separateness of the adolescent from the adult, a we–they stance. They are seen as being different from us. In order to have an empathic understanding, we need to put ourselves into what the adolescent is experiencing, to sense what it is like to go through turmoil, and we need to be ready to deal with our then growing awareness of how we felt back in our own adolescence. To do so, there has to be a theoretical change in our understanding of the adolescent's activity in therapy. Instead of the therapist seeing himself or herself as the object of the drive, the therapist must come to understand that the adolescent is having a loss of cohesiveness and is very frightened and vulnerable—the therapist needs to be able to experience that with the adolescent. Our understanding of our patients will be completely different then, as I will describe in the following illustration:

A patient in analysis came to the office and tore a subscription form out of one of my magazines. The patient was not going to discuss this with me, and when I asked what was the meaning of the tearing off of the subscription form in the magazine, he was not able to explain his behavior. I recognize that I was annoyed, maybe at the patient for not wanting to answer me, or maybe for his tearing the magazine as if he had intentions to tear me apart. Not until much later was I able to change my understanding of the patient. Instead of looking at what he was doing to me, as the object of his aggressive drive, I started understanding that for a long time my patient had been reading that magazine as a way of keeping himself together while he was waiting for me. One day the magazine, which was old, was removed from the waiting room by my cleaning woman and was replaced by new ones. My patient had lost his transitional object and was desperately looking to regain what he had lost. A few days before the incident described, he had written down the address of the magazine intending to order it, but he did not do so. He felt that tearing off the subscription form might facilitate his accomplishing what he needed so badly—to keep himself together. I was wrong in believing that he was being aggressive toward me; he was only attempting to keep himself together during the process.

That brings us to the topic of empathic listening. The question is often asked, does the self-psychologist have a kind of empathy different from the one that we have had up to now? Kohut (1984) answered that question as follows: We have a different theory now, one which permits us to understand some aspects of our patients in a depth and breadth that was not possible before.

> If a patient tells me how hurt he was because I was a minute late or because I did not respond to his prideful story of success, should I tell him that his responses are unrealistic? Should I tell him that his perception of reality is distorted and that he is confusing me with his father or mother? Or should I rather say to him that we all are sensitive to the actions of people around us who have come to be as important to us as our parents were long ago and that, in view of his mother's unpredictability and his father' disinterest in him, his perception of the significance of my actions and omissions has been understandably heightened, and his reactions to them intensified? Clearly, it is the second response that provides the patient with a more accurate assessment of that aspect of reality with which we deal in psychoanalysis. And to insist that we should tell him otherwise—that we should tell him with even the faintest trace of disapproval that he confuses the present and the past, that he mixes us up with his parents, and the like—is as misguided as to insist that our painters should go back to the medieval style and paint distant objects the same size as near ones [p. 172].

The theory has changed, and that permits us to understand behavior in a different way from the way we have understood it in the past, as in the example that I gave previously about my patient.

A classic example of this is Freud's treatment of Dora (1905), the first treatment of an adolescent patient. As we review it now, it is amazing to us that the creator of psychoanalysis was not able to empathize with the feelings of this adolescent female. Because Dora had been bothered by repressed drives, Freud was able to overlook the facts—that Dora had been sexually abused and that she was being used by adults for their benefit—without consideration of her feelings, and that she was overwhelmingly anxious and apprehensive.

Therapist and Patient as a Contextual Unit

Another important contribution of self-psychology in the treatment of adolescents is seeing the patient and therapist as a contextual unit. This implies that in the reconstruction of our formulations, we include how the adolescents are reacting to the way that we are perceiving them. If at times we fail to be empathic, we will see an adolescent who has become suspicious, distrustful, feels the room has been bugged, and who is slightly paranoid. That is the time for us to look at the contextual unit of the patient and therapist. We need to know what transpired in the previous session, why the patient felt so misunderstood that he or she is falling apart like Humpty Dumpty and needs to be put back together. This concept of looking at our involvement in the reactions of patients has been present throughout many years of psychotherapy and understood by most therapists. Self-psychology greatly enhanced its significance by utilizing empathy as the chief focus of the psychotherapeutic process.

I would like to further illustrate the psychotherapeutic process with the following case presentation: Peter lost his father when he was 16 and his mother when he was 17. His father died of an acute myocardial infarction; his mother, after a long illness, died of cancer. Peter remembers how he was afraid to go out in the evening lest he would come home and find his mother dead. This went on for a long period of time. At the time that he came for treatment, his girlfriend had broken off their relationship because she had begun dating somebody else. Peter had recently tried to kill himself. After many months of treatment he started showing his vulnerability about the break-up with his girlfriend. He could not resist his impulses to call her, to maintain contact with her. He desperately needed to pass in front of her house, always wondering if her new boyfriend would be there. Even though this produced a number of painful experiences for him, he could not stop himself from being driven to maintain contact with her. In his desperate need, he lent her his car, so she could go out and at times give rides to her new boyfriend, while Peter was taking public transportation, even to come to his therapy sessions. When this procedure did not bring about the desired restoration of his self-cohesion, he became angry with her, especially when she was late in returning his car. Many times Peter would not leave his house because his girlfriend might call him. It was a similar pattern to his not accepting the trauma of his mother's death, and not being able to leave the house while she was sick with cancer because he feared she might die. He could not bear to lose these selfobjects. The main treatment processes for Peter were the therapist's understanding of these fragmentations and of his desperate need to be in contact with the girlfriend, and the therapist's realization that the resultant behaviors should not be put down or attacked, for Peter was doing the best that he could to keep himself together. The explanation of this behavior, along with his therapists's empathic stance, proved most therapeutic for Peter.

I wish to emphasize that empathy has become a glorified word in our field today. I do not believe that empathy has a curative power in itself, but rather, it is a way to listen to what is going on in the patient. The real working through of adolescent psychopathology is through a process very similar to the one that Freud formulated. Freud said that the patient forms a libidinal attachment to the therapist, resulting in the formation of a transference in which the disappointments and frustrations that occur in the therapy reactivate the disappointments and frustrations in the patient's past history. Working through these in the transference is essential for the amelioration of the problems and for the potential cure for these patients. The same applies to self-psychology. The patient comes, needing mirroring for his grandiosity, or an idealization of the therapist. The abrupt de-idealizations that occur in the therapy bring about fragmentations and some working through and reconstruction of those earlier experiences of empathic failure and de-idealization, thus enabling the patient to reconstruct his past and to change his future. Aristotle (n.d.) said that adolescents "have high aspirations; for they have never yet been humiliated by the experience of life" (p. 18). What he is saying is that adolescents have the quality of grandiosity because they have not yet experienced the realities of frustrations and defeats that all adults have experienced. Many of our patients need our help in working through their reactions to the inevitable failures in life, so that they can control their grandiosity and set more mature goals for themselves.

I wish to take a fresh look at the separation-individuation process. Separation-individuation is described in classical theory as a need for self-sufficiency, autonomy, liberty, and freedom from parental figures. I believe that the separation-individuation process focuses on autonomy, whereas self-psychology focuses on the need for selfobjects throughout life. Growth implies the maturation of selfobject relationships.

The adolescent needs parents who are worthy of admiration, can admire and respect the uniqueness of the adolescent, and can recognize the adolescent's need to assert himself or herself, and to become a person with an autonomy of his or her own. If the parents are not able to encourage the adolescent's self-strivings because of their own grandiosity, the adolescent will continue to look for archaic selfobjects to help him or her to maintain self-cohesiveness.

At this time, I would like to describe some aspects of my own adolescence and young adulthood. Separation does not need to be a loss that is insurmountable. Separation could be the transition to a new world. For example, I was born in a small town in Cuba, but I decided to find a new land and a new scientific belief. I wanted to become a psychoanalyst, leaving what was familiar to me to take a new voyage, a new trip, a new discovery. I experienced this not as a loss, but as an opportunity for self-development, even though I was losing the familiarity of what I had known up to that time. This particular voyage has continued throughout my life and throughout my professional career as an analyst, and as a past president of this society. Most of all, I am very proud to have been fortunate enough to receive the prestigious Schonfeld Award. It represents to me recognition of my ability to relate to the members of ASAP with joy and satisfaction and gives me a feeling of accomplishment among my peers.

The Maintenance of Narcissistic Equilibrium

If I were to specify what I believe is the main task of the transition from adolescence to adulthood, I would say it is regulation of self-esteem, the maintenance of narcissistic equilibrium. To do that, adolescents need to reconstruct the past, and to own that past as their own historical truth. For this to be accomplished there is a great need for parental understanding of the process, and for the encouragement of the transition toward adulthood. Without parental encouragement, this task tends to be truncated, and the adolescent feels empty and depleted.

During adolescence, there is also a reactivation of the grandiose self, which needs considerable mirroring from the parents. There is concomitantly a tendency to idealize the parents, and a tendency to react with narcissistic rage when the idealization fails abruptly.

As Nathan and I have described (Lage and Nathan, 1991), one of the most important tasks of adolescence is finding other adolescents who are like themselves. The need for this feeling of alikeness does not only appear in adolescent development, it continues throughout life: in finding a twin to write a book, in finding a tennis partner, in finding colleagues. We continue all our lives needing mature selfobjects that will work with us in accomplishing our goals. To me, the most significant contribution of self-psychology is its emphasis on the idea that we continue to need people throughout our lives as an integral part of our ongoing development.

315

Summary

I do not see a clear line of demarcation between adolescence and adulthood. I believe that the developmental processes of childhood and adolescence continue throughout our lives. We always need selfobjects to mirror us, to be admired by us, and to give us a feeling of alikeness. Hopefully, as we develop, the selfobjects we seek will be more mature and less archaic.

Our struggles with our own developmental processes interfere with our roles as therapists for adolescents. We fear the reactivation of our adolescent struggles, which hampers our empathic listening to our patients, and makes it difficult for us to see the therapist–patient contextual unit. It is necessary for therapists to work through these impediments so that their adolescent patients can be helped to reconstruct their life history and proceed with their development. Both therapists and patients need to be on voyages of self-discovery.

REFERENCES

Aristotle (n.d.), In: *The Universal Experience of Adolescence*, ed. N. Kiell. Boston, MA: Beacon Press, pp. 18–19, 1964.

Blos, P. (1977), When and how does adolescence end: Structural criteria for adolescent closure. *Adolescent Psychiatry*, 5:5–17. New York: Aronson.

Freud, S. (1905), Fragment of an analysis of a case of hysteria. *Standard Edition*, 7:7–122. London: Hogarth Press, 1953.

———— (1930), Civilization and its discontents. *Standard Edition*, 21:64–145. London: Hogarth Press, 1961.

Kohut, H. (1984), *How Does Analysis Cure?* ed. A. Goldberg & P. Stepansky. Chicago: University of Chicago Press.

Lage, G. A. & Nathan, H. K. (1991), *Psychotherapy, Adolescents, and Self-Psychology*. Madison, CT: International Universities Press.

Pumpian-Mindlin, E. (1965), Omnipotentiality, youth, and commitment. *J. Amer. Acad. Child Psychiat.*, 4:1–18.

Schwaber, E. (1983), Psychoanalytic listening and psychic reality. *Int. Rev. Psychoanal*, 10:379.

Settlage, C. F. (1972), Cultural values and the superego in late adolescence. *The Psychoanalytic Study of the Child*, 27:74–92. New Haven, CT: Yale University Press.

16 THE PSYCHOTHERAPEUTIC PATHWAY TO ADAPTIVE INDIVIDUATION FOR ADOLESCENTS CONFRONTING CONFLICT

PAUL V. TRAD

Families that experience conflict when one child reaches adolescence often benefit if all members of the household enter psychotherapy. During such treatment, family members are made sensitive to the paradox of development—the continual alternation between states of intimacy and autonomy. For optimal functioning the family must learn to balance both forces in order to avoid enmeshment, which swallows individuality, or estrangement, which isolates family members emotionally. A case history demonstrates how this goal can be met by dynamically juxtaposing family, group, and individual psychotherapeutic principles.

Although most family therapists concur about the awkward nature of adolescence—the kinds of developmental tasks a teenager must accomplish and the difficult metamorphosis anticipated by those tasks—treatment of the social and psychological ills that may manifest during the teenage years tends to be divided among several radically different modalities. That is, a troubled teenager may well be referred to a number of separate treatment formats—individual therapy, peer group interaction, and family therapy—with no appreciable synergistic advantage to counter the fragmentation of care that results.

An upsurge in treatment modalities has occurred as therapists have recognized the inherent paradoxical nature of the developmental process. Maturational change results in more sophisticated skills, which promote autonomy, but these skills also enhance intimate communication with others. This paradox is experienced more keenly at adolescence than at any other stage of life. The adolescent straddles the border between two realms—childhood and adulthood—yet can be fully at home in neither. Developmentally advanced skills, coupled with increased pressure from academic and social environments, preclude escape into a world of games and pretend, the domain of the child; yet the teenager remains too inexperienced and untested to shoulder the full responsibilities presented by the grown-up world. Indeed, adolescence is a period of transition. The teenager's personality structure necessarily undergoes revision as he or she formulates an identity separate from that of other family members.

The adolescent's negotiation of the chasm between intimacy and autonomy in some respects parallels the individuation efforts of the infant a decade earlier. As with that transition, in many cases, the task is achieved with little disturbance to the family structure. However, the teenager's struggle to extricate himself or herself from the protective domain of home life can also result in a litany of problems that bring the child to the attention of the therapeutic community—conduct disorder, school truancy, substance abuse, and teenage pregnancy.

The tendency to recommend multiple treatment formats in these cases has generated its own problems. For example, if different therapists are involved, the teenager and family members may be obliged to establish multiple allegiances. The ensuing competitive interests and divided loyalties can divert family members from working together to resolve common issues. Moreover, multiple treatment formats squander resources that may ultimately lead to deficiencies.

On the other hand, certain psychological dynamics become evident only when the entire nuclear family attends a session, whereas other kinds of conflict surface primarily when the child is observed interacting with a peer group. Thus, theorists have become increasingly convinced of the value of psychotherapeutic integration—that is, the flexible combination of various formats based on patient need and established efficacy.

As noted by Goldfried, Wiser, and Raue (1992), the fragmentation that has characterized adolescent psychotherapy has resulted in neither an accurate nor an effective means of diagnosing and treating disorder; yet no single orientation enjoys success with a variety of psychological problems. Integration seeks to unify approaches by identifying common elements. An eclectic approach that encompasses diverse concepts and treatment options is more apt to lead to comprehensive and potentially effective treatment strategies.

An integrated form of treatment involves the entire nuclear family. Its goal is to help the family achieve equilibrium as a social unit as each family member attains adaptive individuation. In each session the therapist uses strategies derived from a variety of formats to help each family member adjust to the paradoxical needs for both intimacy and autonomy. Specifically, the therapist helps family members devise strategies for the expression of intimacy when trends toward individuation threaten to isolate them emotionally and, conversely, facilitates strategies for the display of autonomy when patterns of enmeshment begin to restrict adaptive modes of functioning.

The following case example illustrates this integrated method. The focus of treatment was a teenage girl determined to become pregnant in opposition to her family's wishes. Preliminary analysis, however, suggested that both family and group strategies were warranted. For example, family members displayed some dysfunctional interactions that intimated problems in establishing boundaries with each other, as well as maladaptive patterns that suggested members' difficulty in formulating adaptive relationships with peers.

By drawing on both strategies, along with techniques more common to individual work, the therapist was able to note the transition from one mode of interaction to the other: family to group and group to family. He used three markers to identify when a transition had occurred: 1) the family members' expressive cues, that is, mannerisms that served as outward signs of psychological distress and indicated a need to modify the mode of interaction; 2) analysis of narrative content, which evidenced shifts from intimacy to autonomy and vice versa; and 3) the therapist's own countertransference feelings, which allowed him to predict and explain the reasons underlying a family member's shift in functioning.

Researchers have verified that impressions based on brief observations of expressive cues—mannerisms that employ movement, speech, and gesture: facial expression, body postures, vocal intonations, and so forth—are generally accurate (Albright, Kenny, and Malloy, 1988; Funder and Colvin 1988; Ambady and Rosenthal, 1992). By analyzing these cues in conjunction with the content of the patient's narrative and countertransference feelings, the therapist can gain sufficient insight into the patient's behaviors and attitudes.

Case History Example

PRESENTING PROBLEM

Julia T., aged 14 years and 9 months, was referred for treatment by her parents who complained that in the year prior to presentation their daughter had become increasingly rebellious and uncontrollable.

Among the many concerns they voiced were Julia's overt sexual relationship with her boyfriend, the abortion she had obtained without their knowledge several months earlier, and her expressed wish to become pregnant again and to raise a baby despite their fervent protests.

Both parents reported that, in retrospect, their daughter's behavior had changed at approximately the time of the abortion. She had begun to cut classes and her grades had fallen. She had also become irritable and gloomy, in stark contrast to her usual "sunny disposition." Two months after the abortion, Julia became pregnant again, but within several days of realizing her condition, she had a spontaneous miscarriage, verified by a gynecologist. She told her boyfriend about both pregnancies. She also confided in her older sister, but only about the second pregnancy. Despite Julia's request for confidentiality, her sister told their parents, who became concerned and took Julia to a therapist for two sessions. However, when Julia's mother learned that her daughter had not given up her wish to have a child, she insisted that the entire family seek evaluation at a different facility.

Julia is the youngest of three children. Her brother Michael is eight years her senior; her sister Lois is five years her senior. At the time of presentation, both siblings attended college and were living in the parents' home. Julia's parents had been married for 25 years. Both mother and father described the relationship as "solid" and "stable," but Julia's mother added, almost as an aside, that "there have been some rocky times." According to the parents, Julia achieved all developmental milestones in a timely fashion. From the time she was young, she had been "very independent." As an example, the mother reported that on Julia's first day of school, "I was the one who started crying, not Julia." She added that Julia continued to assert her independence through elementary school. Both parents described Julia as being "defiant," "stubborn," possessed of "a temper," and able to get what she wants by being "pushy." The mother voiced some reservations about her daughter's "independent" disposition, whereas the father regarded it as a "sign of strength." He noted, "I have great hopes for her. Maybe someday she will run her own business." On the heels of this comment, the mother stated, "Of course I'm also proud that Julia's a leader," but added that Julia's "nurturing qualities" should be mentioned as well. For example, she said, since nursery school her daughter has adopted and cared for stray pets. At the time of presentation, Julia was continuing to date the boy who got her pregnant. Of this boyfriend, the parents stated, "He's nice, but we think she can do better." Julia was apparently popular with her female friends, although they didn't entirely understand her desire to become pregnant. According to Julia, "They are surprised I want a baby. They say only poor girls do that and they think it will ruin my chances for a good career."

FAMILY HISTORY

The parents, Vincent and Janet, had met at a school dance 26 years earlier. They had dated for six months, at which point Vincent entered the Navy. Two months later, they were married. Vincent, an electrical engineer, was, at the time of presentation, an executive with a large corporation, having "worked [his] way up through promotions" over a period of 16 years. Prior to the marriage, Janet had been an executive secretary; after marriage, she took care of the house and children. Recently she had taken a part-time job at a clothing store "more out of boredom than a need for money."

The mother reported that her three pregnancies were all planned and had progressed normally. After some hesitation, however, she acknowledged that two years before Julia's birth she had terminated a pregnancy. She had been in a car accident in which the fetus sustained severe injuries, and her doctor had recommended abortion. She was opposed to this course of action because the procedure violated her religious beliefs, but her husband convinced her that raising "a deformed infant would not be fair" to their two older children. "I finally gave in and did what my husband wanted," Janet said, but added that not long afterward she became "extremely angry" with her husband for insisting that she terminate the pregnancy.

Both parents agreed that Janet became pregnant again almost immediately after the abortion in an effort to resolve the "bad feelings" between them. Despite the success of that pregnancy and the birth of their third child, Julia, they agreed that "a barrier went up between us." They remained on good terms, but periodically, Janet said, became "furious with one another," at a level of rage they had not experienced before the car accident.

Following the abortion, Janet confessed that she acted out her resentment against her husband "by refusing to have sex" or coercing him to buy her "expensive gifts." Vincent said he began to feel that he was responsible for "destroying the marriage" and tried to be a "perfect husband." The couple separated on two occasions for brief periods, but then got back together because, as Janet explained, "we really care about each other." Both parents expressed happiness at the birth of Julia; the father regarded his daughter as "a replacement for the aborted child," and the mother considered her a "special child." Ironically, Julia's pregnancy appeared to revitalize the abortion issue between the couple.

During the few years before Julia's abortion and miscarriage, a number of significant deaths occurred in the extended family. First, Janet's brother, a former drug addict, was hospitalized with AIDS and died within a few months. Janet, who knew only that her brother had used heroin "long ago," was "shocked and devastated" by these events. Julia, who was close to this uncle, had also appeared shaken, especially when she visited him during the final weeks of his life. During the same period, Janet's father died of a heart attack. Julia was close to this grandfather as well. Like the rest of her family, she knew that her grandfather had condemned her uncle's involvement with drugs and subsequent death from AIDS.

Vincent's family background was not as stable as his wife's. His parents were divorced shortly after he was born and he spent the first five years of his life in foster homes. When he was six years old, he moved in with his maternal grandmother, who raised him until adulthood. Vincent reported that his mother, since deceased, had had psychiatric problems. He had few memories of her. His father was an alcoholic who had died more than 25 years earlier.

The parents described their oldest child, Michael, 22 years old, as "very serious and organized." Michael was in graduate school, preparing for a career in the FBI. He was often angry with Julia because she was "irresponsible." The second child, Lois, 19 years old, was described as being "flighty and emotional." The father fought with her constantly. The relationship between Lois and Julia, previously tranquil, had recently deteriorated in light of Lois's disclosure of Julia's pregnancy history to their parents.

The details of this case history strongly indicate that although Julia had become the expressed focal point of the family's attention, dysfunctional patterns affected every member of the family and the interrelationships between them. For example, the mother's abortion prior to Julia's birth continued to reverberate as an unresolved source of tension that not only affected husband and wife, but had broadened to encompass the children.

The therapist surmised that by expressing a desire to become pregnant, Julia might, on some level, have become an agent through which her mother could work through the ambivalence she continued to feel about her own abortion. He also noted the parents' contradictory views of Julia's independent nature, which suggested an unspoken conflict between the couple. Finally, apparently minor pieces of information—the mother's dissatisfaction with the first therapist and the sister's disclosure of Julia's miscarriage after Julia had requested confidentiality—suggested that the family might be experiencing a form of enmeshment that hindered adaptive functioning. The therapist, therefore, hypothesized that the entire family would benefit from treatment. He chose to use an integrated approach that would interpret patterns of family interaction by way of different treatment modalities. That is, he opted to use principles commonly applied in family therapy, such as enmeshment and the intergenerational transmission of psychopathology, and to supplement them with principles such as cohesion and universality, which are generally part of group therapy. His assumption was that family members would alternate in using maladaptive forms of these phenomena as they attempted to negotiate the balance between autonomy and intimacy. As indicated, he also used three indicators derived from the strategies of individual interpretation to discern points of transition between family and group functioning: the expressive cues manifested by family members; analysis of their narrative content; and countertransference feelings. Shifts from one mode of interaction to another were harbingers of conflict. They suggested that either intimacy or autonomy had reached a crisis point.

APPLYING FAMILY PRINCIPLES TO THE TREATMENT OF A TEENAGER

The rationale behind family therapy is perhaps best expressed by Bowen (1966). The essential dilemma confronting a family is the constant attempt to balance two ostensibly contradictory forces—the force that promotes individuality and autonomy and the force that promotes togetherness or fusion. Thus, the primary thrust of many family techniques is to teach family members how to individuate and separate in order to assert their unique personalities, as well as how to be close without smothering the individuality of other family members (Abel, 1983).

The family's continual effort to establish a balance between emotional sharing, on the one hand, and independent exploration, on the other, is held to derive from the paradox of development each person encounters during early life. An infant's mastery of the environment is fueled by the acquisition of new skills, which in turn enables the infant's progressive acclimation to the challenges of the external world. But the infant is equally concerned with establishing an intimate relationship with the caregiver. Indeed, the child's capacity to function autonomously develops in concert with the capacity for more sophisticated forms of expressing intimacy. The intrapsychic conflicts that arise from this paradox are believed to emerge during interpersonal relationships, especially those within the family (Abel, 1983). As family members experience too much closeness and intimacy, an acute sense of loss of self triggers a shift to behaviors and attitudes that promote greater autonomy; similarly, when autonomy becomes too pronounced, the individual seeks to reexperience the emotional closeness of the family. Thus, when examining a family's relational patterns, the family therapist will usually look for either enmeshment and fusion (that is, a maladaptive version of closeness) or estrangement (that is, a precocious version of autonomy). The primary goal of family therapy is to help the family members achieve an equilibrium between these two modes of functioning. From such a balance, relationships gain unequivocal emotional boundaries with the possibility of moving back and forth between close involvement and loneliness (Skynner, 1981).

One of the preeminent forms of family treatment is systems theory. Systems theory posits that the etiology of psychological conflict is not within the individual but is symptomatic of an imbalance in the family system, the emotional exchange that governs the individual's life. A rectification of this imbalance requires that family members devise an accommodation between their emotional and cognitive perceptions. Emotional perception moves an individual to respond to the environment by way of identification with others; cognitive perception moves an individual to respond by way of differentiation. The extremes of these two responses are, respectively, fusion and isolation (Minuchin, 1974). Dysfunctional families tend to exhibit either of these two extremes: They may be overly dependent on one another and thus susceptible to sharing dysfunctional patterns, or, conversely, they may maintain rigid boundaries and isolate themselves from each other, their extended relatives, and the community (Bowen, 1978).

Family systems theory proposes several intervention techniques, all of which serve to alert family members to the structure they have adopted and to motivate necessary change. Specifically, a therapist may have to interrupt a parent who speaks for a child, encourage a withdrawn or silent family member to speak, or control a disruptive child who makes constructive change impossible. Beels and Ferber (1969) have recommended three additional interventions: directive ("from above"), detached ("from the side"), and enmeshed ("from below").

When the therapist intervenes "from above," he or she modifies the structure of the family by actively intervening, giving advice, rendering praise or criticism, or modeling more adaptive behavior for family members. When the therapist intervenes "from the side," he or she remains neutral but devises instructions or tasks that make it impossible for the family to continue dysfunctional patterns. When the therapist intervenes "from below," he or she submits to the control of the family and becomes enmeshed in the family dynamics. From this posture, the therapist plays the role of "child," "patient," or "scapegoat." The family is often so jarred by the therapist's adoption of this demeanor that they may be jolted back to a more objective perspective.

In several respects, intervention "from below" resembles a technique recommended by Bowen (1966): Where a family has learned to diffuse volatile emotions between two of its members by creating a triangle, the therapist inserts himself or herself as the third point in that triangle.

A review of the nominal complaint voiced by Julia and her family suggested that the teenager had come to embody a key conflict between the parents—namely, their failure to achieve marital reconciliation after the mother's abortion. Julia's expressed desire to have a baby indicated that she had somehow merged her mother's needs with her own. To assess the level of family differentiation here, the therapist encouraged the family members—parents Vincent and Janet; siblings Lois, Michael, and Julia—to interact in a relatively unfettered fashion. The only prompt provided by the therapist was to ask Julia to explain her parents' response to her wish to become pregnant.

Therapist: (*Directing the question to Julia*) I wonder if you could clarify your perceptions as to how your parents reacted when they first learned about your pregnancy.

Julia: (*Looks down, hair falls in face, with embarrassment in her voice*) I have to think. (*Silence. She appears to be in a world of her own. The adolescent begins playing with a strand of hair, apparently absorbed by this activity. As she twists her hair, she continues to turn away from her parents.*)

Therapist: It would be helpful to tell us about your parents' reaction.

Julia: Well, my father, he wasn't so nice. (*Giggles and covers her mouth. She rolls her eyes and stares at the ceiling. She also adopts a scornful expression, directed at her father, and begins edging her chair toward her mother.*) He started yelling right away and giving orders the way he usually does. He told me if I get pregnant again, he'll send me away and put the baby up for adoption. (*She pauses again and seems to laugh. She is now next to her mother and has crossed her legs in the same position as her mother. It is as if mother and daughter are challenging or confronting the father.*)

Therapist: Can you explain why you find that funny?

Julia: I don't think it's funny. It's just . . . well, we don't take my father too seriously. (*These words are said cryptically, as if "we" has special meaning*)

Therapist: Who doesn't take your father seriously?

Julia: My mom, for one. When she found out I wanted to get pregnant, she seemed really happy. We even looked at some cribs at the mall. My mom told me that if I got pregnant, I wouldn't have to give the baby up for adoption. She would help me raise the baby. (*Julia now stares in open defiance at her father. Almost immediately, her mother interjects*)

Mother: Julia, stop it. You know that's not what I meant. I just want you to be happy. I don't want you to disobey your father.

Julia: (*Anger in her voice*) So now you take his side.

This exchange provided insight into the level of differentiation in this family and enabled the therapist to begin understanding the "family-as-a-whole" (Richter, 1974). First, Julia's sense of identification with her mother was strong, even fierce in its degree of emotional loyalty. Her psychological loyalty was reflected in the expressive cues she manifested, from which the therapist discerned a special alliance between mother and daughter. The teenager sat within inches of her mother's body. Each had her legs crossed facing one another, as if obliterating other family members entirely. While speaking, Julia would occasionally establish eye contact with her mother. Finally, when Julia's mother interrupted her daughter, she placed her hand on Julia's arm, and the teenager responded by immediately becoming silent. It was as if the two had a special language and were accustomed to communicating with one another using only gestures. The implication was that the mother had funneled her own hostility through her daughter. Julia had, in effect, become her mother's "mouthpiece."

In contrast, Julia's father sat at a distance from the other family members, as if in self-imposed exile. His arms were crossed on his chest and one leg leaned against the knee of his other leg. He even tilted backwards in his chair, creating more physical distance from the other family members. To a trained observer, this form of physical configuration suggested that the only strategy family members had for separating from one another was distancing (Skynner, 1987). The family members were capable of achieving separation, but at the expense of breaking up the blurred boundaries they shared. As a result, the family member who broke away became the "scapegoat," ostracized by the others as the father was here.

Given the closeness between Julia and her mother, and the parallel isolation of the father, the therapist was intrigued by the mother's ultimate effort to reunite the family, as if she could not tolerate any family member breaking away from the undifferentiated mass. This effort at reunification became evident when the teenager's anger at her father surfaced. As if threatened by the direct expression of hostility, Julia's mother then chastised her daughter. These behaviors suggested to the therapist an "undifferentiated family ego mass" (Bowen, 1978). Family members displayed a pronounced lack of individual differentiation in this situation. Moreover, the patterns of enmeshment revealed that the family diffused emotional tension by creating a triangle.

According to Bowen (1966), triangles occur when the tension between two family members becomes untenable. At that juncture, a third family member is "triangled in," which alleviates the high level of emotion—at the price of the emotion's direct expression. Thus, family members can continue affective subterfuge. In this particular case, the subliminal conflict between the parents was the unresolved issue of their third, unborn, child. Whenever this conflict threatened to erupt between them, they triangled Julia in, and she siphoned off some of the emotional volatility. This mode of triangulation dissipated tension, but the process also exacted a toll from the family. First, the technique no longer worked. Julia could not absorb enough tension and the parents were beginning to experience their own hostility. Second, Julia had begun to resent playing her part in the triangle; in an effort to assert her own individuality, she was now, in adolescence, acting out her parents' conflict.

As the therapist recognized the draining repercussions of the enmeshed patterns of interaction in the family—and, in particular, on Julia's attempts to help the family members differentiate adaptively— he sought to interfere "from below," by assuming the role of the scapegoat in the family. In this regard, the therapist spoke for Julia, as an advocate. To assume this role, he sat close to Julia and imitated her posture and gestures. He also maintained eye contact with Julia, somewhat to the exclusion of the other family members. In this fashion, the therapist indicated a special allegiance with the teenager.

Therapist: I get the feeling that Julia's perspective is not completely understood. It's really hard to be Julia in this family, isn't it?

Mother: (*The therapist's comment has caught her attention.*) What do you mean? (*She looks startled.*)

Therapist: I hear from Julia that you continually change your mind. First you seem excited about her getting pregnant, but then you criticize her for having sex with her boyfriend. No wonder she is confused.

Mother:	You mean I send mixed signals?
Therapist:	That's one way to describe it.
Father:	That's the perfect way to describe it. Come on, Janet. You know that's the way you behave. That expression, "It's a woman's prerogative to change her mind," that's my wife. (*This final comment has been directed to the therapist. The father gestures with his hands, as if in frustration.*)
Mother:	(*Glares at husband*) That's not fair.
Father:	It isn't? Why don't you tell the truth, Janet.
Mother:	I should tell the truth? All right. (*Scornful tone enters her voice*) Maybe I change my mind so much because in the end we wind up doing what we want anyway.
Father:	You're not making any sense.
Mother:	Oh yes I am. What about the abortion?
Father:	What abortion? Julia's abortion?
Mother:	No, my abortion. Our abortion. For once be honest. You wanted me to have that abortion. I just did it to please you.
Father:	That's unfair. You wanted it as much as I did. Now you just won't forgive me. Just like you blame your father for not accepting your brother. You always have to blame someone, Janet. Why don't you take responsibility for yourself, for a change.
Lois:	Stop fighting. I can't take this.
Julia:	(*Sobbing*) Please don't be mad at Daddy anymore, Mommy.

Therapist: It seems that Julia's wish to become pregnant has a lot of meaning for this family.

Following this session, the family members became more amenable to discussing themselves as individuals. Julia spoke more about school activities and referred less to becoming pregnant. She also expressed a desire to study architecture. From this session on, both parents seemed to have acquired a more mature capacity to address one another's concerns. For example, the father reported, "I listen to Janet much more and I don't try to impose my views on her anymore. Also, I give her credit. She seems more receptive to my point of view, and I appreciate that." Janet conveyed a similar change in perspective. "A lot of the anger I had for Vinnie seems to have gone away. I know he encouraged me to have the abortion, but now I understand his motives better. And, ultimately, it was my own decision to have the procedure."

These comments, as well as Julia's change in attitude, suggest that the family was devising adaptive strategies for differentiating from one another. Indeed, these comments indicate that the family had begun to achieve differentiation, which, as Skynner (1987) indicates, is manifested by defined and secure identities that, in turn, permit adaptive levels of closeness and intimacy. Another sign of differentiation—a willingness to assume individual responsibility—was also present.

At approximately this time, during an individual session, Julia reported a dream to the therapist. In the dream, Julia is lying in bed, her infant on one side, her mother on the other. Suddenly her mother begins gasping for breath. Julia becomes frightened but is able to remain in control. She attempts to help her mother breathe, but finally her mother "slips away." The dream suggested that Julia was also beginning to differentiate from her mother. She was separating from her and confronting the pain and anxiety that attended such separation.

TRANSITIONS BETWEEN GROUP AND FAMILY PRINCIPLES

Although Julia's family eventually extricated themselves from patterns of enmeshment, the process of achieving an optimal level of functioning may be quite challenging for a therapist. The psychotherapeutic process itself may spark paradoxical patterns (Abel, 1983). That is, family members may attempt to defuse the powerful emotions generated in the therapeutic encounter by displaying an extreme form of individuation and autonomy, until the individual boundary to which each group member has retreated leaves him or her feeling isolated (Goffman, 1974). At this point the family members will again seek the security of emotional entanglement. If the family is organized around an undifferentiated family ego mass, the individuals will be caught in a vicious cycle between these two extremes: They will become fused with the emotional turmoil being experienced by other family members or they will experience isolation and estrangement. In order to sever this pattern, the integrative therapist may attempt to promote adaptive principles of group interaction such as cohesion, which allows each family member to be close without reasserting the negative pattern of fusion.

The therapist may do this by making family members sensitive to periods of transition between the extremes of isolation and entanglement. These periods of transition are akin to episodes of developmental crisis when new skills are consolidating. If the individual is willing to acknowledge the nature of the strong emotions that have been evoked during this time, it is possible to motivate a genuine change in psychological perception and behavior.

The following excerpt reveals how this process works.

Father: (*Responding to Julia's explanation of why she wanted to have a baby.*) Wait a second. We keep rehashing this theme and get nowhere. I will not allow Julia to have a baby. Julia, do you understand me? Erase that idea from your mind!

Mother: (*Sarcastically*) That's right, order her around. That's exactly what you did with me after the accident. You gave me an ultimatum: Have the abortion or else.

Father: Oh stop it, Janet. You were just as responsible for that decision as I was, so stop complaining.

Mother: Was I? Is that how you see it? I guess you don't remember who was driving the car?

Father: So that's it. (*Raises voice*) You just can't forgive me, can you?

331

Julia: (*Places hands over ears*) Stop yelling. I can't stand it. That's why I want to leave home. You're always yelling. Why don't you listen to yourselves or listen to me for a change!

Therapist: We need to think about some of the things everyone just said. I think we now have some insight into why Julia has been behaving in such a disruptive fashion and keeps saying she wants a baby.

Mother: (*Sighs deeply*) I have something to say. I feel like I've been hit with a bolt of lightning. (*Makes eye contact with husband and leans in his direction*) I never realized how much pent-up anger I still have for Vinnie about my own abortion. I didn't realize until this minute. And I also just realized that I resent the fact that Vinnie thinks of Julia as the "replacement" for the baby we lost.

Therapist: Would you like to say anything else about the resentment?

Mother: Yeah! Please realize I'm sort of talking off the top of my head, but I know this may sound crazy . . . but, it's almost as if I want Julia to get pregnant and have a baby to hurt Vinnie. To finally make him understand how I felt when I got the abortion.

Father: Whew! I knew it hurt you, Janet, but I never knew how much.

Therapist: Julia, do you have a reaction to your parents' comments?

Julia: It makes me feel weird. I hate it when my parents fight. I always feel like somehow it's my fault, even though I know deep down inside that I have nothing to do with whatever it is they are fighting about.

Therapist: Did you know your mother had an abortion before you were born?

Julia: Yes! Whenever she gets angry at my father she mentions
              it. I tell her, "Mom, enough already." I even wish there
              was something I could do. My dad is really not so bad.
              I know I complain about him, but he's really a good
              father, so I don't know why my mother doesn't let him
              off the hook about it.

Therapist: Maybe you're trying to help get your father off the hook
              by becoming pregnant yourself. It's your way of giving
              your mother back the baby she lost through the abortion.

Julia: (*Deep in reflection*) Hmmm.

Father: Janet, I honestly didn't understand how deeply the
              abortion affected you. If I had known . . . well, I can't
              say I would have changed my mind, but I would have
              tried to be more considerate of your feelings.

Mother: I appreciate your saying that.

Throughout this session, the therapist was attempting to make the
family members more aware of the emotions they were experiencing
in the "here and now." Working in the "here and now" means focusing
on the patient's contemporary experience as the psychotherapeutic
process unfolds (Slife and Lanyon, 1991). Although the content of
treatment may involve the "there and then" of the past, the process of
therapy occurs in the "here and now" of the patient's feelings,
attitudes, and relationships. As much as possible, therapeutic attention
is confined to the temporally present and spatially proximal which
permits the therapist to call attention to the direct experience of an
emotion when it occurs. A focus on past experience is one step
removed from this immediacy. In effect, the patient needs to have an
immediate experience, rather than be offered an explanation.

The following excerpt demonstrates how the therapist directed the
family members' attention to immediate awakened emotion during
episodes of transition.

Therapist: Julia, it would be helpful if you could share with us how
              you feel when your parents say these kinds of things.

Julia: (*Shrugs and turns away*) I don't know.

Therapist: I have a feeling you feel strange when they talk about you as if you weren't there.

Julia: So why should I express my feelings. They won't listen anyway.

Father: I'll listen, Julia. (*sounds sheepish and looks down at palms of hands as if embarrassed*) I guess I haven't been doing a lot of that lately.

Julia: I'm glad you can admit it. Sometimes I feel like your servant. The only thing you tell me to do is get soda or the newspaper. You order me around, then you fight with Mom. So now I'm supposed to tell you how I feel? I don't believe you'll listen to me.

Mother: Julia, we both want to help you, we truly do. It's not easy for your dad and me to come here either. We're not used to letting out our emotions either. Please try to understand.

Julia: (*Suddenly sobbing*) Then why do you always fight . . . and talk about the dead baby. (*Turns to face father*) Daddy, I am not a replacement for the dead baby. I don't want to be a replacement, so stop calling me that. (*Turns to face mother*) And Mommy, I'm not your baby either.

Mother: Julia, you're right. We just didn't allow you to express yourself before because we were so preoccupied with our own problems. But we're really sorry.

Father: Julie, you know you're mother's speaking from the heart. We love you so much, baby . . .

Julia: Dad, I'm not your baby!

Father: Right. (*Laughs*). Understand, Julie. It's not so easy being a parent. Your mom and I will really try to change. Not just because it will help you, but for ourselves. We really do care about each other. The anger doesn't really represent how we feel.

As suggested by this excerpt, whenever the therapist senses that strong emotion has been generated, it is important to apply pressure gently but firmly, to help the family member express and acknowledge the nature of the emotion. In this manner, tension may be overcome and differentiation initiated.

The following excerpt presents the other side of this transitional episode. As noted, nondifferentiation of the family ego mass may be followed by an extreme level of autonomy that threatens to sever all ties within the family. At this point, the family members will make an effort to reassert a family configuration. This kind of transitional episode presents the therapist with another opportunity to make family members aware of the behaviors and emotions they are displaying.

Therapist: What happened during the past week?

Mother: Guess what. I've enrolled in school.

Therapist: Tell us about it.

Mother: I never graduated from college, but it was something I always wanted to do. I'm finding it a little scary to get back into the swing of things, but I'm managing.

Julia: (*Glances down, picking at nails, says in sarcastic tone of voice*) Don't you feel a bit old, Mom? I mean, it's ridiculous!

Mother: Okay, Julia. Let's have it. What's wrong now?

Julia: (*Sullenly*) Nothing.

Father: Come on, Julia. We all agreed that at least during the sessions we would express our feelings openly and honestly.

Julia: All right. Quit nagging. (*Continues looking down, but stops picking nails*) At first I liked the idea of Mom going to college. But now she's never there when I get home from school.

Mother: What? Julia, I'm flabbergasted. You used to complain that I was always around, watching your behavior. You even said you wanted me to get a job like your friends' mothers. I thought you didn't want me around. Now you say you do. I'm confused.

Julia: I guess . . . well, it's hard to think of you as a person besides your being my mom or Dad's wife. You know, as a separate person with your own personality. Now you have new friends and sometimes I'm scared you'll . . . leave us.

Lois: Mom, you know Julie has a point. I'm not scared you will leave us, but sometimes I feel as if I'm in competition with you and that you are not really our mother anymore.

Therapist: Everybody seems to be responding to a natural evolution that is taking place in the family.

Father: What do you mean by an evolution?

Therapist: Well, Janet has always been the mother and the wife in this family. Those are her two roles, the roles that have been assigned to her and the roles everyone accepts. But recently, this family underwent some changes. We saw how Janet and Vincent sometimes triangled Julia between them to avoid facing certain issues. When that happened, we said everyone's emotions got tangled up. Well, we managed to untangle things. Now Janet is beginning to assert a different aspect of her personality. Julia extricated herself from her family's emotional entanglement, and maybe now it's Janet's turn.

Mother: That's right. I won't stop being your mother. It's a role I love and cherish.

Therapist: Julia, it may not be easy to accommodate to your mother's changing role, but in some respects it resembles the kind of change you underwent recently.

Julia: You mean when I stopped trying to have a baby.

Therapist: Yes. Everyone in the family continues to change and grow, not just you, but your parents as well.

Julia: Actually, that makes me feel good when you say it like that.

From the insight this family gained during treatment they were able to learn strategies for balancing their needs for intimacy and dependency with countervailing needs to differentiate and assert individuality.

APPLYING GROUP PRINCIPLES TO THE TREATMENT OF A TEENAGER

Perhaps the key word for understanding adaptive family functioning is *equilibrium*. Family members need to learn how to balance intrapsychic and interpersonal conflicts that arise with other family members. As family therapy techniques teach family members how to differentiate from one another, the therapist should be alert to nascent feelings of alienation. Dysfunctional families often lack a forum within which to experiment with intimacy, and they become emotionally stifled.

At this juncture, family members need to begin expressing their emotions as individuals in a more overt fashion. This is when the principles of group therapy become relevant to the therapeutic process. When a certain level of autonomy and exploration have been attained, individual members need to recapitulate the configuration within the family. During this process, it is as if the family members were functioning as a group. Within the group setting, each individual carries a special "frame," a mode of organizing experiences that determines how the individual will respond in a given situation (Goffman, 1974). Families in which the power of the undifferentiated family ego mass has been defused or in which the estrangement between family members has been overcome, must begin to become reacquainted with one another and to unconsciously reassert a family system.

The adage that characterizes group therapy is "The sum is greater than the parts." When group principles are applied, the therapist is exposed not only to the perspective of each family member as an individual, but also to the dynamic that comes to govern the family as a group.

Group principles are designed to motivate patients to modify their maladaptive patterns and to experiment with new behaviors (Fromm-Reichman, 1950; Bloch and Crouch, 1985; Colijn, Hoencamp, Snijders, Van der Spek, and Duivenvoorden, 1991). The process attempts to generate feelings of hope, universality, and altruism among the family members. That is, each individual is encouraged to have faith in the treatment, bolstered by other group members; to recognize that others have the same or a similar problem and need not face psychological fears alone; and to develop the capacity to "feel for another." As the family members begin to reestablish a structure, they tend to disclose the conflict that lies at the core of family discord by recapitulating the primary family configuration. Every group tries unconsciously to form some sort of family system (Abel, 1983), and this tendency is increased when the group members do in fact belong to the same family. A group generally assigns the parental role to the therapist, and each individual regards him or her as either malevolent or benign. As the group members come to feel more comfortable, they express more feelings—positive and negative—and begin to act as they would in their own families of origin.

In a family therapy context, the therapist, as the figure of authority, assumes the parental role and the family members act like siblings. In this way, a family encounter with strong transferences and powerful emotions from childhood are resurrected. Socializing techniques, such as imitative behaviors and interpersonal learning, also surface in the group context. By offering family members the opportunity to devise examples of more adaptive behavior, the family members, removed from the constricting roles that have characterized interaction within the family, may feel more capable of experimenting with new roles.

Finally, a primary goal of the therapist who uses group principles will be to promote a sense of cohesion among family members. In contrast to enmeshment, which is a maladaptive form of interaction, cohesion enables family members to share a particular perspective

338

without overshadowing one another as individuals. Indeed, if the group approach is to succeed, all family members need to share a common reference point that unites them in a joint endeavor. Group effectiveness will also diminish to the extent that one family member has a unique problem that distances him or her from the other members of the group (Hulce, 1960).

As the therapist applies group principles to interpreting the dynamics of the family unit, he or she must recognize the point at which family members relinquish the pursuit of autonomy and begin unconsciously to define their own system (Abel, 1983). This is an opportunity for the therapist to help mold a new family structure, with different strategies for effecting intimacy and autonomy. As the therapist becomes aware of this transition, he or she should interpret the relational patterns as they emerge. For example, the therapist should encourage family members to express their emotions—positive and negative—candidly. If "sibling rivalry," "triangulation," and/or "enmeshment" arise they should be addressed. During this process, a more attuned awareness will become evident in the family members. They have managed to overcome the debilitating patterns of enmeshment and are now attempting to devise systems of interaction that will enable them both to assert their needs for autonomy and to return to the family for emotional sustenance when necessary.

Of course, some families have difficulty expressing balanced and appropriate emotions to one another. After they overcome patterns of enmeshment, they may be hesitant to renew their engagement in emotional interaction. Other families have never communicated with one another emotionally. During the group phase of the treatment, the therapist will attempt to rectify these impasses by helping family members to establish adaptive contact with one another.

This process is illustrated in the following excerpt. Three months after the last excerpted exchange, Julia's maladaptive behavior patterns had remitted and the teenager no longer expressed a desire to have a baby. However, as she began to form an alliance with her father—a new configuration in the family—both Julia's sister and mother exhibited distressed responses. Significantly, as the session began, Julia and her father had taken chairs at one side of the treatment room. They were separated from the other family members, mother, Michael, and Lois, and their body gestures—crossed legs, bodies tilted back, adjacent arms touching—suggested closeness and compatibility.

However, the therapist needed to verify that this new closeness did not signify a means of excluding the other family members.

Therapist: Why don't we continue the discussion from last week. Julia was telling us about her application for the special summer project for students interested in architecture.

Julia: (*Animated*) My teacher thinks I have a chance to make it. There are only five openings from the entire city, but my teacher will sponsor me. Also, my Dad is helping me write the proposal. (*Julia flashes her father a broad smile and establishes eye contact with him. Notably, Julia and her father are sitting close together, their chairs touch, and both have crossed their legs in a similar fashion. Now Julia moves her chair even closer to her father.*)

Mother: (*Mumbles*) Too fast, Julia. (*Sighs deeply*)

Therapist: We can't hear you. Remember the agreement we have? You can express any emotion you want, but you have to share your feelings with everyone in the group.

Mother: There. You said it! (*Glares at therapist*) We're not a family anymore. You've turned us into a group of people and all of us are going our separate ways.

Lois: It's true. Our family wasn't perfect when we started to come for these sessions, but at least we all knew where we stood. Now it's . . . chaotic!

Father: Wait a second. I don't feel that way. Not at all. And I'm a member of this family, too. In fact, for the first time in a long time I really feel like I am a member of the family and I feel close to Julia. Maybe you two are just jealous. I used to be the odd man out, but now it's you, Janet.

Julia: Wait a second. Daddy, I like what we have now. I mean I can talk to you and you take me seriously. But I don't want us to be close only if Mom and Lois are left out.

Father: Julia, you're right. Janet, I'm sorry. So much has changed in these last few weeks. I see Julia so differently.

Therapist: I think what has happened is that all of you have gained new perspectives on the roles that you used to play in the family.

Julia: But I didn't like the role I used to play.

Therapist: That's true, and now that's changed. Each of you has become more of an individual. You've each been flexing your muscles and flying alone for a while. Now it may be time to come together again as a family, but in a more adaptive way than before.

Michael: How do we do that? (*Laughs nervously*) After all, we don't have a very good track record in this family.

Therapist: Maybe we should talk about how all of you want to structure your family.

Julia: You mean we can redo our family?

Therapist: Not entirely. But you can express to each other the kinds of emotional responses you expect from each other and the role each of you expects to play in the family.

During this session, family members were challenged to reexamine their family's structure. Optimal family functioning exhibits certain characteristics, which a therapist may need to point out and facilitate as interaction between the members occurs (Skynner, 1987). One such characteristic is an affiliative attitude to human encounter. In contrast to an oppositional attitude, which is characterized by distrust and withdrawal, an affiliative attitude is manifested when family members display an open, outreaching, and trusting stance toward one another.

341

A second characteristic of optimal family functioning is each member's respect for the separateness, individuality, autonomy, and privacy of the others. The opposite of this quality is the tendency for family members to speak for one another, which is encountered in enmeshed family configurations.

Communication in an optimally functioning family is honest and direct, in contrast to confused, evasive, and restrictive forms of communication.

Another characteristic of an optimally functioning family is the display of boundaries between the desires of the individuals within the family and the roles allocated to them in the family system. In this regard, a firm parental coalition should be evident, with power shared equally between the parents. Dysfunctional families, in contrast, display coalitions in which a parent and one child form an alliance that ultimately causes an imbalance in the family structure. This kind of imbalance was apparent in the parent–child coalition established between Julia and her mother.

The exercise of control in an optimally functioning family is flexible. Family members are able to work through problems by negotiation within the basic parent–child hierarchy, as opposed to adopting rigid patterns and unchangeable rules.

Family members are also secure enough to engage in spontaneous interaction characterized by positive feelings and to express negative emotion when appropriate. They attempt new modes of interaction, appear to derive pleasure from experimenting with behaviors, and abandon stereotypical responses. High levels of initiative are also characteristic of these families. In essence, family members appear eager to learn about each other. They ask questions of one another and express interest in one another's lives without being intrusive. They seem enlivened by family interaction.

Moreover, when a family is functioning adaptively, the open and unfettered flow of emotions is manifested in the expressive cues displayed by the family members. Specifically, family members do not hesitate to make direct eye contact, vocal intonations are soothing, and a listener will acquire a sense of vocal reciprocity. That is, family members listen to one another without interruption. Physical touching behavior between family members will also be appropriate when it occurs. In addition, family members will use their bodies as domains of communication by leaning toward one. another, smiling, and displaying open gestures with their hands. These expressive cues promote the adaptive interactive patterns that characterize groups, such as cohesion and universality, as well as the adaptive interactive patterns that characterize families, such as maintaining a balance between differentiation and intimacy.

Finally, optimally functioning families do not fear the unique gifts of their members. Each family member is encouraged to achieve his or her optimal level of functioning.

Some of these qualities were displayed by Julia's family after they had been in treatment for several months. The following excerpt indicates that the family had realigned itself in a more optimal fashion than before.

Therapist: Everyone is smiling today. Would you like to share your feelings?

Mother: We came to a big decision earlier this week.

Father: We are taking a trip to Europe this summer, the entire family.

Mother: It's something my husband and I planned before our marriage. Then the kids came along and things got away from us.

Father: But we've decided not to put it off any longer.

Mother: Besides, now we have a special reason to go. Julia was selected to participate in that special summer program, so she gets to spend two weeks in Italy. We will join her there afterwards and continue traveling as a family for two more weeks.

Lois: We are very happy about everything. This is a trip that has been discussed in my family ever since I can remember. But now that we all get along-we can finally communicate—it will be wonderful to go together.

Michael: We've even made plans to find our family village near Scotland.

Therapist: Which side of the family is from Scotland?

Father: My side. I've never been interested in my family history before . . . given my background and all. I guess I was ashamed that my parents weren't able to raise me and I was raised by my grandmother. But lately, I stopped feeling so sensitive. It is my family and I should try to learn about them. My son, Michael (*Places arm on Michael's chair*) helped me to design a family tree. Now I'm excited about going.

Mother: We may even find some long lost relatives!
End of dialogue

As this excerpt suggests, the family members appear to have restructured their family along more adaptive lines. Emotions are expressed openly and family members are no longer threatened by each other's individuality; indeed, they appear to welcome signs of individuality.

Conclusion

Adolescence is an intense developmental period for teenagers even in optimal family circumstances. In essence, the adolescent is challenged to assert an individual identity that is separate from the identity enjoyed in the home. In addition, the adolescent needs to rebel, to a certain extent, from the family. When the teenager's transition to adulthood creates too much dysfunction, the entire family may be experiencing a conflict that has been displaced onto the teenager. One technique for resolving the conflict is to have all family members attend psychotherapy. During such sessions, the therapist may use, in a flexible fashion, techniques derived from family, group, and individual treatment modalities. Juxtaposing these strategies clarifies, perhaps for the first time, the nature of the interaction within the family.

In particular, principles of family therapy are helpful for understanding the degree to which family members are functioning as an undifferentiated family ego mass. Family members may be using strategies such as triangulation and scapegoating to avoid confronting powerful emotions. Principles derived from group therapy, on the other hand, clarify whether family members are asserting patterns of autonomy adaptively. Here the therapist should be sensitive to the levels of cohesion and universality family members express for one another.

This chapter presented the case of an adolescent with a history of two previous pregnancies, one of which was aborted and one of which ended in miscarriage. At the outset of treatment, the teenager expressed a wish to have another infant and, this time, to raise the child. Both parents were vehemently opposed to their daughter's plan. Psychotherapy for the entire family revealed that prior to the adolescent's conception and birth, the mother had herself undergone an abortion because she had been in a car accident that had harmed the fetus, and her teenage daughter was now acting out her conflict.

Psychotherapy enabled the family to better differentiate from one another, as well as to learn how to express individual needs. In particular, the therapist highlighted episodes of transition between intimacy as autonomy. Focusing on the emotions generated during these transitions enabled family members to achieve a more adaptive mode of interaction. In addition, they became more adept at using expressive cues to convey emotions to one another in an unfettered manner.

REFERENCES

Abel, T. M. (1983), Comparisons between group and family therapy. In: *Group and Family Therapy*, ed. L. R. Wolberg & M. L. Aronson. New York: Brunner/Mazel, pp. 185–199.

Albright, L., Kenny, D. A. & Malloy, T. E. (1988), Consensus in personality judgements at zero acquaintance. *J. Per. Soc. Psychol.*, 55:387–395.

Ambady, N. & Rosenthal, R. (1992), Thin slices of expressive behavior as predictors of interpersonal consequences: A meta-analysis. *Psychol. Bull.*, 111 256–274.

Beels, C. C. & Ferber, A. (1969), Family therapy: A view. *Fam. Proc.*, 9:280–318.

Bloch, S. & Crouch, E. (1985), *Therapeutic Factors in Group Psychotherapy*. Oxford: Oxford University Press.

Bowen, M. (1966), The use of family theory in clinical practice. *Comp. Psychiat.*, 7:345–374.

——— (1978), *Family Therapy in Clinical Practice*. New York: Aronson.

Colijn, S., Hoencamp, E., Snijders, H. J. A., Van der Spek, M. W. A. & Duivenvoorden, H. J. (1991), A comparison of curative factors in different types of group psychotherapy. *Internat. J. Group Psychother.*, 41: 365–378.

Fromm-Reichman, F. (1950), *Principles of Intensive Psychotherapy.* Chicago: University of Chicago Press.

Funder, D. C. & Colvin, C. R. (1988), Friends and strangers: Acquaintanceship, agreement, and the accuracy of personality judgment. *J. Per. Soc. Psychol.*, 44:107–112.

Goffman, E. (1974). *Frame Analysis: An Essay on the Organization of Experience.* Cambridge, MA: Harvard University Press.

Goldfried, M. R., Wiser, S. L. & Raue, P. J. (1992), On the movement toward psychotherapy integration: The case of panic disorder. *J. Psychother. Prac. Res.*, 1:213–224.

Hulce, W. C. (1960), Psychiatric aspects of group counseling with adolescents. *Psychiat. Quart.*, 34(Supp.):307–313.

Minuchin, S. (1974), *Families and Family Therapy.* Cambridge, MA: Harvard University Press.

Richter, H. E. (1974), *The Family as Patient.* New York: Farrar, Straus & Giroux.

Skynner, A. C. R. (1981), An open-systems, group-analytic approach to family therapy. In: *Handbook of Family Therapy*, ed. A. S. Gurman & D. P. Kniskern. New York: Brunner/Mazel, pp. 39–84.

———— (1987), *Explorations with Families.* London: Methuen.

Slife, B. D. & Lanyon, J. (1991), Accounting for the power of the here-and-now: A theoretical revolution. *Internat. J. Group Psychother.*, 41:145–167.

PART IV

INTERVENTIONS
FOR VIOLENCE
AND TRAUMA

17   INTERVENING AGAINST VIOLENCE
IN THE SCHOOLS

MARK D. WEIST AND BETH S. WARNER

Violence was not even mentioned as a problem in schools in 1949, when a survey of high school principals in the United States documented "lying" and "disrespect" as their most serious concerns (Hennings, 1949). Since this early survey, however, school-based violence has progressively increased, spiraling in the late 1980s and early 1990s. Violent incidents within schools include verbal threats and taunts, harassment, physical assaults, destruction of property, thefts, and may even include sexual assaults, rapes, and homicides (Bybee and Gee, 1982; Nuttall and Kalesnick, 1987; National School Boards Association, 1993).

It is important to note that, in many cases, this school-based violence is merely one aspect of the brutality that youth experience in their homes and communities, either as witnesses or direct victims. Particularly for youths living in the inner city, school-based violence can be seen as exacerbating emotional, behavioral, and cognitive difficulties related to other violence exposure (Shakoor and Chalmers, 1991). In this paper, we briefly review statistics underscoring the scope and magnitude of school-based violence and related community violence, and discuss its impacts on youth. We then provide guidelines for decreasing school violence, and for developing mental health interventions for youth exposed to violence in their schools and communities.

School-Based and Community Violence and Youth

In the 1992–93 academic year, the National School Boards Association (NSBA; 1993) conducted a survey of over 2000 school districts in the U.S. on violence in schools. Over 90% of administrators responding to the survey indicated their view that violence had increased in their schools in the past five years. The most common problems reported by school districts were student on student assaults (78% of districts), carrying of weapons by students (61% of districts), and student on teacher assaults (28% of districts). As expected, school districts from urban areas reported the highest levels of violence in the past year, with 93% reporting student on student assaults, 91% reporting weapons found on students, 39% reporting a shooting or knifing, 25% reporting a drive-by shooting, and 18% reporting a rape, with each of these incidents occurring on school property.

The increasing use of weapons by youth is central to the violence problem. The 1990 Youth Risk Behavior Survey, a nationwide, school-based assessment of high school students, revealed that one of five students in grades 9 through 12 carried a firearm, knife, or club at least one time during the month prior to the survey's administration (Centers for Disease Control, 1991). The NSBA (1993) estimated that 135,000 American children carry guns to school each day. In the period between 1986 and 1990, 71 people were murdered with guns at school, 201 people were severely wounded, and 242 people were held hostage (Center to Prevent Handgun Violence, 1990).

Statistics on violence exposure for children and adolescents in schools are reflective of a more general problem in their communities. For example, in two pertinent studies from Chicago, Bell (1987) found that 31% of elementary and middle school students had witnessed a shooting, 34% had seen a stabbing, and 84% had seen someone "beaten-up." Shakoor and Chalmers (1991) assessed a group of African American youths ages 10 to 19 and found that a startling 75% of boys and 70% of girls surveyed had seen someone shot, stabbed, robbed, or murdered.

The above is not a complete review of the scope and magnitude of the problem of violence and youth in the U.S. However, it does highlight a significant problem that appears to be worsening in recent years. We now turn to a brief discussion of the impacts of violence on youths in schools.

Impacts of Violence on Students

Exposure to violence has significant emotional, behavioral, and cognitive effects on students. In general, youths who are most exposed to violence show high levels of internalizing and externalizing behavioral difficulties, attentional and cognitive problems, with concomitant failure in school and later social and occupational adjustment. Major effects of violence exposure are reviewed in the following:

FEAR

Pervasive fear is perhaps the most salient impact of violence on youth. Menacker, Weldon, and Hurwitz (1989) surveyed students in three middle schools in Chicago. Over one-half of the students reported feeling unsafe in school, with these fears contributing to poor school performance. Bybee and Gee (1982), in an early and comprehensive review of school violence reported, "about 3% of students are afraid at school most of the time" (p. 104) due to school-based violence.

Fears about personal safety often translate into behavioral changes. School avoidance, refusal, and phobias may develop in students in reaction to violence exposure. Bybee and Gee (1982) reported that about 16% of students avoided places at school (e.g., restrooms, cafeterias) because of safety concerns. Avoidance is also seen in the form of skipping classes or the entire school day (NSBA, 1993; Nuttall and Kalesnik, 1987). Hranitz and Eddowes (1990) reported that around one in ten absences among inner city junior and senior high school students were related to their expressed fears of being assaulted.

In addition to contributing to school avoidance, fear of violence in schools may serve as a catalyst for youth to become violent. For example, almost one-third of a sample of middle school students from Chicago reported carrying weapons to school related to fears of violence (Menacker et al., 1989).

TRAUMATIZATION SYMPTOMS

A number of investigators have documented symptoms of posttraumatic stress disorder (PTSD) in children and adolescents who have witnessed or been victimized by violence (Hilton, 1992; Terr, 1979). Many PTSD symptoms exert indirect and direct effects on the school performance of youth affected by violence. Nightmares and other sleep disturbances lead to fatigue during the school day. Hyperarousal and hypervigilance contribute to attentional and concentration difficulties, as do preoccupations about harm to self and others. Truancy and dropping out of school may result from avoidance of situations and other stimuli associated with the violence, particularly when violence has occurred on or near school property.

In addition to these traumatization symptoms, Pynoos and Nader (1988, 1990) suggest other reactions to trauma in children. These include disturbed grief and loss reactions, as reminiscing about the lost person is impeded by images of his or her violent death. Second, separation anxiety may occur as traumatized youth worry excessively about family members and have difficulty being apart from them. Finally, exacerbation or renewal of prior symptoms may occur, as adjustment difficulties from earlier traumas can reemerge with subsequent violence exposure.

DEPRESSION AND "FUTURELESSNESS"

Studies have documented that children who are exposed to high levels of violence are likely to develop symptoms of depression (Fitzpatrick, 1993). These symptoms may include severe hopelessness characterized by an inability or unwillingness to consider the future, and the perception of a shortened life span, a phenomenon termed "futurelessness." This kind of hopelessness in inner city youth shockingly manifests itself in stories of adolescents and even children, who are not planning for college or future occupations, but for their funerals. A sense of futurelessness is fueled by sensitivity among urban youth to the deaths of their friends and associates from violence, as well as the awareness of how many of their contemporaries do not make it. In the schools served by our School Mental Health Program, most adolescents have lost at least one friend or family member from violence. One of us recently assessed a 15-year-old black male who had lost four friends to violence in the past year; when asked about his goal for his life in five years, he reported, "to be buried in Western Cemetery" to escape the past and ongoing pain in his life. This story gives poignant meaning to the statistic that black males in the 15–24 age range have the highest rates of violent death and incarceration of any group (Centers for Disease Control, 1990).

Impacts on Cognition and School Performance

As we have discussed, symptoms of traumatization may impact school performance. In addition, it has been documented that young people who fear for their personal safety have concentration problems and an impaired ability to absorb classroom material (Gorski and Pilotto, 1993). Further, among children and adolescents who have witnessed excessive violence, general negative effects on cognition and memory are commonly shown (Nuttall and Kalesnik, 1987; Shakoor and Chalmers, 1991).

In relation to the random and frequent violence they contend with, many urban youth show an external locus of control, feeling that they have no influence over events in their lives. This contributes to feelings of futility about school, perceiving that it will not make a difference for them. Consequently, many urban youth give up on school before they reach high school or in their early high school years, a problem underscored by drop out rates in many urban school districts that exceed 50% (Rhodes and Jason, 1990).

This brief review emphasizes the many ways in which exposure to violence can negatively affect the emotional/behavioral and school adjustment of children and adolescents. As the problem of violence exposure and youth has increased in recent years, so have efforts to assist youth in schools in coping with violence. We turn now to a review of methods of intervening against violence in the schools.

Interventions

School administrative staff have traditionally had the main responsibility for handling the problem of school-based violence. In general, schools that have fair and clear rules that are implemented firmly and consistently, provide adequate supervision of students, and have an engaged and active teaching staff tend to have relatively lower rates of school-based violence (National School Boards Assn., 1993). Most school administrative approaches for reducing violence strive to meet these objectives.

Historically, mental health professionals have not played a role in finding solutions to interpersonal violence in schools. In recent years, however, the role of mental health professionals in addressing the impacts of violence on youth in schools has increased considerably with the expansion of school-based mental health services: the placement of clinical therapists in schools who provide services that attempt to replicate those available in community mental health clinics. These services include focused mental health evaluations, individual, group and family therapies, and referral for more intensive services.

These services are distinguished from mental health services traditionally offered in schools—via school psychologists and social workers—
by their emphasis on treatment and availability to all students, not just
those in special education. Placement of clinical therapists in schools
began in the late 1980s, and since then there has been almost an
exponential growth in these services. For example, in Baltimore in the
1989-90 academic year, mental health programs operated in eight
schools; in 1993-94 these programs operated in over 30 schools, and
in 1994-95, there were programs in over 60 schools. Such local growth
is congruent with regional and national trends (Flaherty, Weist, and
Warner, 1996). In the program for which we are responsible, we
provide mental health services to children and adolescents in 15
elementary, middle, and high schools, which represents an increase of
nine schools in the past three years. Importantly, development of these
mental health programs in schools has facilitated the design and
implementation of programs to address violence. Programs take a
number of different approaches, which we now review.

CURRICULUM-BASED APPROACHES

The most widely used interventions are curriculum or educational
approaches. These programs are typically implemented by educators
with input from mental health professionals. They target the general
student body and students who are at risk for aggressive behavior.

Prothrow-Stith (1987) has developed and implemented a structured
10-session violence prevention curriculum for use with urban adolescents that has received considerable national attention. The curriculum
is designed for teachers to use in the classroom as an educational tool,
but appears appropriate for use by facilitators in other settings (e.g., by
health and mental health professionals in clinic settings). Initial
sessions provide information on the types of violence in society,
statistics on violent behavior, and risk factors for violent and homicidal
behavior, including use of weapons and substance abuse. These are
followed by sessions focused on anger, and its precipitants, physiological and behavioral concomitants, and destructive versus constructive
methods of anger expression. Concluding sessions in the curriculum
focus on alternatives to getting into violent interactions, with an
emphasis on conflict-resolution techniques. Preliminary findings
indicate that the program is effective in reducing conflicts between
students (Prothrow-Stith, 1991).

PRESENTATIONS ON VIOLENCE

We have recently begun classroom presentations on violence to students in middle and high schools. In half-hour presentations, teams of two professionals (ideally of different race and gender, and from different disciplines) review with students the problems of violence, its effects, ways of reducing it, strategies to avoid involvement in it, and how to cope with its aftereffects. These presentations are interactive, with presenters posing a series of questions to the students about each aspect of violence to get them involved. Also, role-play techniques are briefly used to highlight conflict mediation approaches. At the end of the presentations, students are provided with a resource list of all staff in the building (school administrators, psychologists, social workers and counselors) who can assist them in dealing with violence. These presentations have been very well received by the students, who have responded with high levels of animated, and usually appropriate, discussions. Following these presentations we have observed increased numbers of students seeking out school professional staff for help in handling problems related to violence.

ORGANIZED RESPONSES TO CRISES

As in most city schools, an unfortunate problem that appears to be increasing is distress experienced by students when one of their schoolmates is killed in the community. In most of our high schools, there will be at least one student death from violence each year, and depending on the popularity of the student and the nature of his or her death, negative effects in the school can be significant. For example, after such an incident, many students will be found crying in classrooms and hallways, while others express anger over the incident and may respond by leaving school or yelling at teachers, and still others appear detached and reclusive. Not only the students but also the teachers and other school staff are usually quite distressed over the violent death of a student.

As a result of our experiences, we have developed an approach (Warner, Weist, and Crouch, 1995) designed to assist students and staff in coping with such incidents. Core elements of the approach are: 1) formal announcement of the death of the student by the principal over the loudspeaker and 2) availability of group counseling. In the announcement, the principal simply informs the student body of the

355

death (without specific details), requests a moment of silence, and then announces classrooms where counselors will be available to students who wish to talk about the loss of the student and feel in need of support. Teams of two counselors, of various disciplines including psychology, social work, and guidance, are then available in designated classrooms at specified times for group sessions that occur two to three times weekly for two or more weeks.

Groups are limited to seven or eight students, and may include males and females, or be comprised of students of the same gender (we have not discerned that either arrangement is better). During the initial group meeting, students are usually at the level of wanting to learn about the incident and sharing information that they have. It is useful for counseling staff to share whatever formal information that is available; for example, counselors distributing copies of a newspaper article creates a basis for discussion of what happened. Variably, during these initial meetings, students cry and express sadness and anger over the loss of the student, and counselors encourage such emotional expression. As such, foci in this initial meeting are usually limited to information sharing, and at times, also include free emotional expression by students. Subsequent sessions guided by counselors include continued emotional expression, bereavement activities such as sharing stories about the deceased student, developing and reinforcing coping skills, fostering reciprocal social support for group members, and discussions on survival skills and avoidance of violence. Most groups run for between four and six sessions, at which point students usually appear brighter and reinvolved in their normal routines. However, in many instances, groups express their desire to continue meeting and evolve into more general support groups.

PEER MEDIATION PROGRAMS

Peer mediation techniques are increasingly being used by school systems as a means to decrease levels of conflict and violence. In peer mediation, students designated as mediators are called in as neutral parties who help guide the resolution of conflict when students are unable to solve their own disputes successfully. For example, in Johnson and Johnson's (1994) program in a suburban high school, a group of peer mediators were taught to identify and define conflicts, use negotiation skills to reframe disputes as conflicts of interest, and to facilitate "perspective taking" and problem solving in other students.

The program resulted in clear decreases in conflicts between students, and many students used aspects of the program in situations at home.

Similar programs at all grade levels, and in urban, suburban, and rural school districts have been found to be highly effective in reducing conflicts between students, disciplinary infractions, and referrals to the principal. Generally, such programs show particular benefits for the peer mediators, who evidence increases in prosocial behaviors and decreases in antisocial behaviors (Johnson and Johnson, 1994).

PROGRAMS FOR YOUTH
HIGHLY EXPOSED TO VIOLENCE

Our literature review revealed few comprehensive group therapy programs geared toward witnesses to violence. In one exception, Dyson (1990) reported that a school-based group therapy program, concurrent with individual therapy, resulted in improved academic and behavioral adjustment for six inner city African American adolescents who had been chronically exposed to violence, particularly in the home. The group program, which was viewed as complimentary to the adolescents' individual therapy, taught participants nonaggressive ways of coping with provocative situations, fostered feelings of acceptance and belonging among members, and led to enhanced feelings of self-esteem and perceived mastery over conflictual situations with others.

In the 1993–94 academic year, we implemented a school-based group therapy program for adolescents exposed to high levels of violence. The intervention consisted of eight structured group therapy meetings and was implemented with ninth and tenth grade students from two Baltimore high schools (six females from one school, and five males from another). Initial group sessions focused on discussion of violence, for example, its prevalence in urban areas, and sharing by group members about violence they had experienced or to which they been exposed. This was followed by sessions in which the cognitive, emotional, and behavioral reactions to violence exposure were reviewed. Group members were then assisted in developing strategies to address the impacts of violence on them, and they were provided with direction on obtaining additional assistance as indicated. In the final phase of the group, members learned conflict mediation and general survival skills to reduce the probability that they would become victims of or witnesses to violence. From preintervention to postintervention, group members showed decreased internalizing symptoms such as depression and anxiety. We are beginning efforts to conduct more controlled studies of such group programs for youth exposed to high levels of violence.

INDIVIDUAL AND FAMILY INTERVENTIONS

It is beyond the scope of this paper to review the range of approaches that we use in the provision of individual and family therapies to youths exposed to violence. However, these therapies are provided in schools, which improves their accessibility to many youths who need them. Briefly, our treatment efforts build upon the theoretical model of Pynoos and Nader (1988, 1990) and target four key areas as discussed earlier: PTSD symptoms, grief and loss, separation anxiety, and renewal of symptoms. Key features of therapy with traumatized youth include encouraging emotional expression, normalizing emotional reactions, and educating about the recovery process, decreasing cognitive distortions regarding the safety of self and others as well as attributions of responsibility for the violent incident, facilitating use of social support from family, friends, and others (e.g., teachers, coaches), and assisting families in providing a supportive and nurturant atmosphere that protects the child from further harm, in which grief and bereavement reactions can be expressed. For some youths, these approaches are used in combination with psychopharmacological treatment, which is facilitated by psychiatric consultants who work in our program.

Concluding Comment

Exposure to violence in communities and in schools is increasing for adolescents, particularly for those from urban areas. In reaction to such exposure, youths present a range of cognitive, behavioral, and emotional problems, as well as becoming violent themselves. While the problem of violence exposure and youth has grown in recent years, so has our ability to respond to it, with the progressive, and rapid, development of intensive school-based mental health services— augmenting existing school psychology and social work services— throughout the U.S. We have highlighted a number of interventions against violence in the schools including administrative, curriculum-based, didactic, crisis intervention, peer mediation, and psychotherapeutic programs. Unfortunately, few schools are implementing more than one of these programs, and some do not have any programs to address violence (NSBA, 1993). Intuitively, we would assume that multifaceted approaches, including numerous elements as above, would be the most effective in addressing violence and its effects in schools. However, this remains an empirical question; our literature review revealed only a few studies (e.g., Dyson, 1990; Prothrow-Stith, 1987, 1991) involving assessment of the treatment impacts of violence interventions. Clearly, there is significant need for increased clinical and research efforts to prevent and address the impacts of violence in children and adolescents.

REFERENCES

Bell, C. C. (1987), Preventive strategies for dealing with violence among blacks. *Comm. Ment. Health J.*, 23:217–228.

Bybee, R. W. & Gee, E. G. (1982), *Violence, Values, and Justice in the Schools*. Boston, MA: Allyn & Bacon.

Centers for Disease Control (1990), Homicide among young black males - United States, 1978–1987. *Morbidity and Mortality Weekly Reports*, 39:869–873.

Centers for Disease Control (1991), Weapon-carrying among high school students. *J. Amer. Med. Assn.*, 266:23–42.

Center to Prevent Handgun Violence (1990), *Caught in the Crossfire*. Washington, DC: Center to Prevent Handgun Violence.

Dyson, J. L. (1990), The effect of family violence on children's academic performance and behavior. *J. Natl. Med. Assn.*, 82:17–22.

Fitzpatrick, K. M. (1993), Exposure to violence and presence of depression among low-income African-American youth. *J. Consult. Clin. Psychol.*, 61:528–531.

Flaherty, L. T., Weist, M. D. & Warner, B. S. (1996), School- based mental health services in the United States: History, current models and needs. *Comm. Ment. Health J.*, 32:341–352.

Gorski, J. D. & Pilotto, L. (1993), Interpersonal violence among youth: A challenge for school personnel. *Educat. Psychol. Rev.*, 5:35–61.

Hennings, C. (1949), Discipline: Are school practices changing? *The Clearing House*, 13:267–270.

Hilton, N. Z. (1992), Battered women's concerns about their children witnessing wife assault. *J. Interpers. Violence.*, 7:77–86.

Hranitz, J. R., & Eddowes, E. A. (1990), Violence: A crisis in homes and schools. *Childhood Ed.*, 66:4–7.

Johnson, D. W., & Johnson, R. T. (1994), Constructive conflict in the schools. *J. Social Iss.*, 50:117–137.

Menacker, J., Weldon, W. & Hurwitz, E. (1989), Community influences in school crime and violence. *Urban Ed.*, 25:68–80.

National School Boards Association (1993), *Violence in the Schools.* Alexandria, VA: National School Boards Association.

Nuttall, E. & Kalesnick, J. (1987), Personal violence in the schools: The role of the counselor. *J. Counsel. Devel.*, 65:372–375.

Prothrow-Stith, D. (1987), *Violence Prevention Curriculum for Adolescents.* Newton, MA: Education Development Center.

——— (1991), *Deadly Consequences.* New York: HarperCollins.

Pynoos, R. S., & Nader, K. (1988), Psychological first aid and treatment approach to children exposed to community violence: Research implications. *J. Traumatic Stress,* 1:445–473.

——— & ——— (1990), Children's exposure to violence and traumatic death. *Psychiat. Annals,* 20:334–344.

Rhodes, J. E. & Jason, L. A. (1990), A social stress model of substance abuse. *J. Consult. Clin. Psychol.*, 58:395–401.

Shakoor, B. H. & Chalmers, D. (1991), Co-victimization of African-American children who witness violence: Effects on cognitive, emotional, and behavioral development. *J. Natl. Med. Assn.*, 83:233–238.

Terr, L. (1979), Children of Chowchilla: A study of psychic trauma. *The Psychoanalytic Study of the Child,* 34:547–623. New Haven, CT: Yale University Press.

Warner, B. S., Weist, M. D. & Crouch, J. (1995), School–based crisis intervention in response to violence. Unpublished manuscript.

18 THE GAME'S THE THING: PLAY PSYCHOTHERAPY WITH A TRAUMATIZED YOUNG ADOLESCENT BOY

STEVEN M. WEINE*

In the last few years, there has been a growing interest in the effects of psychological traumas. Across the disciplines of psychiatry, psycho-analysis, psychology, sociology, literature, history, and film making there is an increasing awareness of the contemporary significance of trauma and an enhanced desire to learn more about its impact on human life.

The new urgency and priority being given to traumatic experiences is also having an impact upon established patterns of psychotherapeutic understanding and practice. In recent years we have seen the emer-gence of new psychotherapeutic treatments for children and adults with histories of childhood trauma, including cognitive-behavioral tech-niques (Foa, Steketee, and Rothbaum, 1989) and trauma-focused group psychotherapies (Herman, 1992). At the same time, we are finding that the existing body of psychotherapeutic knowledge and skills provides a valuable foundation for clinical treatment of posttraumatic conditions in children, adolescents, and adults.

The case of a traumatized early adolescent boy whom I treated with psychotherapy illustrates some particular ways in which play psycho-therapy may be used in the treatment of a traumatized individual. The adolescent had struggled with intense, overwhelming feelings that stemmed from a history of abuse and neglect, further complicated by his entering adolescence. This therapy pushed me toward the limits of my psychotherapeutic knowledge, causing me to experience milder

*The author would like to acknowledge gratefully the comments and suggestions of Daniel Levinson, Al Solnit, David Carlson, Syd Phillips, Ira Levine, Charles Gardner and Daniel Becker.

versions of his affective storms: uncertainty, hopelessness, guilt, and hate. The challenge we shared was to create a means of joining together in a psychotherapeutic process that best addressed his developmentally and psychopathologically determined treatment needs. He, however, was too old to participate in the imaginative play games of younger children, which form the basis for the therapeutic work in child psychoanalysis and explorative child psychotherapy. Yet, he was equally unwilling to enter into a relationship with me based primarily on our talking to one another as might an older adolescent or adult.

The treatment I devised for this adolescent, who was more prone to "doing" than "talking," illustrates the uses of both traditional and novel play psychotherapeutic approaches. The treatment approach was strongly shaped by the traditional concepts of psychoanalytic play therapy (Solnit and Newbauer, 1987). The treatment also involved extensions and adaptations of those concepts into novel modes of play. The unique solution we discovered involved using competitive athletic games as the major psychotherapeutic activity.

Structured games, such as competitive athletic games, are often perceived as having a marginal place in contemporary psychoanalytic play therapy. It is often felt that these games are too rigid and unimaginative to serve as a pathway to the inner world of the child or adolescent. The play of structured games is not usually thought of as having any particular value in psychotherapeutic work outside of the initial phases of engagement. It is sometimes thought of as a part of resistance to the analytic process of achieving insight. Yet, through this case, I discovered that the play of structured games could have a central role in a psychotherapeutic treatment of a severely traumatized young adolescent. The case is also a testimony to the important contributions made by psychoanalytic play therapy in the treatment of trauma-related conditions.

The psychotherapy took place on a long-term inpatient unit for treatment-resistant adolescents. Individual psychotherapy was part of a multidisciplinary treatment that included family therapies, group therapies, milieu therapy, substance abuse therapy, art and music therapy, occupational and recreational therapy, and pharmacotherapy. (This report will cover only the individual psychotherapy.) I met with the boy three times a week for 45 minutes over a period of one year. I participated in monthly treatment team meetings and received weekly supervision from a psychoanalyst supervisor.

Case Report

Sam, an African American boy in the eighth grade, was admitted at age 13 and received over one year of inpatient treatment. Long-term hospitalization was arranged after short-term hospitalizations proved ineffective in treating his increasingly severe behavioral problems.

Sam is the only child born to an unwed single late adolescent woman from a working-class background. Shortly after the birth, his father told Sam's mother that he wasn't ready to be a father, and he has never been a consistent presence in Sam's life. Sam's mother, Joanne, is the oldest of a sibship abandoned by their father in childhood. She had been responsible for providing for her siblings and cousins, who were reportedly involved with drugs, alcohol, and destructive interpersonal relationships.

Joanne raised Sam in the housing projects of a large northeastern city, though she always aspired to give him a better life. To support her and Sam's "little family," she worked hard to earn money and create stability. She proved able to lift them out of poverty and into the middle class. She loves Sam, feels connected to him, and strives to provide for him and to make time for them to be together. Early in her son's life she had substantial difficulty in providing enough sustenance, nurturing, and protection for him. Throughout his life, Sam was left with a bewildering succession of unsuitable sitters or with Joanne's cousins, who exposed him to sex, drugs, violence, and physical beatings. At age 4, Sam was sodomized by a baby-sitter. Though his mother took Sam to the emergency room and had him begin counseling, the fact that she did not insist he continue in therapy against his wishes and did not press charges against the perpetrator has often disturbed Sam. Further, his counseling was interrupted because "he wouldn't talk," and his mother thought "he would forget about it because he was so young." Joanne has also had difficulty controlling his exhibitions of temper and has tended to react to Sam's outbursts by engaging him in vicious verbal and, at times, violent physical struggles, before collapsing in guilt and despair.

Sam had problems in nursery school, and Joanne received numerous complaints that he needed to be the center of attention. He had a good year in kindergarten and he liked his teacher, but in first grade he hated his teacher and was disruptive, oppositional, inattentive, and was often sent home. Second and third grades were marred by more of the same behavioral problems. In the fourth and fifth grades, Sam was placed in residential treatment, which neither he nor his mother felt was of any benefit.

For sixth grade, Sam's mother enrolled him in another school, and had him see the school psychologist. He spent much of his free time with high school–age peers, telling them that he was 15 years old, staying out late at night, openly disobeying his mother, stealing from her, fighting, using and dealing drugs. That year he was arrested for shoplifting and criminal mischief. Because Joanne was increasingly unable to "handle" Sam, she brought him for his first hospitalization six months prior to the current admission.

INITIAL PSYCHOLOGICAL EXAMINATION

Sam underwent initial psychological examination upon admission. Tests administered were Projective Drawings, Thematic Apperception Test, Sentence Completion Test, Rorschach, and Object Relations Inventory. Sam's personality was organized at a high borderline level with marked dysphoria and anxiety, pronounced aggressivity, vulnerability to perceptual distortions, and lapses into paranoid ideation and autistic logic. He relied on oppositionality, avoidance, and paranoia to defend against severe dysphoria and fears of being abused. His object relations were poorly integrated and malevolent. Sam lived with an abiding conscious sense of failure, fright, and loneliness, and less consciously, badness, that he covered with a defiant stance. Representations of maternal figures were consciously available and helpful to him, and less consciously vulnerable, unstable, disappointing, and distant. Representations of paternal figures were markedly negative, though not completely condemned: there was a conscious wish to have a loving father, though this was more often than not met with rejection and disappointment. Cognitive performance was within the average range.

The examiner found Sam attentive, reflective, and motivated—abilities that make him well suited for individual psychotherapy—but with the qualification: "What he needs help with most, at this point, is connecting his feelings with his conduct. Acutely aware of each, he does not appreciate the full extent of their interrelatedness. Combining activities with talking during therapy times will facilitate these connections, as well as respecting his strengths and what he needs to feel safe."

STEVEN M. WEINE

THE PSYCHOTHERAPY

Sam and I began our first therapy session sitting together in my office and talking. He recited his problems in a manner as calculated as reciting a multiplication table: "I've got depression, drugs, alcohol addiction, anger, fights, family problems, and two kinds of abuse," a remarkable but canned account. Just before our time ran out, he said: "I'm not comfortable with you. I trust women better. I had some past experiences of abuse by men."

In our second session, also in my office, Sam sat quietly. Twenty minutes later he said, "Today's been a really bad day. I cut my finger and banged my head. I bruised my arm and I got a bloody nose." He asked if we could play ping pong, something he did with a former therapist, and I agreed, thus beginning a shift toward play.

In our third session, he again sat silently in a chair in my office. After our talking hit a dead end, he spotted a cactus plant on a small table beside his chair: "That's neat." Not a second later, he conspicuously plucked a leaf from my plant as if he were stripping an artichoke. "Oh, I'm sorry. Really I am." He straightened his oversize frame against the chair back. "I didn't mean that. Really I didn't." I said, "What happened there?" Sam: "I was just playing with it. I like your plant, really I do. Really." He seemed terrified of immediate repercussions, perhaps that I would explode and beat him up for killing my plant. It was no wonder that thereafter he would say or do anything to avoid returning to my office. Not only did he refuse to meet in my office, but Sam also found talking with me completely intolerable. Thus, from the start, it seemed that talking would not be an effective way to make contact with Sam. He demanded to meet in the front lounge of our unit, the hospital courtyard, or the hospital gym, and insisted on spending our sessions playing ping pong, tossing a football, or shooting baskets. I was reluctant, however, to make a structured game, such as ping pong, a regular part of our therapy. I was concerned that this seemingly rigid and unexpressive form of play would overserve defensive functions and ward off or hide the aggressive and libidinal fantasies that I presumed Sam needed to explore and work through in his therapy. Still, it felt as if I had little choice but to go along with Sam's insistence upon playing games in our therapy if I wanted us to interact at all.

Those first months of our play were characterized by escalating cycles of stimulation and aggression. A cycle began with Sam's cautious approach to me, followed by some friendly play that became increasingly strained by hostile behavior, and climaxed in outbursts of rage. When Sam lost control of himself, what began as "just a game" took on catastrophic dimensions and completely disrupted the play. At first these cycles lasted only a session, then a string of sessions, and then they eventually extended to a few weeks' duration. Each cycle brought a shift in games: when ping pong proved too much to bear, we turned to basketball, then cards, then back to ping pong, then back to cards, then back to basketball. Each new game was enough like starting over to allow Sam to regroup after a venomous outburst, and yet, the cycles were similar enough to allow me to consider silently each event as part of a growing, patterned process about which we were becoming increasingly aware.

For the first month we played fiercely competitive matches of ping pong. As the unequivocal ping pong champion of his unit, Sam was surprised to find me a competitive rival. When I'd return his slams, he'd say: "I can't believe you got those. That's luck!" He became very irritated when he fell behind or lost, and his irritation and frustration would, at best, interfere with or, at worst, totally disrupt our play. He expressed his aggression in nearly every game: throwing the paddle, breaking the ball, swearing, fighting with another kid, fighting with me. I tried to keep Sam's play under control by setting limits: "Sam, if you slam your paddle again, then we will not be able to play." Sometimes limit setting would work because Sam really didn't want to stop playing, and other times, when he was already too far gone, it only sparked even more extreme agitation.

Playing these games with Sam forced me to confront in supervision my own conflicts concerning competitiveness. The games also raised questions of psychotherapeutic technique. If I were to beat him whenever possible, as I would if it were strictly a competitive game, then I would have been needlessly adding to his frustrations. Yet, when I played under my ability level, Sam could easily spot when I wasn't trying hard enough and would experience this as an insult to his athletic abilities. I had to be in the game enough to make it believable and invigorating, but detached enough from competitive zeal to remember the game was a vehicle for therapy. Thus, my goal in the competitive play was not to win, but to use the experiential context of the play to help Sam attend to his present bodily experiences, perhaps to recover traumatic memories, to master his hate, and to tolerate close contact. Because Sam had a way of bringing out the killer in me, I found that it was a constant struggle to keep the goals of the therapy in mind and to realize that this was not "just a game," but also a play therapy.

Over time, I began to notice that in his play Sam sought higher and higher levels of stimulation. For example, Sam situated himself on whichever side of the ping pong table other kids were congregated and let himself get revved up by the others in the middle of a game. He seemed completely unaware of his state of agitation and unable to put the brakes on. At these moments, our play inevitably collapsed. I tried to notice when his play first began to deteriorate and then say something like, "Gee, Sam, you seem frustrated from the way you tossed that ball away from me." A preemptive stance such as this was occasionally effective in heading off an explosion and refocusing Sam on the play.

I found it remarkable how often Sam became overstimulated in our play. Once after missing an easy point he became so enraged that he slammed his paddle down and walked out of sight. Perhaps he went to the bathroom and would soon return, I thought. A few minutes passed, and there was no sign of Sam. Not in the back lounge, not in the bathrooms, not in his bedroom, not in other patients' rooms. A staff member said to try his closet. When I swung open the doors I found Sam cowering in a closet barely larger than his hefty frame, afraid that I would do something horrible to him. I asked him to step out of the closet, but he was unable to tolerate being in the same room with me and walked away. Experiences such as these were extremely frustrating and exasperating and tested the limits of my self-control. Later, in a calmer state, I wondered if that was the very point of such interchanges.

By insisting that we play hour after hour of ping pong, cards, football, checkers, and basketball, Sam proved a tenacious teacher. He taught me to regard competitive games as a powerful therapeutic activity. Through the playing of these games, he made it necessary that I attend to his bodily experiences and made it possible for me to understand the ways in which he used his body to represent and communicate internal dramas. Thus, Sam helped me free myself of the concept that talk was the exclusive therapeutic activity and competitive play an undesirable defensive filler. I came to see that competitive play served Sam and me well as a transitional phenomenon, involving multiple representative and expressive modes, including the verbal, lexical, and enactive. Playing games became the medium for accomplishing what the psychological testing recommended—a means of letting feelings and conduct, thought and action flow into one another, connect, and become integrated. Thus, playing games became the main activity of our sessions even though there were still moments when I doubted whether our play accomplished anything at all. Old habits die hard.

Our play demonstrated again and again how overstimulated Sam became in our sessions. I surmised that his subjective experience of the overstimulation was feeling a fear of being horribly attacked by me as well as a fear that he might destroy or obliterate me. At the very least, our play provided an activity that fortified Sam's defenses enough that he was able to tolerate our meetings. Playing games also helped to elaborate patterns of overstimulation marked by sadism and masochism and approach and avoidance that characterized Sam's interpersonal relatedness. Playing games, however, had not yet elaborated the fantasies underlying such behaviors so that he and I might understand and gain mastery over these intensely charged inner dramas.

At one session, three months into our work, Sam asked if we could play racquetball. He led me up to the basketball gym, and we began playing racquetball. He kept the score. When Sam discovered that he couldn't dominate or obliterate me in racquetball, just as he had also hoped to do in ping pong, his frustration mounted. At first by accident, then by design, he had us transform our manner of play: instead of playing between the two most proximate walls, we began to hit the ball against the full length of the basketball court. Sam invented a new game: one player tried to hit the ball as hard as possible—"kill it"—against the front wall with the object of having it bounce against as many walls and corners as possible until the energy of the initial slam had dissipated. We took turns "killing" the racquetball. During this play Sam relaxed and spontaneously told me about his experiences playing racquetball with his mother ("She's all right") and with a male psychiatric assistant ("He got me in the balls").

This racquetball game is a good example of a qualitative shift that occurred in our play after three months. Sam and I began to invent play situations that permitted the active parallel expression of our mutual feelings of overstimulation and were maximally capable of absorbing both his and my aggressive discharges. Standing side by side, pounding the racquetball into the far wall, we enacted identificatory processes that were extremely useful to Sam in controlling his feelings of overstimulation. He identified with the part of me capable of aggressive discharge but also identified with my capacity to "let it out" in a controlled and modulated way. This example was the first noticeable step in a process of internalization whereby Sam used my greater capacities for control and modulation to form new structures of internal control over his behaviors, thoughts, and emotions.

In a session shortly thereafter, Sam, sitting at a table in the front lounge, surprised me by putting some of his experiences into words. He said, "I'm mad at my mother. For putting me away." I said, "She put you away?" He said, "Yeah you know. Like put me in here instead of letting me stay home." I said, "Do you miss being home?" He said, "Sure. Doesn't everybody?" I said, "I suppose but in different ways." He said, "Well I miss my pets." I said, "You've never told me about your pets." He said, "So . . . My favorite is Rex. He's a pit bull. I like taking him for walks. Like I was out with Rex one day and I had him off his leash in this park. I let him run around without a leash so that he can be free and stuff. And sometimes there's other dogs there and, like, he will get into fights. One day there was this other dog and Rex killed him." I asked, "He killed him?" He said, "Yeah you know what he did? He bit him, like, right on the nose." I felt extremely disturbed by this sadistic act and confused by the juxtaposition of love and disdain for animals, and said, "Oh my. Sounds horrifying." He said no. I said, "No? Well, then what was it like for you?" He said, "I didn't mind. 'Cause the other dog was really natty and stuff." I asked: "Natty?" He answered: "Yeah, like he didn't have a home. Like nobody took care of him and shit. So, like, it didn't matter what happened." I felt intimidated and frightened by this boy and his dog, and as if I'd met them in a dark alleyway, I kept my emotional distance.

I do not know for certain what made Sam talk that day. I do know, however, that it came at a time when he was feeling increased rapport with me through our play and safe enough to share with me some of his thoughts and feelings. I thought how much this was like Shengold's (1989) "rat people" who associated to the rat imago in psychoanalytic sessions. Sam's story revealed both the identification with the pit bull as a cannibalistic killer as well as the terrifying wish for the passive role that is so characteristic of victims of childhood trauma. If this was Sam's way of telling me to keep away, then it was at least a more developmentally advanced way of protecting himself than he had shown previously through violent enactments.

Sam and I played lots of games, but none served the psychotherapy as well as basketball. There are a number of reasons why basketball was an excellent vehicle for our therapy. First, basketball was something that Sam liked and played well. I too like basketball and am a good enough player. Thus, basketball made it possible for me to empathize with Sam, and for Sam to identify with me, no small accomplishment. I believe that our mutual love of the game helped sustain our capacities to play when threatened by overwhelming floods of hate and aggression. As we played it, hour after hour, basketball became a very sensuous experience. Our play permitted the expression of a great deal of aggression—charging, defending, blocking shots— yet we maintained fairly rigid limits for when to say "that's enough." Of course, to win in our basketball play also required a soft touch, quick moves, and agility. Basketball also afforded an excellent mode of discharge; there was a bathroom into which Sam would plunge for such purposes when overstimulated.

On the basketball court, Sam and I played Twenty-one, Around the World, One on One, and on occasion we just shot baskets. Twenty-one[1] was far and away Sam's favorite game to play with me. It was as physical as One on One, yet punctuated by free throws. In Twenty-one, Sam could assume his overwhelmingly preferred bodily orientation with me: his backside to my frontside. Around the World[2] by contrast, offered a respite from the close physical contact of Twenty-one.

---

[1]In Twenty-One, one player shoots a free throw while the other is positioned for a rebound; make it and you get one point and shoot again; miss it and the ball is up for grabs by either player. The player who them makes the shot successfully is awarded two points and goes to the free throw line. The first to reach 21 points wins.

[2]In Around the World, the players take turns at shots from designated spots around the perimeter of the three-point lane. To win, you must go all the way around and back again. On each turn you get one shot; if you make it, then you move on to the next position; if you miss, then you may either stay on the same position and wait for your next turn or take a "chance" shot. If you miss your chance shot, then you go all the way back to the first position, but if you make your chance shot then you go on to the next position.

The basketball play was at times unbearably aggressive and hateful. Sam was ruthlessly competitive. He'd stop at nothing to come out on top. The rules changed as fast as the score. A well-placed elbow, toe crunch, eye jab, trip, shove and slap—all flagrant fouls—were his strategic core. When he fell behind, which he couldn't stand, his powers of self-control fared as poorly as a house of cards in a hurricane. He'd whip the basketball at the walls, clock, backboard, and me. Burp, fart, and scream. Lock himself in the bathroom for ten minutes. Let the water run and flush the toilet over and over.

Eventually, I found interventions that helped Sam to become more settled. At times, I'd make an issue of how stimulated I was getting. I said, "Gee, Sam, I'm feeling really sweaty, overheated, revved up. I feel like I need to slow down before ward group." Comments like this had a decisive impact; he calmed down and was able to continue in our play. In the very next session, Sam approached me in the front lounge: "We have to go up to the court today. We just have to." "Oh, we do?" "Yeah, because I feel really hyperactive, and I need to go up there and work it all out." I said, "You notice that you are hyperactive." "Yeah, like all itchy and stuff. Like I have all this energy in my body that I have to run around and get out." We played three great games of Twenty-one in which he won the tiebreaker. On the way down, we talked not just about how the games went and about how good it felt to "let out" all that hyperactivity.

In our basketball play, as in the racquetball game, I let myself become stimulated to a manageable degree, thus embodying a facsimile of what I imagined Sam's subjective experience to be. I then purposely drew Sam's attention to my agitated condition to indicate how I judged for myself what subjective experiences were tolerable and what were intolerable, and how I set about reshaping and delimiting my states of excitement or agitation so as to maintain control and stay on task. Sam willingly participated in this interactive process. He identified with my struggles to control my own bodily experiences and readily let this inform his own experience of himself. This intervention had supportive aspects, as it helped him to gain more control over his aggressive impulses, improve his level of functioning in his basketball play, and feel better about himself. This manner of play drew him out of his entrenched sadomasochistic pattern of relatedness with me and forged more cooperative and friendly modes of being with another.

About six months into our work, Around the World was all we played for a time. Sam had not won once in two weeks, and it was tearing him apart. The more he lost, the more he wanted to win, and the more he wanted to win, the more desperate his play became. One day he said, "I'll chance again." I replied, "Are you sure you want to do that? It doesn't seem to be working too well for you." He said, "Shut up. It's only a fuckin' game." He missed his chance, as he almost always did and then asked, "Do you know about Death?" I asked "Death?" Sam said, "Yeah, it's after chance. You miss it, and you are totally out. You know, like dead." I: "Sounds pretty extreme." "What are you, too much of a baby? It's only a fuckin' game." I agreed to Death and watched him die, again and again and again.

A turning point occurred in the next session when I made a decisive intervention in our play of Around the World. I said, "I'm not sure if you notice what keeps happening here. You make as many or more shots than I do, but you lose because you chance." Sam said, "Shut up. I don't want to hear it. I can do whatever I want. You can't tell me how to play. It's my therapy." I said, "Yeah, sure, but I think that it's something you might want to know about yourself so that you could play better." Sam said, "I don't want to hear about it." I won twice more and felt I could not let this go on, so I said, "Let's try an experiment. How about if you play like me and don't take any chances, and I'll play like you and chance it every time?" Sam agreed. He made a lot and missed a lot, but because he couldn't chance, he made steady progress for the first time ever. I made tons of shots and came close to winning but inevitably choked and went back to zero.

After the umpteenth miss, I was fed up. I said, "Fuck." He said, "What was that you said?" I said, "I guess that it was something like what you would say." He saw me falling apart and himself maintaining the lead and smirked, "Oh, I see what you're trying to show me. That it pays to be patient and not to rush."

I saw that Sam was making use of my more fully developed capacities to cope—tolerate frustration and delay gratification—given to him in this session, on loan. With some reluctance, I accepted his passivity in giving in to frightening overstimulation. I offered to stop the charade, but he insisted that we continue for 20 grueling minutes until he finally won.

I tried to make Sam more aware of how his body feelings affected his play. Here, Sam wanted to continue to play; he explained how anger helped him with his play, "It's good that I get angry because when I'm angry I play better." I said, "Huhh. That's interesting. How so?" He said, "Because when I'm angry I want it more, and when I want it more I play better." I asked, "Well, then what do you think about how you have been playing thus far? You seemed plenty angry but you were missing lots of shots that I know you can make." He said, "That's because l was getting angry that you were getting so lucky and making all these lucky shots while I'm having a bad luck day on the basketball court. That's all. So, are we going to play or not?" After Sam beat me fair and square in a rigorous contest of Twenty-one, I asked, "What do you think was different about that game that you were able to play so much better and beat me?" He responded, "Nothing. I just played better." I said, "Yeah, you did play better, but how'd you do it? It seemed to me that you might have been less upset and angry than before and that when you are less upset, you play better." He said, "No, I was even more angry than before. It's just that I held it in." "You held it in?" He said, "Yeah, instead of letting it all out and yelling and throwing the ball and stuff, I just held it in." I asked, "How were you able to do that?" He answered, "I just made my mind up, that's all." I responded, "That's good that you are able to hold your anger in. I saw how it helped you to play better." He said, "Yeah."

In the next session, I met Sam in the front lounge, and he went off to get the basketball. He had with him a white teddy bear with a "Merry Christmas" red stocking on it. He brought the bear to his room and then brought it along with him to our session, the bear in one hand, the basketball in the other. On the way I asked, "Who've you got there?" He responded, "It's a bear." I asked, "Does it have a name?" He said, "No, not really. I got it from someone." He seemed reluctant to say any more than that he got it from Beth, a fellow patient for whom Sam had a fledgling romantic interest, and set the bear on the drinking fountain in such a way that it could oversee our play.

Sam suggested that we play one game of Twenty-one, then play Around the World, and talk as we play. Our game of Twenty-one was spirited and competitive. He played superbly and beat me without cheating. We then played Around the World. His play continued to be excellent. He even showed great restraint in not taking chances and cautioned me against chancing it when I felt the temptation. He talked about his family therapy. Sam said that he and his mom couldn't take passes last week because she had been in New Hampshire with her boyfriend. After Sam brought that up twice, I asked, "Mike?" He was surprised and asked, "How did you know?" I said, "Jody [the family therapist] told me that. But I guess it's something that you and I haven't talked about." He said, "Yeah." I said, "I don't know much about him. Do you feel comfortable telling me more about him?" He said, "Sure. . . He is a really nice guy." I asked, "You have gotten to know him?" He answered, "Yeah, I've known him for about eight or nine months." I said, "You said he's moving to New Hampshire." He said, "Yeah, that's because he got a job there. He's a security guard. A really good security guard. He had a job near here, but he, like, was looking for more of a, a better job, like a promotion. . . ." I said, "A career." He said, "Yeah, that's it. So he took this new job." I asked, "What's that going to be like with him being farther away?" He said, "I don't know. No different really. He used to live about 45 minutes from where we lived. Him and my mom will keep seeing each other. . . . He's real fast. A real fast runner. He works out and stuff and is like a black belt in tae kwon do. He's really strong and fast. That's what makes him a good security guard. If you're not so fast then you're in lots of trouble. I mean like if you steal something and you're not fast and he catches you. . . man. . . ." I said, "He sounds real strong." "Yeah." I asked, "Is he like a scary person to be with for you?" He said, "What do you mean?" I said, "Well, with being so strong and big as you say?" He said, "No, he's really a teddy bear." I said, "A teddy bear?" "Yeah." We finished the game. Sam won and said, "That's the first time I beat you." I said, "How about that." He said, "I think it's 'cause I didn't chance a lot." I said, "You think that made a difference?" He said, "Yeah."

In our next session, Sam began, "Are you Mark's doctor?" He went on to tell me, "You have got to do something about Mark. He has a hormone problem. He wants it too much." Sam told me that Mark had been flashing Julie and asking her "Don't she want it?"

For Sam, I was now a benign enough presence that he could share with me his concerns about his mother, her boyfriend, and about another boy's frightening sexual behavior. I could detect the presence of a benevolent, nurturing, and protective figure in Sam's recounting of his mother's teddy bear of a boyfriend, and in his new experience of trusting me to do something about Mark. The fact that Sam was here asking me to protect him from a boy who was sexually out of control resonates with his history of having no one to protect him from being sexually assaulted by a teenage boy and physically assaulted by his uncles. He seemed to have achieved enough distance from the intense sadomasochistic experiences and to have become capable of experiencing men anew as viable allies. The long-sought opportunity for Sam and me to talk about his experiences was at hand.

In a subsequent session, which I began by telling Sam about my upcoming vacation, I broke into some good basketball play to share thoughts which had been on my mind for months, but which I felt suddenly pressured to share. I said, "Sam, I have something tough to bring up with you. If you don't feel like talking about it, then you can tell me and we do not have to. I have been thinking a lot about our play together, especially how it has at times been pretty rough. I am aware from what you have told me and what your family therapist told me, that with your cousins you have also played rough and that sometimes that became abusive. I wondered if you noticed some similarities between what has happened in our play and between you and your cousins." He appeared devastated, and said, "I don't want to talk about that. It was very different." I said, "I can understand that it would be very difficult to talk about with me." He evaded and I pursued until I was chased away by choruses of "I don't fucking want to talk to you! Go away, Steve!" I was impressed that instead of engaging me in an overstimulating struggle, as he had many times before, this time Sam sought distance from me. Still I felt bad for having disrupted our play and awful for having hurt Sam, and used my supervision to understand just why I had done so.

I approached Sam numerous times before our next session, but he would not let me come near. When we finally met in session, I explained, "Sam, I think I made a mistake in our last session. I spoke to you about the abuse issues because that has been very much on my mind and I think it's important. However, I think it was wrong for me to bring it up as I did. As I remember it, we were talking about my leaving for vacation. I think I brought it up because it was hard for me to talk about leaving." He accepted my words and did not challenge my understanding. We then resumed our basketball play.

In a basketball game a few sessions later, the ball careened off the backboard's side and ricocheted into the near corner of the gym. I was stuck there in foul territory out of my shooting range. Sam had me cornered. Whichever way I flexed, he reacted as if my neurons were telling his neurons which way 1 would move before my muscles got the cue. There was only one way out. I nodded upwards—as if to aim and shoot—and got Sam off his feet, slyly bounced the ball on the floor between his tree-trunk legs, sprung past his left side, and stepped toward the ball, which I hoisted up to sink a lay-up. Sam squinted and stomped. He didn't believe what had just happened. He did not, however, lose control. Sam could now appreciate a good move, even if he lost on account of it. Instead of retaliating, Sam wanted to learn from me. "How'd you do that? What a move. I can't believe it." Later, when I was on the foul line, Sam bounced the ball through his legs. Another day, when a bit more confident, he bounced it between his legs and then slid past me. Weeks later, after he had become the master of the between-the-legs-bounce, he split my legs as I had split his and stepped up to the hoop for an easy lay-up.

Another day, Sam showed me his best move. He had seen Michael Jordan do it on TV as the Chicago Bulls won the N.B.A. World Championship series. He made me learn the move. You start at the top of the key by tossing the ball three or four feet down court. You charge after it and dribble only once more as you head in for a lay-up. But you double fake pump instead, pass below the net, and flip the ball backwards into the hole without using the backboard. He had me do it again and again until I could make the shot just like he could.

I ended my work with Sam when I completed my one-year training appointment. In the last weeks of our therapy, termination issues and themes became the major part of our play. Sam invited me to join him and another male staff member on a basketball team for a hospital tournament. For the first time, we had brought our basketball play out of the closet and were playing together as teammates. Winning the tournament seemed an invigorating demonstration, for both Sam and me, of how working with another man could yield valuable shared accomplishments, and that what he had gained through playing in our sessions could be put to use in the world outside of our therapy. In this last phase of the therapy, Sam had us shift our interactions from the play activities we were by then used to practicing to activities that came closer to the boundaries that our play shared with his world. For example, Sam often began sessions telling me how well he had played in a basketball game with others and about the great shots he made, as if he were saying again that he was able to practice what we had learned together, even without me around. He even introduced a number of new games into our play and had us move out to the courtyard—a transitional space between the hospital world and the external world. Sam repeatedly kicked the ball out of the hospital courtyard to have a passerby fetch it and toss it back over the courtyard wall.

REPEAT PSYCHOLOGICAL EXAMINATION

Sam underwent a repeat psychological examination after one year of intensive treatment to aid in discharge planning. Tests administered were the WISC-R, Thematic Apperception Test, Rorschach, and Object Relations Inventory. Sam was engaging, thoughtful, and cooperative. His personality was still organized at the high borderline level; however, there was significant progress in his ego development, including greater capacity to test perceptions and interpretations; enhanced conscious appreciation of his tendency to distort when distressed; reliance on higher-order defenses such as repression, intellectualization, sublimation, and avoidance; and the use of mirroring and twinning to define himself and others.

Sam's experience of himself and others was overall far more controllable, predictable, and benevolent. His experience of himself was overall positive, and included some negative attributes, an appreciation for his own psychological complexity, and a higher regard for the importance of relationships with others in his self-definition. His view of paternal figures was significantly different: men were powerful, assertive, playful, helpful; he was less likely to "write them off"; he perceived the possibility for more benign and nurturing relationships with men; he had a conscious yearning for a father, stating, "Everybody needs a father to help him grow up and become a man."

At the time I left the hospital, one year after my work with Sam began, he was preparing for discharge to a residential treatment facility. Sam told me that he knew he still had a lot to get out of treatment, but agreed with the treatment team that he was now at a place where he could continue to learn about himself and to develop in his life and treatment outside of the long-term setting.

Discussion

THE BOY WHO COULD NOT PLAY

The psychotherapy opened with Sam letting me witness some of the severe disturbances in psychological functioning that are a result of the marked early-life traumatization he suffered. For Sam, being alone with his therapist, a man, brought on a sudden reexperiencing of intolerable discomfort, danger, and mistrust, associated with past traumas. Initially, Sam showed some faint capacity to verbalize these intense negative affects. In time, however, he revealed a far more pervasive tendency toward somatization; experiencing the discomfort in his body apparently without much ideational connection to current stresses or past traumas. This bodily reexperiencing was further extended into the interpersonal realm through physical enactments, such as the episode when Sam damaged my office plant and then feared I'd kill him. The inner dramas he repeatedly enacted were stark sadomasochistic themes—either Sam was dominating me or being dominated by me—characteristic sequelae of childhood abuse.

The degree and breadth of Sam's presenting psychological difficulties are in accord with the marked intensity and frequency of traumatic events Sam experienced across multiple developmental epochs: one episode of sexual abuse in early childhood; one episode of physical abuse and repeated episodes of the loss of caregivers in late childhood. Trauma of this frequency, intensity, and scope must be considered a major etiologic factor for his difficulties in adolescence, even though Sam did not meet the criteria for Posttraumatic Stress Disorder. One might see this presentation as an example of Lenore Terr's Type II childhood traumas, where prolonged and repeated traumas may result in conduct disorder, personality disorder, depression, and somatization (Terr, 1991).[3] Still, childhood trauma need not be the exclusive factor accounting for Sam's psychological difficulties. Consideration should also be given to other contributing factors such as disturbances in temperament, or family interactions, as well as comorbid psychiatric disorders. My case discussion will focus on the traumas as the predominant etiologic contributant to his difficulties.

There were times, as in our very first session, when Sam was able to distance himself, albeit momentarily, from the brewing storm within, enough to stay in the verbal realm. The tremendous defensive effort he made, however, also appeared to have the effect of shutting down vital

---

[3]The presentation is also consistent with the diagnosis of disorder of extreme stress, which has been proposed for adult survivors of multiple, prolonged, and repeated childhood traumatization (Herman, 1992).

and spontaneous aspects of his self. The result was similar perhaps to what Winnicott has called the "false self" (Winnicott, 1965) and what Shengold refers to as a "hypnotic living deadness" (Shengold, 1989). It was also reported to me that in contrast with the portrait of Sam in the therapy I have presented, there were in fact times in his relations with same-age or younger peers or with other staff, particularly women, when he was capable of being friendlier and more compliant. If Sam, like some individuals, was able to maintain this distant, but nonetheless verbal, characterologic style, then, one potential pitfall of a predominantly talking therapy would be to address only his more compliant part-self, and to miss the more troubled parts within.

In the psychotherapy meetings with me, however, Sam experienced not too little, but far too much. Sam had little capacity to contain the "affective storm center" (Shengold, 1989) within. He could barely prevent the eruptions of aggressive and libidinal impulses from invading the most routinized everyday activities. This was clearly evident in Sam's way of playing games during sessions, which, as I have described, often brought us to the brink of sadomasochistic violence. Without the inner capacity to contain these intense negative affects and control his violent behavior, Sam was unable to play. As the therapist, I too was at risk of perpetrating a countertransference reaction to Sam's aggressivity that would have further damaged a fragile therapeutic alliance.

Clearly, Sam had a great need to develop more awareness and understanding of the psychological difficulties that he tended to enact. Thus, initially I tried to give Sam enough opportunities to verbally reflect upon and talk about his bodily experiences and physical enactments. I naively hoped that Sam and I would proceed stepwise in the psychotherapy: recognizing, labeling, ordering, and exploring his often violent and turbulent experiences until he achieved sufficient insight to gain mastery over his self. Yes, there were some extraordinary moments when Sam was inexplicably able to find "the words to say it" (Cardinal, 1983). The story of the killer pit bull kept my hopes alive temporarily that Sam could achieve insight through verbal analysis of his experiences. Soon enough, I learned that by going further or faster toward talking than Sam was prepared to go, I only brought on the feelings of too-muchness that were at the center of his traumatic reexperiencing and severely weakened the therapeutic alliance. Unable to rely primarily on talking with one another, Sam and I badly needed another way of being together in the psychotherapy. A comment by Winnicott provided a signpost for a more fitting direction for the psychotherapeutic treatment: "If the patient cannot play, then something needs to be done to enable the patient to become able to play, after which the psychotherapy may begin" (Winnicott, 1971).

THE ASPECTS OF PLAY IN COMPETITIVE ATHLETIC GAMES

The currents of the psychotherapeutic process shifted when I turned my attention from the talking interspersed at the margins of the games we played onto the playing of the game itself. Playing became the central element of the psychotherapeutic experience. The shift from a predominantly verbal psychotherapy geared to enhancing insight to a predominantly play psychotherapy centered on advancing development is central to the theory and practice of psychoanalytic play therapy with children. With this adolescent boy, the concepts and techniques of psychoanalytic play therapy were extended from the play of imaginative games in psychoanalytic play psychotherapy with school-age children and adapted to playing the competitive athletic games more suited to his chronological age.

In concert with this shift, I paid careful attention to the establishment and maintenance of a transitional space for the psychotherapeutic process. Winnicott described the transitional space as "an intermediate area of experiencing to which inner reality and external life both contribute" (Winnicott, 1971, p. 2). In this space, unlike many other realms of experience, no challenge is presented to the relating of inner and outer experience. Winnicott believed that the transitional space defined the space for play within which play, art, religion, and psychotherapy may happen.

The actual physical spaces where the play of competitive athletic games occurred were conducive to the emergence of the experiential "transitional space" described by Winnicott. The gym, where most of the meetings occurred, was enough a part of the hospital to be a place where treatment might occur, yet far enough removed to become our own potential space. Being in the gym would give Sam the feeling that he could have me to himself, a feeling otherwise hard to come by on a bustling adolescent ward. More importantly, being in the gym gave Sam a place when he could play as he desired and invite me to join with him in the play. Had we remained in my cramped office, we never would have been able to play together in his way, nor reap the therapeutic benefits of that play.

Because basketball had been a central part of Sam's life since latency and had long had a place in my life, it was an excellent activity for the making of a transitional phenomenon. I was good enough at basketball and the other games we played to be able to sustain the play where Sam could not. At the same time, I could also focus on subtle intrapsychic and interpersonal aspects of the play experience. Over time, I could see how the play, though bound by formalities and rules, could nonetheless function as a rich mode of expression of Sam's inner world. Also, I was able to appreciate how I could communicate my own ideas about Sam within the expressed context permitted by the play. I do not think that we would have been as successful in constructing a transitional space of this sort had there not been an activity such as basketball, so well known to both Sam and me.

Sustaining the therapeutic process required that I be active in multiple dimensions: joining in the games, observing his behavior, silently interpreting his feelings, and always providing experiences for new developments in his thoughts, feelings, and actions. Throughout much of the play, words were used sparingly, largely as a secondary marker of predominantly nonverbal exchanges. When Sam and I were playing together at our best, we arrived at transformations in our ways of interacting with each other from both the spontaneous play of the games and mutual agreement. At times, such as the Around the World game, when we tried the "experiment," our play was an intensive, shared, contained experience that offered special opportunities for learning about oneself.

THE THERAPEUTIC FUNCTIONS OF PLAY

Winnicott taught: "Psychotherapy has to do with two people playing together" (Winnicott, 1971, p. 38). Thus, the psychotherapy proceeded by my using competitive athletic games as the predominant means for playing together with Sam. In this approach, I did not seek to terminate the play or let the play erode so that it might be replaced by talking. Instead, I worked toward sustaining the play of competitive games as the major therapeutic activity. I did not seek to step out of the boundaries of the play to make interventions. Instead, I tried to make changes that lay within the unique interactive modes of experience brought to us through play. There were times, however, when out of misjudgment or impatience, I did interrupt the play with verbal comments, with little clinical benefit.

The play was a window onto Sam's inner life. By means of playing basketball Sam allowed me to enter into his world in a way that talking would not allow. The basketball play brought Sam's bodily experiences into center court. One might even say that the play made it possible, figuratively speaking, for Sam to bring his pit bull along. No one in his life had sufficiently helped Sam to tame the ferocity of this animalistic internal figure. This unique psychotherapeutic situation facilitated Sam's bringing the beast into therapy. We soon discovered that my office, with its fragile objects and relaxed tones, could never handle it. The gym, on the other hand, lent itself to this kind of therapy rather well. I did not, however, make verbal interpretations to help draw Sam's attention to the existence of a pit bull within. The therapy did not help Sam achieve any such insights.

The play served other important therapeutic functions. The playing of competitive games gave Sam repeated opportunities to experience the inner affective storm in an interpersonal context well suited to his developing new approaches. Up in the gym we encountered the dog. We took the leash off and practiced putting it back on. We learned how to talk him down. Rather than directly comment on Sam's thoughts, feelings, or behaviors, which Sam would have found unacceptable, I helped Sam create a space where he could try out new solutions. We helped Sam to get more of a hold on his pit bull.

I have described examples of Sam's highly contradictory behavior, either from one session to another, or from his being with me in our sessions to his being with others outside of our sessions. In some instances Sam's self seemed to be under the sway of the pit bull and its victim, whereas at other times, one sensed the presence of gentler animals like bunny rabbits and teddy bears in his experience of his self and others. When Sam's behavior was being enlivened by the killer pit bull he seemed unable to bring the other parts of his self to bear upon his experience—to mediate, temper, or restrain the overwhelming aggression. When Sam was being more of a teddy bear, the aggressive parts of his self—the pit bull—were nowhere to be found. These contradictory behaviors or so-called splits in the self are highly characteristic of adolescents and adults traumatized as children. The play of competitive games provided Sam with experiences for reorganizing these aspects of the self into a more balanced and cohesive self to better regulate these severe behavioral difficulties. He learned to bring the considerable ego strengths lodged in the gentler figures to bear upon the more sadomasochistic figures, thus beginning a self-organization capable of healthier relatedness.

I doubt this could have ever happened had I not been able to join Sam in play. It was only through fully entering into the play that I was able to come up with such interventions as the "experiment" in Around the World. Winnicott's words reflect a deep appreciation for the necessity of the therapist's play: "Psychotherapy is done in the overlap of two areas of playing, that of the patient and that of the therapist" (Winnicott, 1971, p. 54).

THE DILEMMAS OF THE THERAPIST

I hope I have not conveyed the sense that I knew with confidence that this was the most useful psychotherapeutic approach for this troubled adolescent. To the contrary, prior to this I was accustomed to conducting psychotherapy with adults in an office sitting in chairs, talking and listening. Initially, I chose to play competitive athletic games because it seemed the only way to engage Sam, a doer and not a talker. Over the course of our year's work, I lived with tremendous uncertainty, confusion, worry, and guilt for using competitive athletic play instead of talking as a vehicle for psychotherapeutic work.

I was plagued by questions about how I was working with Sam. Was what we were doing together therapy, or was it just playing basketball? Was I playing games to avoid verbally confronting Sam? Was I indulging Sam's aggression as others had? Would this turn out to be yet another traumatic experience with a man? Did I have a leash on my countertransference—my own conflicts around competitiveness and aggression in our play? How should I conduct our play? Should I let him win or should I win if I could? Why weren't we talking? Why weren't we addressing his depression? And these were only some of the questions for which I didn't always have a ready answer.

The very nature of our play—physical, sensual, nonverbal, aggressive, formal—put it at risk of collapsing as a therapeutic endeavor if either he or I transgressed the boundaries of play therapy and, at one extreme, "just played a game" or, at the other extreme, allowed for no play at all. For example, there were instances, as illustrated in my account of the psychotherapy, when I had difficulty containing the feelings our work stirred in me and broke into the play with an impatient and rigid need to make Sam talk. Yet, as our work progressed, I found that Sam and I had established enough of a therapeutic alliance, primarily through our play, that we were able to tolerate such disruptions and work out an understanding of them through a flexible intermingling of talking and doing in the psychotherapy.

The dilemmas inherent in psychotherapeutic treatment with this enacting adolescent made for a constant struggle to reconcile a number of opposing tendencies: a struggle of character styles, between Sam's tendency toward unreflective doing and my tendency toward talking and analyzing; a struggle over how to guide Sam's activities in therapy, between letting Sam use his body to interact physically with me and pushing Sam to talk about and reflect on his experience; and a struggle overseeing my own experience in the therapy, between letting myself become involved in potentially overstimulating enactments, and maintaining distance, awareness, and understanding over actions and impulse. I believe that the psychotherapy worked well because Sam and I discovered, through the play of competitive games, a way of being together that intermingled, bridged, balanced, and lessened these opposing tendencies.

The experience of providing the psychotherapeutic treatment expanded my understanding of psychotherapeutic approaches to the treatment of adolescents who have suffered childhood and adolescent traumatic experiences. Psychoanalytic play therapy provided a useful conceptual context for developing a psychotherapeutic approach most suitable for this adolescent boy. The approach did not involve reaching for verbal recollection of past traumatic experiences or more recent traumatic reexperiencing, all of which would have been intolerable to the patient. Sam was nowhere near ready to put his traumatic experiences into words, given how he felt them to be far too much to bear in his body. An approach directed at helping him gain more awareness of and control over his bodily experiences and physical enactments was needed. The concepts of psychoanalytic play therapy guided my efforts to derive a novel therapeutic approach involving the play of structured athletic games. Further experience with this approach is needed to identify its applications, benefits, limitations, and dangers.

The Developmental Gains of the Patient

Over the course of our work together, Sam was progressively able to reshape the psychological sequelae of marked childhood traumatization.

He was able to make significant connections between feelings and conduct; thought and action; his gentler side and the pit bull within. He gained substantial control over the hateful emotions that so colored his experience, thereby showing a greater capacity for genuine and modulated relatedness. This was evidenced in Sam's improved capacity for age-appropriate competitive athletic play and in the stories he told in our session, such as that of his mother's boyfriend being a teddy bear. There was also an overall improvement in his level of functioning at school, in his family, and on the hospital ward. The repeat psychological examinations described the significant progress in Sam's ego development and his capacity for object relatedness. During our therapy, Sam's world opened up. There were now helpers and heroes and nurturers and friends, where before there were too often just predators and prey. There was now play, be it basketball, ping pong, or Koosh, where before there was only evasion and capture. Sam was now freer to join in normal developmental processes of early adolescence, which for this young boy included the joy of working up a good sweat, win or lose, with another guy on the basketball court.

When I completed my clinical placement on the long-term inpatient unit and ended the one year of psychotherapeutic work with Sam, I shared his sense that he had indeed come a long way but that he still had far to go. I was encouraged by the significant changes I witnessed in Sam's enhanced capacity to play better. Yet, would this newly gained fluidity of his self and its psychic structures be sustained and flow into a more healthy "adolescent reassemblage of psychic components" (Blos, 1979)? Or would Sam's experience take a more disturbed form of either compulsive repetition of the traumatic experiences or staunchly defended but deadened existence? Certainly, Sam would have the best chance of sustaining a more normal developmental path if his hospital stay were followed by his living in an environment that was consistent, stable, nurturing, and respectful. I took some optimism in noting that his mother had made significant progress in family therapy and was better prepared as a mother and that Sam was to be discharged to a good residential treatment facility. I also felt that Sam needed further psychotherapeutic treatment to help him achieve greater control over and build more awareness and understanding of the psychological difficulties that he tends to experience in his body and to enact. Though I could not then know how Sam would fare, I was certain that I and the others involved in his treatment had given him a second chance to come to terms with the damaging sequelae of the abuse and neglect he suffered as a young boy. Developmentally speaking, he had elevated his game.

REFERENCES

Blos, P. (1962), *On Adolescence: A Psychoanalytic Interpretation.* New York: Free Press.
———— (1979), *The Adolescent Passage.* New York: International Universities Press.
Cardinal, M. (1983), *The Words to Say It.* Cambridge, MA: VanVactor & Goodheart.
Foa, E., Stekette, G. & Rothbaum, B. (1989), Behavioral/cognitive conceptualizations of post-traumatic stress disorder. *Behav. Ther.*, 20:155–176.
Herman, J. (1992), *Trauma and Recovery.* New York: Basic Books.
Shengold, L. (1988), *Halo in the Sky: Observations on Anality and Defense.* New York: Guilford.
———— (1989), *Soul Murder: The Effects of Childhood Abuse and Deprivation.* New Haven, CT: Yale University Press.
———— (1991), A variety of narcissistic pathology stemming from parental weakness. *Psychoanal. Quart.*, 60:86–92.
Solnit, A. J. & Neubauer, P. B., eds. (1987), *The Psychoanalytic Study of the Child, 42.* New Haven, CT: Yale University Press.
Terr, L. (1991), Childhood traumas: An outline and overview, *Amer. J. Psychiat.*, 148:10–19.
Winnicott, D. W. (1958), Transitional objects and transitional phenomena. In: *Collected Papers.* New York: Basic Books, pp. 229–242.
———— (1965), *The Maturational Processes and the Facilitating Environment.* New York: International Universities Press.
———— (1971), *Playing and Reality.* London: Tavistock.

PART V

SPECIAL SECTION ON TRAINING

19 REPORT OF THE ACCREDITATION COUNCIL ON FELLOWSHIPS IN ADOLESCENT PSYCHIATRY

RICHARD ROSNER

The By-laws of the American Society of Adolescent Psychiatry (ASAP) state that:

> The Accreditation Council on Fellowships in Adolescent Psychiatry serves as a semiautonomous component of ASAP responsible to the House of Delegates through the Executive Committee and governed in accordance with its own Bylaws. The Council identifies post-psychiatry-residency fellowship programs in adolescent psychiatry; establishes and periodically revises Standards for Fellowship Programs in adolescent psychiatry; surveys programs to determine conformity to these Standards; encourages the development of Fellowship programs in adolescent psychiatry; and stimulates and encourages teaching and research in the field of adolescent psychiatry. The Council Chairperson(s) is an ex-officio member of the House of Delegates.

In accordance with the recommendations of ASAP's Task Force on Specialization in Adolescent Psychiatry, chaired by the late Richard Marohn, M.D., a Task Force on Fellowships in Adolescent Psychiatry, chaired by John Meeks, M.D. was created. Dr. Meeks was succeeded as chair of the Task Force by Richard Rosner, M.D. In May 1993, the Accreditation Council on Fellowships in Adolescent Psychiatry was created as the successor to the Task Force on Fellowships in Adolescent Psychiatry. The initial Board of Directors of The Accreditation Council included: Richard Rosner, M.D. (president), Lynn Ponton, M.D. (vice-president), Robert Weinstock, M.D. (secretary), Lloyd Wells, M.D,, (treasurer), Michael Kalogerakis, M.D., Marshall Korenblum, M.D., Edward Leatherman, M.D., Donald Swanson, M.D., and Sidney Weissman, M.D. There were three consultants appointed to the Council: Lois Flaherty, M.D., John Looney, M.D., and John Meeks, M.D.

The Accreditation Council on Fellowships in Adolescent Psychiatry (ACFAP) sends three documents to programs that inquire about potential accreditation of a Fifth Post-Graduate Year (PGY-5) fellowship in adolescent psychiatry. These documents are appended to this article:

1. A brief explanation of what the ACFAP is and how its accreditation processes operate.

2. An extended statement, "Special Requirements for Programs in Adolescent Psychiatry," drafted similarly to such documents prepared by the Accreditation Council on Graduate Medical Education (ACGME) for other psychiatric subspecialties that offer Added Qualifications training. The statement makes reference to the ACGME's Residency Review Committee (RRC) for psychiatry, demonstrating how adolescent psychiatry could be integrated into the accreditation processes currently in place, at such time as the ACGME recognizes adolescent psychiatry as a subspecialty.

3. An explicit statement of the criteria used by the ACFAP to evaluate programs that seek accreditation, called "Standards: Special Requirements for Programs in Adolescent Psychiatry."

The accreditation process occurs in two parts. First, an applicant program completes a program survey form, designed to assess whether or not the program is in substantial compliance with the ACFAP's *Standards*. If the applicant program appears to be in conformity with the *Standards*, the director of the program is so notified. Second, a site visit to the applicant program is scheduled, to determine whether or not the program actually has the faculty, facilities, and didactic and clinical training that it claims to have, and that the faculty and actually do what they claim to do. If the site visit demonstrates that the applicant program is in substantial compliance with the council's *Standards*, has what it claims to have, and does what it claims to do, then the director of the program is advised that the program has qualified for full accreditation. When appropriate, provisional accreditation may be granted to applicant programs.

The council recognizes that programs certified by the Accreditation Council on Graduate Medical Education's Residency Review Committee on Child & Adolescent Psychiatry meet the standards of competence expected of subspecialty programs in adolescent psychiatry.

The original ASAP Task Force on Specialization in Adolescent Psychiatry understood that the hallmarks of a subspecialty include:

1. An established and sizable organized body of practitioners.
2. A body of scientific and clinical data and skills that are unique to the field.
3. A body of literature that embodies a representative and substantial portion of those unique data and describes or otherwise sets forth those unique skills.
4. An appropriately recognized credentialing organization to certify the quality of the subspecialty training programs.
5. Subspecialized fellowship training programs designed to impart the unique data and skills to physicians seeking entry into the field.
6. An appropriately recognized credentialing organization to distinguish between those who claim competence in the field and those who successfully demonstrate the competence.

The established and sizable organized body of practitioners is the American Society for Adolescent Psychiatry itself. As of June 1990, ASAP had 1475 members.

The body of scientific and clinical data and skills that are unique to the field are exemplified, in the United States, by the series of annual programs presented under the auspices of ASAP. Alternatively, it might be more accurate to say that the data and skills are actually embodied in the practitioners of adolescent psychiatry and are best exemplified in their practice.

The literature in which the data and skills are set forth is varied, too extensive to be cited here, but readily found by a computer search of the literature on adolescent psychiatry. It includes *Adolescent Psychiatry: the Annals of the American Society for Adolescent Psychiatry,* and *The Journal of Youth and Adolescence,* sponsored by ASAP.

The credentialing organization to certify the quality of the subspecialty training programs is the Accreditation Council on Fellowships in Adolescent Psychiatry, sponsored by the American Society for Adolescent Psychiatry.

The existence of subspecialty fellowship training programs devoted exclusively to adolescent psychiatry was addressed by the Accreditation

Council on Fellowships on Adolescent Psychiatry. On one hand, the council encouraged the formation of new programs in adolescent psychiatry by the model for such programs set forth in its *Standards*, and by the recognition it offered to programs that complied with that document. On the other hand, the council sought to identify existing programs that either offered or were willing to offer a Fifth Post-Graduate Year in adolescent psychiatry. In 1994, the council first surveyed all psychiatry residency programs. At that time seven programs were identified as being willing (subject to funding availability) to provide one year of postresidency, fellowship training in adolescent psychiatry. They were:

1. Foothills Hospital, Calgary, Alberta, Canada
2. University of North Dakota, Fargo
3. University of Arkansas
4. University of Cincinnati
5. University of Oklahoma
6. South Illinois University
7. State University of New York at Stony Brook

The Council will periodically re-survey the existing psychiatry residency programs to determine the availability of PGY-5 training in adolescent psychiatry.

The credentialing organization to identify those practitioners who have demonstrated their competence in the subspecialty is the American Board of Adolescent Psychiatry (ABAP), founded in 1989. Like the ACFAP, the ABAP is a product of the recommendations of the ASAP Task Force on Specialization in Adolescent Psychiatry. Although sponsored by ASAP, the ABAP is a separate and autonomous corporation, operating in accordance with its own bylaws. The first president of the board was Sidney Weissman, M.D. The board was established to offer a route to certification for psychiatrists with special competence in treating adolescents, but who have not sought training in the treatment of children. The ABAP recognizes that psychiatrists certified by the American Board of Psychiatry & Neurology in Child & Adolescent Psychiatry meet the standards of competence expected of subspecialists in adolescent psychiatry.

Notwithstanding the substantial facts that support the *de facto* existence of adolescent psychiatry as a subspecialty, formal *de jure* recognition of the field has been withheld. The American Psychiatric

Association (APA) has not yet recognized that adolescent psychiatry is a distinct subspecialty, that training in applied clinical adolescent psychiatry does not have to be linked to training in applied clinical child psychiatry; the APA only recognizes the combined field of child and adolescent psychiatry as a subspecialty. The American Board of Psychiatry & Neurology (ABPN) has thus far declined to offer a subspecialty examination for Added Qualifications in Adolescent Psychiatry; the ABPN only offers an examination for Special Qualifications in Child & Adolescent Psychiatry. The Accreditation Council on Graduate Medical Education has so far declined to certify PGY-5 training programs devoted solely to adolescent psychiatry; the ACGME only certifies programs in combined child and adolescent psychiatry. While there may be some legitimate professional disagreements regarding the value of recognizing an additional psychiatric subspecialty generally. there can be no argument specifically but that adolescents are in need of mental health services from psychiatric practitioners who have the requisite specialized knowledge and skills essential for working with teenagers. The subspecialty of adolescent psychiatry exists regardless of whether or not the APA, the ABPN, and the ACGME countenance its existence, in much the same way as the former Soviet Union existed without diplomatic recognition during its early history, and communist China existed for decades without recognition as a legitimate government by the United States, and Israel existed for many years without recognition by its Arab neighbors.

The main obstacles to the recognition of adolescent psychiatry as a separate subspecialty are best understood in terms of organizational inertia, vested interests, and economics. It is the position of ASAP that the needs of adolescents should take precedence over proprietary, political, and pecuniary concerns. Geriatric psychiatry, forensic psychiatry, and addiction psychiatry have received formal recognition, but adolescent psychiatry continues to wait. In the case of geriatric psychiatry, there were already subspecialty examinations in Geriatric Family Medicine and Geriatric Internal Medicine; the subspecialty of geriatric psychiatry had to be recognized if psychiatry was not miss out on its share of Medicare funds. In the case of forensic psychiatry, there was competition from certified subspecialists in forensic psychology and no competitive opposition to the field from within organized medicine. In the case of addiction psychiatry, there was again an incentive to create psychiatric specialists who could compete for government funds to combat drug abuse. Adolescent psychiatry faces opposition to its subspecialty status from within psychiatry. General psychiatrists, who may have had only minimal training in adolescent psychiatry, do not wish to be perceived as less qualified to treat adolescent patients than those who specialize in adolescent psychiatry. Child and adolescent psychiatrists do not want to have to compete for teenaged patients with specialists in adolescent psychiatry. This potential competition for adolescent patients is a mistake. There are more than enough teenagers in need of care, albeit a shortage of money to pay for such care. General psychiatrists, child and adolescent psychiatrists, and specialists in adolescent psychiatry must work together, rather than against each other, if there is to be any hope that the government and managed care will address the psychiatric needs of teenagers.

There is a discrepancy between the number of adolescents in need of mental health services and the number of psychiatrists trained and motivated to work with teenagers. The 1995 report of the Carnegie Council on Adolescent Development, *Great Transitions: Preparing Adolescents for a New Century* states in its Executive Summary that:

Since 1960, the burden of adolescent illness has shifted from the traditional causes of disease to the more behavior-related problems, such as sexually transmitted disease, teenage pregnancy, motor vehicle accidents, gun-related homicides and accidents, depression leading to suicide and abuse of drugs (alcohol and cigarettes as well as illegal drugs). Instilling in adolescents the knowledge, skills, and values that foster physical and mental health will require substantial changes in the way health professionals work and the way they connect with families, schools, and community organizations. At least three measures are needed to meet these goals. The first is the training and availability of health providers with a deep and sensitive understanding of the developmental needs and behavior-related problems of adolescents.

The American Society for Adolescent Psychiatry offers the opportunity to set aside parochial personal interests in favor of serving the teenagers of our nation. ASAP provides an opportunity for general psychiatrists and for child and adolescent psychiatrists who are interested in working with adolescents to have access to current knowledge and to increase their clinical skills in adolescent psychiatry. ASAP provides a local and national forum where colleagues can meet, network, and advocate on behalf of adolescents generally and adolescent mental health specifically.

The Accreditation Council on Fellowships in Adolescent Psychiatry is one of the means through which ASAP seeks to accomplish its goals. The council's *Standards* and its accreditation processes are designed to foster the education of subspecialists in adolescent psychiatry who will address the mental health needs of young people today and in the future.

Council on Fellowships in Adolescent Psychiatry

The Council on Fellowships in Adolescent Psychiatry (CFAP) is a component of the American Society for Adolescent Psychiatry.

The function of the Council includes the creation of Standards for Fellowship Programs in Adolescent Psychiatry, the dissemination of those Standards, and the evaluation of whether or not a specific program that has applied for accreditation is substantially in compliance with those Standards.

Applications for accreditation should be directed to:

Council on Fellowships in Adolescent Psychiatry
American Society for Adolescent Psychiatry
4340 East West Highway, Suite 401
Bethesda, Maryland 20814–4411

Upon receipt of a request for evaluation for accreditation, the CFAP will provide a copy of its Standards and a copy of the Program Survey form to be completed by the Director of the Program to be evaluated.

The Council will review the Program Survey form and advise the Director of the program being evaluated as to (a) the fact that the Program appears to be in substantial compliance with the Standards, so that a Site Visit to the Program is indicated for the purpose of completing the evaluation, or (b) the fact that the Program does not appear to be in substantial compliance with the Standards, so that it might appropriately be strengthened and apply for future re-evaluation for potential accreditation.

At a mutually convenient time, the Council will arrange with the Program being evaluated for Site Visitors to come to the Program to complete the evaluation. The reports of the Site Visitors will be reviewed by the Council and the Director of the Program will be advised as to (a) the fact that the Program appears to be in substantial compliance with the Standards and qualifies for Full Accreditation, or

(b) the fact that the Program does not appear to be in substantial compliance with the Standards, so that it might be appropriately strengthened and apply for future re-evaluation for potential accreditation. Where applicable, Provisional Accreditation status will be granted.

SPECIAL REQUIREMENTS FOR PROGRAMS
IN ADOLESCENT PSYCHIATRY

I.   Introduction

This outline presumes that an adolescent fellowship would follow an accredited three-year general psychiatry residency, i.e. be a fifth postgraduate year (PGY5). Thus, the suggested program does not include clinical experience with adults or younger children, which will have been part of the general psychiatry training. Instruction in the normal development of younger children will be included, however, since this can be directly linked to the didactic material on normal adolescent development. Similarly, adolescent psychopathology with an earlier onset would be dealt with in didactic seminars from its beginnings, although the emphasis would be placed on its manifestations during adolescence.

The present curriculum represents what can realistically be included in one year. A longer period of training would allow for a more comprehensive and more intensive experience. Since what a given training program can offer will depend on factors such as the quality and depth of its faculty and the components of clinical rotations that are locally available, it is understood that not all that is suggested can be necessarily provided.

A.   Definition of the Subspecialty

Adolescent psychiatry is that area of psychiatry which focuses on prevention, diagnosis, evaluation and treatment of mental disorders and disturbances seen in adolescents. An educational program in adolescent psychiatry must be organized to provide professional knowledge and a well-supervised clinical experience.

B. Duration and Scope of Education

1. The training period must be at least 12 months in duration following successful completion of an ACGME-accredited psychiatry residency.

2. Training in adolescent psychiatry that occurred during general residency training will under no circumstances be counted toward meeting this requirement.

3. Training is best accomplished on a full-time basis. If it is undertaken on a part-time basis, the 12-month program must be completed within a two-year period.

4. Prior to entry in the program, each trainee must be notified in writing of the required length of training for which the program is accredited. The required length of training for a particular individual may not be changed without mutual agreement during his/her program unless there is a break in his/her training or the individual requires remedial training.

C. Educational Goals and Objectives

1. Adolescent psychiatry programs must provide advanced training for the trainee to acquire expertise as a consultant in the sub-specialty. Programs must emphasize scholarship, self-instruction, development of critical analysis of clinical programs, and the ability to make appropriate decisions.

2. Clinical experience must include opportunities to assess and manage adolescent inpatients with a wide variety of psychiatric problems. Trainees must be given the opportunity to provide both primary and consultative care for patients in both impatient and outpatient settings in order to understand the interaction of adolescent development and disease, as well as to master techniques of assessment, therapy, and management.

3.   The program must include training in the biological and psychosocial aspects of adolescent development, psychiatric assessment of adolescents and their families and the diagnoses of psychiatric disorders beginning in adolescence.

4.   There must be a focus on multidimensional biopsychosocial and functional concepts of treatment and management as applied both in inpatient facilities (acute and long-term care) and in outpatient clinics and community settings such as detention facilities, day treatment settings or at home. There must also be emphasis on the medical and iatrogenic aspects of illness as well as on sociocultural, ethical, and legal considerations, etc., that may affect or impinge on psychiatric management.

II.   Institutional Organization

A. The program must be administratively attached to and sponsored by a core residency program in psychiatry that is fully accredited by the ACGME (exception may be made for existing general psychiatry programs that have been comprehensively reorganized and reaccredited as provisional programs). The program must function as an integral part of the psychiatry residency.

B. The presence of trainees in adolescent psychiatry must not dilute or otherwise detract from the didactic or clinical experience available to general psychiatry trainees. The RRC shall approve the size of the trainee complement. Any changes in trainee complement require prior approval by the RRC.

C. The training program must take place in facilities that are approved by the appropriate state licensing agencies and, where appropriate, by the Joint Commission on the Accreditation of Healthcare Organizations.

D. There shall be a clear educational rationale for the inclusion of each participating institution.

E. There must be current, written affiliation agreements specific to the provision of training in adolescent psychiatry between the sponsoring institution of the adolescent psychiatry program and each of its participating institutions. These agreements should specify:

1. Program goals and objectives and the means by which they will be accomplished.

2. The resources and facilities in the institution(s) that will be available to each trainee.

3. Information on professional liability insurance, fringe benefits, and vacations.

4. The duties and responsibilities the trainee will have in each institution.

5. The relationship that will exist between adolescent psychiatry trainees and the trainees and faculties in other programs as appropriate.

6. The supervision each adolescent psychiatry trainee will receive by the faculty in each institution.

III. Faculty and Staff

A. Program Director

The Program Director should be an active clinician and must devote sufficient time to the program to ensure achievement of the educational goals and objectives. The program director should be primarily based at the main program teaching site. The program director must be:

1. Certified by the American Board of Adolescent Psychiatry or have equivalent qualifications in adolescent psychiatry.

2. Appropriately qualified by training and experience in psychiatric education and administration.

3.   Participate in scholarly activities appropriate to the profession such as local, regional and national specialty societies research, presentations, and publications.

B. Program Director Responsibilities

The program director will be the person who has primary responsibility for the administration of the program and should be assisted and advised by a training committee that shall include the program director of the general psychiatry program and a trainee. The program director shall be responsible for:

1.   Supervising the recruitment and appointment process for applicants, including compliance with appropriate credentialing policies and procedures. No applicant who has completed a general psychiatry residency in another program shall be appointed without written communication from the prior program director that verifies satisfactory completion of all educational and ethical requirements for graduation.

2.   Monitoring the progress of each trainee, including the maintenance of a training record that documents completion of all required components of the program as well as the evaluations of performance by supervisors and teachers. This record shall include a patient log for each trainee, which shall document that each trainee has experienced all clinical experiences required by the Special Requirements and the educational objectives of the program.

3.   Monitoring the quality of all didactic and clinical experiences, including the collection and review of periodic written evaluation by the trainee of all such experiences and supervision.

4.   Maintaining all other training records, including those related to appointment, the departmental processes regarding due process, sickness and other leaves, call responsibilities, and vacation time.

5. Providing to each trainee the written goals and objectives for each component of the program upon beginning that aspect of training.

6. Providing written descriptions of the departmental policies regarding due process, sickness and other leaves, call responsibilities, and vacation time to all trainees upon appointment to the program. All trainees must be provided with written descriptions of the malpractice coverage provided for each clinical assignment.

7. Placing a statement in the training record of each trainee upon completion of the program that documents the satisfactory completion of all program requirements.

8. Notifying the RRC promptly of any major changes in the program or its leadership.

9. Preparing timely, accurate program information forms and related materials in preparation for review by the Residency Review Committee.

10. Reporting to the Residency Review Committee by September of each year the name of each trainee in the program.

C. Number and Qualifications of the Physician Faculty

1. There must be a sufficient number of qualified physician faculty to maintain a quality didactic and clinical educational program. In addition to the program director, there must be at least one other faculty member who is an experienced adolescent psychiatrist preferably certified by the American Board of Adolescent Psychiatry (or its equivalent).

2. These individuals must be additionally qualified by experience in adolescent psychiatry to provide the expertise needed to fulfill the didactic, clinical and research goals of the program.

3. The faculty must devote sufficient time to the educational program in adolescent psychiatry to assure fulfillment of its goals and objectives.

4. The physician faculty should:

   a. participate in the specialty societies of the field, and;

   b. actively participate in clinical and/or basic research.

5. The director of adolescent training at each participating institution shall be appointed by or with the concurrence of the general psychiatry program director.

D. Adolescent Care Team

Adolescent Psychiatry Team members should include representatives from clinical disciplines such as psychology, social work, psychiatric nursing, activity or occupational therapy, pharmacy and nutrition. In addition, it is highly desirable that trainees have access to professionals representing allied disciplines (such as ethics and forensics) as needed for patient care and pedagogical purposes. Regular team meetings should be held.

IV. Facilities and Resources

A. An *Adolescent Impatient Hospital:* The Psychiatry Department sponsoring the program must be a part of or affiliated with at least one adolescent impatient psychiatric unit, which has the full range of services usually ascribed to such a facility.

B. An *Ambulatory Care Service:* The ambulatory care service must be designed to render care in a multi-disciplinary environment such as a clinic or psychiatric outpatient department.

C. *Rotations:* The program must provide opportunities for the trainee to assess and treat adolescents in a variety of settings including juvenile or family court, an adolescent medicine clinic, a day treatment program or a drug and alcohol rehabilitation center.

D. *Ancillary Support Services:* At all participating facilities, there must be sufficient administrative support to ensure adequate teaching facilities, appropriate office space, support personnel, and teaching resources.

E. *Patient Population:* There must be sufficient number and variety of patients in all institutions where training takes place to accomplish the educational goals. This should include not only the spectrum of adolescent psychiatric diagnoses, but also experience with a diversity of patients by sex, socioeconomic, educational, and cultural backgrounds.

F. *Additional Educational Environment:* The program must provide opportunities for the trainee to render continuing care and to exercise leadership responsibilities in organizing recommendations from the mental health team, and in integrating recommendations and input from the consultative medical specialties and allied disciplines.

STANDARDS

SPECIAL REQUIREMENTS FOR PROGRAMS IN ADOLESCENT PSYCHIATRY

Academic Affiliation:
The Fellowship Program in Adolescent Psychiatry should be associated with a residency program in psychiatry that has been accredited by the Accreditation Council for Graduate Medical Education.

Director of the Program:
The Director of the Program should be an experienced adolescent psychiatrist. By the year 1998, the Director should be certified by the American Board of Adolescent Psychiatry, or the equivalent.

Faculty of the Program:
It is important that the Fellow has exposure to more than one practitioner of adolescent psychiatry, so that at least one additional member of the faculty, i.e. in addition to the Director, should be an experienced adolescent psychiatrist. It is not necessary, although it is highly desirable, that the additional faculty person be certified either by the American Board of Psychiatry and Neurology in Child and

Adolescent Psychiatry or by the American Board of Adolescent
Psychiatry.

Supervised Clinical Experiences:
Emphasis should be placed on meeting the educational needs of the
Fellow, rather than on the service needs of the clinical components of
the Fellowship Program. Regularly scheduled, frequent, individual case
supervision of the Fellow's clinical experiences is essential to effective
clinical education.

Basic Components of the Clinical Experiences
    A. In-Patient Experience
    B. Out-Patient (clinic) Experience
    C. Consultation-Liaison Experience
    D. Additional Clinical Experiences:
        1. Juvenile Delinquency and Criminality
        2. Adolescent Risk-Taking Behaviors, for example:
            a. sexual contact
            b. alcohol and drug abuse
        3. Transition to young adulthood
        4. School-related problems, i.e. grades 7 through college
        5. Adolescent Medicine

Didactic Core Curriculum:
The didactic core curriculum presents that body of information and
skills that is to be communicated to the Fellow by means of lectures,
seminars, demonstrations and other formal teaching.

Basic Components of the Didactic Program
    A. Diagnostic Case Conferences
    B. Continuous Case Seminar
    C. Reading Seminar - covering all of the topics listed below
        under the Category of Specialty Content of Adolescent
        Psychiatry

Specialty Content of Adolescent Psychiatry
    A. Normal Development
        1. Developmental tasks of childhood, adolescence and
            young adulthood
        2. Psychosocial development

        3.   Interpersonal relations

        4.   Moral development

        5.   Cognitive development

        6.   Social and cultural influences on development

B. Assessment

        1.   Psychiatric interview of the adolescent

        2.   Family interviewing

        3.   Psychological testing

        4.   Psychosocial assessment, for example: school, peer-relations, work

        5.   Biological

        6.   Medical

C. Psychiatric disorders in childhood, adolescence and young adulthood

D. Sexuality

        1.   Normal sexual development

        2.   Sexual problems

        3.   Sexual abuse

        4.   Pregnancy and parenthood during adolescence

        5.   Sexually transmitted diseases, contraception and abortion

E. Legal and Ethical Issues

        1.   Emancipated minors

        2.   Confidentiality

        3.   Informed Consent for treatment and hospitalization

        4.   Rights to Refuse Treatment and hospitalization

        5.   Juvenile delinquency and the juvenile justice system and adolescents in the adult criminal justice system

        6.   Custody determination and visitation rights

        7.   Status offenses

        8.   Abuse and neglect

        9.   Special ethical considerations in working with adolescents

F. Psychiatric Aspects of Physical Illness

        1.   Acute illness and trauma

        2.   Chronic illness

        3.   Death and dying

        4.   Non-compliance with medical treatment

G. Psychiatric Treatments

        1.   The therapeutic alliance

2. Communication with parents
3. Communication with schools
4. Termination
5. Family Therapy
6. Group Therapy
7. Psychoanalysis and Psycho-dynamic Psychotherapy
8. Behavioral and cognitive therapies
9. Psycho-pharmacological treatment (special considerations with adolescents)

Training in Research:

The Program should provide the Fellow with basic skills in research in adolescent psychiatry, so that the fellow can critically evaluate published research findings in the sub-specialty and is equipped to make some contribution to the scholarly or scientific development of adolescent psychiatry.

The Program should include a research requirement for completion of its course. Suitable research projects include a scholarly review or clinical study suitable for presentation at a scientific program or for publication in refereed journal, participation in on-going externally funded research at a level of effort equivalent to at least two months of full-time work, production of a videotape or film suitable for presentation at a scientific program, production of a practice manual in some specific area of adolescent psychiatry or preparation of an annotated bibliography on a selected topic in the sub-specialty.

The Program must include the resources that would make such research possible. These include, at minimum, access to a major medical library and to at least one behavioral science research resource (e.g. computer processing, a programmable calculator, a one-way mirror observation room, video-tape equipment, endocrine assays, psychotropic drug assays, electroencephalography, or computerized tomography).

Training in Teaching:

The Program should provide opportunities to foster the Fellow's development as a teacher of adolescent psychiatry. Such opportunities should be consistent with the Fellow's acquisition of the essential knowledge and skills of the sub-specialty, so that the bulk of the Fellow's teaching should be scheduled after the Fellow has received basic training in adolescent psychiatry. It is recommended that the

Fellow have exposure to senior teachers in the field, who can provide effective role models.

Among the suitable teaching opportunities are: teaching medical students and residents in general psychiatry, teaching relevant topics to nonpsychiatric physicians.

Further Information:
For further information about the Council on Fellowships in Adolescent Psychiatry or about application for accreditation of specific Programs in Adolescent Psychiatry, contact: Council on Fellowships in Adolescent Psychiatry, American Society for Adolescent Psychiatry, 4340 East West Highway, Suite 401, Bethesda, Maryland 20814–4411.

20 ADOLESCENT PSYCHIATRY TRAINING: GUIDELINES FOR CHILD AND ADOLESCENT PSYCHIATRY RESIDENTS, GENERAL PSYCHIATRY RESIDENTS, AND MEDICAL STUDENTS

ROBERT L. HENDREN, MARIE ARMENTANO, SIMEON GRATER,
EDWIN J. MIKKELSEN, RICHARD SARLES, AND ADRIAN SONDHEIMER

The importance of quality training in adolescent psychiatry is gaining increasing recognition as the problems experienced by adolescents are becoming more severe and widespread. The rates of suicide, substance abuse, depression, eating disorders, conduct disorders, and pregnancy among adolescents have increased at an alarming rate in recent decades. To meet the increasing demand for psychiatric treatment for adolescents, practitioners, hospitals, and various agencies have increased their services for adolescents. Few guidelines exist, however, for training the providers of such services to work with troubled adolescents (Looney et al., 1985; Flaherty, 1989).

This document was developed by members of the Committee on Adolescence of the American Academy of Child and Adolescent Psychiatry. It is designed to identify specific educational and training guidelines in adolescent psychiatry for physicians at various levels of expertise. These include medical students, residents in general psychiatry, and residents or fellows in child and adolescent psychiatry. It is intended to be a general and comprehensive guideline, but it is flexible and open to alteration and new material. Certain training programs may emphasize specific areas. We hope that all programs will use these guidelines to identify weaknesses in their training curricula and strive to improve them, so that the trainees at all levels receive a basic knowledge of adolescent psychiatry. The core of this basic knowledge is an understanding of development from birth onward, and an appreciation of the biological, psychological, and social influences throughout the developmental cycle. Good supervision, including observing and being observed, is an essential part of gaining this knowledge.

The tables that follow throughout this essay list both didactic knowledge and training experiences. Here general psychiatry residents are referred to as residents and child and adolescent psychiatry fellows (residents) are referred to as fellows. The level of knowledge or training ranges from 1 to 3, with 3 being the most sophisticated. The levels are characterized by the descriptors:

1. *Basic level of Knowledge and Training:* has overview knowledge of subject; can recognize symptoms and appreciates need to refer; can answer basic multiple-choice questions.
2. *Intermediate Level of Knowledge and Training:* has working knowledge of subject; can formulate a differential diagnosis and treatment plan an knows where to refer; can implement a basic treatment plan
3. *Advanced Level of Knowledge and Training:* has a detailed knowledge and sophisticated understanding of subject; can implement a specialized treatment plan; can provide teaching and consultation on subject

The accompanying text provides a discussion of each table. The brief bibliography provides reference to papers and books that may be useful to those interested in adolescent psychiatry. It is not intended to be comprehensive and may not include some considered classics.

Normal Development

Normal development serves as a standard by which we can assess and better serve adolescents. By understanding the crucial developmental processes and their sequences we then can ask ourselves about a particular adolescent (see Table 1):

1. What stage of physical, cognitive, sexual, emotional, moral and social development has the adolescent reached?
2. Is the adolescent on target in all the above areas (recognizing the wide range of normal variation)?
3. Are there areas in which the adolescent is delayed or advanced?

TABLE 1
NORMAL DEVELOPMENT

Definition of Adolescence	Medical Student	Resident	Fellow
Biologic Development	1	1	3
Bodily changes	2	1	3
Endocrine changes	2	1	3
Neurotransmitter changes	1	2	3
Genetics/hereditability of physical and personality traits	1	2	3
Psychological Development	1	2	3
Cognitive	1	2	3
Psychosexual	1	2	3
Psychosocial	1	2	3
Moral	1	1	3
Affect regulation	1	3	3
Social Development	2	3	3+
Family	2	3	3+
Peers	2	3	3+
Culture	2	3	3
Society	2	3	3
Institutions	2	3	3+

4. Is the adolescent having trouble mastering one developmental task?

5. Is this an adolescent who is, on the whole, healthy and is experiencing a developmental crisis or is this an adolescent whose previous development has been delayed, distorted or problematic?

The curriculum in normal development must include a working definition of adolescence. All must be aware that adolescence begins with a biological event, puberty, and has a psychosocial endpoint in the assumption of an adult identity. Trainees at all levels should be familiar with the divisions into early, middle and late adolescence and the transition to young adulthood (Offer, 1969).

In the area of biological development, all must have working knowledge of the sequence of bodily changes, including the Tanner (1962) stages (Sexual Maturity Rating). All must be familiar with the endocrine and neurotransmitter alterations that occur prior to and during adolescence. Fellows would know them in detail, including the psychological effects of these changes and the emotional work involved in coping with them, including reactions to early or late development of secondary sexual characteristics. All trainees would be acquainted with the evolving state of knowledge about the roles of genetics, temperament, and the environment in development (Eisenberg, 1980; Bowlby, 1988).

In the area of psychological development, medical students would know that there are changes in cognition, in moral development, and in affect regulation throughout adolescence and would know that the adolescent becomes less egocentric, less dependent on his parents, and more able to have intimate friendships with individuals outside the family and eventually sexual relationships. Psychiatric residents are expected, in addition, to have a specific understanding of cognitive stages of development; for example, Piaget's (1969) stages and his concepts of assimilation and accommodation. General and child and adolescent psychiatry fellows must appreciate the effect of these cognitive changes, or their lack of effect, on the adolescents' emotional growth. In the realm of psychosexual development, general psychiatry residents are expected to understand psychodynamic theories of sexual development. This understanding would include the concepts of latency and the resurgence of sexuality in adolescence with an integration into genital sexuality and an attainment of a full sexual identity. Child and adolescent psychiatry fellows would understand these theories in more depth and would also learn more about developmental problems, inhibitions, psychosexual disorders and variations in gender identity and object choice. Child and adolescent psychiatry fellows would have an appreciation of specific contributions of major figures in the field.

Erikson's (1968) schemata of psychosocial developmental crises and Blos's (1967) concept of the second individuation process of adolescence would be covered at all levels of training in graduated detail as would theories of moral development such as Kohlberg and Kramer's (1969) and Gilligan and Murphy's (1979). Adolescent ego development and its vagaries in terms of an increased ability to tolerate frustration, to delay gratification, and to plan for the future would be emphasized (Freud, 1958; Masterson, 1968). General psychiatry residents and fellows must be familiar with developmental issues in impulse and affect control and the capacity for interpersonal relationships. The curriculum would emphasize the current state of knowledge both about risk factors and about the factors that contribute to resilience, and protect against less desirable outcomes in adolescents.

The intent would be to help developing clinicians appreciate strengths and potentials in our patients, in addition to vulnerability and pathology.

Social development would be covered at all levels of training, but with more depth and more clinical correspondence as the level of training increases. Medical students will appreciate that individuation from the family is an important adolescent task and should understand the impact of peer and family influences on adolescent decision making. Students should be aware that adolescence varies from one culture to another and is prolonged in a complicated and technologically sophisticated culture such as ours. There will be an understanding that adolescents have their own culture and an appreciation of the experience of adolescence varies even in our own culture according to gender, sexual orientation, race, class, and socioeconomic status. There should be an appreciation of the impact of institutions such as school, and, in particular, the impact of school failure in addition to a graduated understanding of all the foregoing. Residents and fellows will have an understanding of the family life cycle and the adolescent's part in it.

All teaching should emphasize interactive effects of biological, social, and psychological areas of development. Residents and fellows will acquire detailed knowledge about the specific impact of learning disabilities and attention problems on school performance, vocational potential, relationships to peers and authority figures, as well as self-esteem.

LIFE STRESSORS

Trainees at all levels should have an appreciation of the effect of life stressors on adolescent psychological development (see Table 2). Stress can enhance development as well as lead to problems with developmental progression. The most significant and common life stressors are outlined in the following sections, along with an overview of the level of specific knowledge that is considered appropriate for each level of training.

SEXUALITY

The development of secondary sexual physical characteristics and sexual desires is one of the most significant factors in the life and development of the adolescent. To a large extent the development of

TABLE 2

Life Stressors	Medical Student	Resident	Fellow
Sexuality	2	3	3+
Divorce/Separation Effects	2	3	3
Adoption and Foster Care	1	2	3
Life Transitions	2	3	3
Shelters—Homelessness, Poverty	2	2	3
Peer Pressure	1	2	3+
Illness and Injury	2	3	3
Physical Abuse and Neglect	2	3	3
Sexual Abuse	2	3	3
Learning disabilities	1	2	3
Mental Retardation	1	2	3
Death and Dying	2	2	3
Exposure to Violence	1	3	3

sexual identity and function, including homosexuality, should be conceptualized within the context of normal development and its vicissitudes. Sexual risks include particular entities such as teenage pregnancy and AIDS, but also behavior and worries such as extreme promiscuity and sexual identity issues.

Medical students should have a good working knowledge of the anatomical and physiological changes that accompany adolescence as well as the normal variations in this development. Medical students should also have an appreciation of the intense psychological turmoil that may accompany the development of sexuality. The psychiatry resident should in addition be well grounded in the physiology of adolescent sexual development and its vicissitudes. Residents should have a more psychodynamically sophisticated understanding of the psychological components of sexual development. Fellows should in addition obtain a detailed knowledge of the physiological changes that accompany adolescence. Their understanding of psychodynamic issues should be sophisticated and should include a detailed knowledge of psychotherapeutic interventions utilized when the sexual developmental process becomes deviant.

DIVORCE/SEPARATION EFFECTS

Parental divorce or separation can have a significant impact on the developing adolescent. The dissolution of the family unit at a time when the adolescent is negotiating his differentiation from that unit can be particularly traumatic. There may also be lingering effects from an earlier parental divorce which may impact on the subsequent adolescent development. Attention should also be given to the particular issues which develop in blended and step families.

The medical student should be aware of the potential impact of parental separation on the adolescent and a general knowledge of the different forms this can take. The resident should have more specific knowledge concerning the general effects on adolescent development, as well as the typical pathological patterns that can occur. The fellow should possess detailed knowledge of the effects of parental divorce or separation on the developing adolescent. He or she should also be aware of the residual effects that an earlier occurring childhood divorce may have on the adolescent. In addition, fellows should possess knowledge of the statistics concerning the frequency and subtypes of pathological developmental outcomes, and of the interventions that have been found effective in preventing or ameliorating these problems.

ADOPTION AND FOSTER CARE

This heading really subsumes two related, but distinct, issues. The first relates to those children who were adopted at an early age and are now entering adolescence. The consolidation of identity that occurs in adolescence can make this a particularly challenging time for the adopted child and the adoptive family. The struggles that develop as part of the transition to independence can also lead to an idealization of the unknown biological family and a denigration of the adoptive family.

The second issus relates to adolescents in foster care who are often those who have been removed from their biological families either because they were abused or because they were unable to be controlled by their families. Thus, they experience the vicissitudes of adolescent development in the context of a new family structure and with unresolved issues with their biological families.

Medical students should be aware of the general statistics concerning adoption and the concept of foster care. They should be aware of the stress that this can place on adolescent development and the common psychodynamic patterns that are seen. Psychiatry residents should have a more sophisticated understanding of the psychodynamic interface between identity formation and adoption. They should also

415

know the accepted criteria for utilizing foster care as well as the pros and cons of foster care placement. The fellow should be able to develop a sophisticated framework for integrating the experience of adoption with developmental theory. They should know the clinical situations in which foster care can be useful as well as the potential negative effects of foster care placement.

LIFE TRANSITIONS

Adolescence itself can be conceptualized of as a major life transition that is comprised of a number of smaller transitions. The first is the physical transition of puberty, which usually coincides with an increase in complexity of social interactions and educational environment. Older adolescents are faced with transitioning out of the parental home environment, leaving high school for college or work, and developing significant relationships outside of the biological family.

Medical students should have a grasp of the magnitude and number of transitions which must be successfully negotiated in adolescence. They should also be broadly aware of the psychological changes which correlate with these transitional phases. Psychiatric residents should have a more sophisticated knowledge of the interface between psychological changes and life transitions. They should also be aware of the more common impediments to the successful negotiation of these transitions. The fellow should have a knowledge of the psychological changes which accompany the transitional phases and a sophisticated knowledge of the common transitional problems, their developmental sequelae, and effective therapeutic strategies for restoring the adolescent to developmental competence.

SHELTERS—HOMELESSNESS, POVERTY

Homelessness itself is obviously a significant stressor. In addition to the instability of the living environment, there are parallel effects on the family unit which may generate additional interpersonal tension within the family. Families are not homeless unless there are extreme financial difficulties and, thus, poverty is almost always a co-stressor.

Medical students should be aware of the large numbers of adolescents who are homeless. They should also be generally knowledgeable of the health risks and psychological stress of homelessness. Students and residents can also be encouraged to do volunteer work at a shelter to gain first hand experience of these problems. Fellows should be able to place the stressor of homelessness into a developmental framework. They should be aware of the broad subcategories of adolescents who run away as well as the physical, medical, and psychological risks that confront them on the street. They should also be aware of the corresponding risks that confront the adolescent who is homeless because his entire family cannot find housing.

ILLNESS AND INJURY

Severe illness or injury can be devastating at any point in the life cycle. The developmental aspects of adolescents can render these individuals particularly vulnerable to negative psychological effects. The principal negative effects are on the adolescent's development of self-esteem, identity, and autonomy. It is also in adolescence that an individual has to come to terms with the realities of long term chronic illnesses such as diabetes.

The medical student should be generally aware of the impact of physical illness and injury at any stage of the life cycle. As a part of this understanding, the medical student will have an understanding of the special vulnerabilities of the adolescent. Psychiatry residents should be generally aware of the developmental considerations that make the adolescent psychologically vulnerable to physical illness and injury. The fellow will possess detailed knowledge of the development and psychodynamic impact of physical illness and injury on the physically, sexually, and psychologically maturing adolescent. He or she will also be experienced in therapeutic approaches which may ameliorate the negative impact of physical illness and injury.

PHYSICAL ABUSE AND NEGLECT

Physical abuse and neglect can have pervasive negative effects on the developing adolescent whether it occurs in adolescence or represents the impact of earlier childhood abuse. The observation that physical abuse and neglect frequently go unreported and unrecognized make it all the more important that trainees be aware of the clues to and effects of abuse, and the requirements for mandated reporting.

The medical student should be aware of the potentially devastating effects of physical abuse and neglect on the developing adolescent as well as the high rate of these assaults. They should also be aware of the important role that pediatricians and primary care physicians have in the detection of abuse. Residents will possess a developmental perspective with which to view the effects of physical and sexual abuse. They should be aware of the more common psychological indicators of abuse which will also make them more able to detect individuals who were formerly abused. The fellow should have a detailed knowledge of the developmental and psychodynamic aspects of physical abuse, and a detailed knowledge of the sequelae of abuse. The fellow will also be knowledgeable concerning therapeutic interventions for abused children.

SEXUAL ABUSE

Medical students should be knowledgeable concerning symptoms that may relate to sexual abuse and the importance of directly asking adolescents about sexual abuse whenever it is suspected. They also should know about mandated reporting and should be generally aware of the psychological manifestations of such abuse. Residents should have a detailed knowledge of symptomatic correlates of past and present abuse. They should know the importance of inquiring about past sexual abuse as a part of their standard work-up and history. They must know the importance of mandated reporting and should be aware of potential psychological indicators and recognized treatment modalities. Given the magnitude and importance of this problem, the fellow should possess a detailed knowledge of the signs and symptoms of abuse, the need for mandated reporting in suspected cases, the psychological sequelae of past and current abuse, prognosis and appropriate treatment interventions. The fellows' knowledge base should be extensive enough that they can assume a leadership role in their community efforts to confront the problem of sexual abuse and be an educational resource to other disciplines, professionals, and community programs.

LEARNING DISABILITIES

Learning disabilities can have multiple impacts on the developing adolescent. There is the direct effect of the disability itself, secondary effects on the development of self-esteem and feelings of competence, and the unfortunate effects of undiagnosed learning disabilities.

The medical student should be aware of the nature and general clinical subtypes of learning disabilities, as well as their frequency. He or she should also be aware of the frequency with which these problems are under diagnosed or misdiagnosed and the psychological

418

sequelae of learning disabilities. The resident should have a working knowledge of the frequency and primary subtypes of learning disabilities. He or she will also be aware of the frequency with which these disorders are underdiagnosed or misdiagnosed, as well as the psychological impact of these problems. The fellow should have a detailed knowledge of the subject of learning disabilities including frequency, clinical subtypes, and psychological sequelae. He or she should also be knowledgeable concerning the diagnosis and remediation of these disorders.

MENTAL RETARDATION

The mentally retarded typically become acutely aware of their deficits in adolescence. This awareness can contribute to developmental arrests and the development of psychopathology.

Medical students should be aware of the impact of cognitive deficits on the process of adolescent development. Residents should have a working knowledge of the interaction between the cognitive deficits of the mentally retarded and adolescent development as this combination relates to the individual, the family, and the broader social context. Fellows will have a detailed knowledge of the developmental aspects of mental retardation as they impact on the process of adolescent development. This knowledge will also include an understanding of therapeutic interventions that may help to ameliorate the development of psychopathology.

DEATH AND DYING

Most individuals will begin to seriously consider their ultimate mortality as part of normal adolescent development. By late adolescence, many will have developed a philosophical-religious perspective that will remain with them throughout their life. For some, this process is accelerated by the death of a parent, loved one, friend, or their own untimely affliction with a potentially fatal disease such as a cancer. These stressors can lead to a variety of pathological outcomes including pathological bereavement, depression, extreme denial, and even suicide.

Medical students should be generally aware of the psychological aspects of normal and pathological bereavement, the psychological stages of the acceptance of death, and potential arrest points in this processes. Residents should have a more sophisticated knowledge of

TABLE 3

Symptomatic Behaviors	Medical Student	Resident	Fellow
Substance Abuse	2	3	3+
Pregnancy and Parenthood	2	3	3+
Violence and Aggressive Behavior	1	2	3+
Recklessness	2	2	3
Physical Self-harm and Suicide	2	3	3
Vandalism	1	2	3
Gang Behavior	1	2	2
Cult Involvement	1	2	2
Runaway	1	2	3
Learning disabilities	1	2	3
Mental Retardation	1	2	3
Death and Dying	2	2	3
Exposure to Violence	1	3	3

the developmental underpinnings of these processes and their psycho-dynamic implications. Fellows should have a sophisticated knowledge of these topics, which include clinical exposure to adolescents who are confronted with the death of a significant other or their own accelerated mortality. They should be prepared to serve as an educational resource to other disciplines and professionals.

SYMPTOMATIC BEHAVIORS

The majority of psychiatric education is syndromic in nature, which is keeping with the current thrust of research and clinical practice. There are, however, a number of symptomatic behaviors of which medical trainees at all levels should be aware (see Table 3).

SUBSTANCE ABUSE

The issue of substance abuse is of great significance to adolescent development even when it does not progress to the point of abuse. Many children will begin to experiment with alcohol and drugs in adolescence. Even if this experimentation does not progress to dependency, it can have serious consequences by increasing impulsive and risk-taking behaviors.

Medical students should be familiar with the statistics concerning the usage of alcohol and drugs by adolescents. They should also be aware of the risk that this experimentation represents both in terms of addiction and the potential consequences of even occasional intoxication. Residents should be aware of the basic usage of alcohol and drugs by adolescents. They should also possess knowledge concerning the risk of addiction and accidents. In addition, they should have an understanding of the developmental considerations that make adolescents particularly vulnerable. The fellow should have a detailed knowledge of the developmental context that makes adolescents particularly vulnerable to experimentation with substance abuse, in addition to basic knowledge of the statistics, risks of usage, and effective prevention.

PREGNANCY AND PARENTHOOD

Adolescent pregnancy places an enormous amount of stress on the mother, as well as the father, whose distress is frequently overlooked. The outcome of teenage pregnancy is multifactorial, but will primarily be determined by the availability of social and family support.

Medical students should be aware of the statistics concerning contraception, adolescent pregnancy, and abortion. They should also have a general understanding of the stresses which confront the adolescent parent. Residents should have a basic knowledge of the statistics relevant to teenage pregnancy. They should also have a general knowledge of the sociological and developmental context of adolescent pregnancy. They should be aware of the stress of adolescent pregnancy and its potential effect on adolescent development. Fellows should have detailed knowledge of the statistics of teenage pregnancy as well as the sociological and developmental context. They should possess a clinical perspective on the stress of adolescent pregnancy and familiarity with the therapeutic interventions that may ameliorate the potential negative effects. Whenever possible, fellows should have direct clinical experience with adolescents who are undergoing the stress of pregnancy or parenthood.

VIOLENCE AND AGGRESSIVE BEHAVIOR

Medical students should have general knowledge about the factors which contribute to aggressive behavior in adolescents. Residents should have a more detailed knowledge of the factors that contribute

421

to aggressive behavior in adolescents and of the developmental and psychodynamic considerations. Fellows will have a detailed knowledge of the biological, familial, societal, developmental, and psychodynamic factors that contribute to adolescent aggressive behavior. Fellows will also possess knowledge of the therapeutic interventions which may ameliorate aggressive behavior.

RECKLESSNESS

The medical student should be aware of the problem of adolescent recklessness and its potential adverse effects on the life of the adolescent. Residents will have a general knowledge of the problem of adolescent recklessness and its potential adverse effects on the life of the adolescent. Fellows will have a detailed knowledge of the physiological, societal, developmental, and psychodynamic contributions to adolescent reckless behavior. They will also have an understanding of the therapeutic interventions that may ameliorate this behavior.

PHYSICAL SELF-HARM AND SUICIDE

While suicidal ideation and attempts are usually the outgrowth of a depressive disorder, there is distressing evidence that serious suicidal behavior can occur in adolescents who do not appear to be severely depressed.

Medical students should be aware of the frequency with which adolescents who do not appear to be overtly depressed attempt to commit suicide. They should also have a general awareness of the factors that contribute to this behavior. Residents will have an understanding of the phenomenon of adolescent suicide as well as of the occurrence rate in those individuals who do not appear to be overtly depressed. Residents will also have a framework for viewing this behavior which includes physiological, sociological, developmental, and psychodynamic factors. Fellows will have a detailed understanding of the factors contribute to suicidal behavior in adolescents who do not appear to be overtly depressed. They will also have a clinical knowledge of the therapeutic interventions that can be utilized when an adolescent with suicidal tendencies is identified, and have information on the risk factors such as cluster suicides, which can help to identify adolescents who are more prone to engage in this behavior.

VANDALISM

Medical students should be aware of the propensity for adolescents to engage in vandalism even when they appear to be developing normally. They should also be generally aware of the factors that contribute to this behavior. In addition, residents should be aware of the psychodynamics of vandalism. Fellows will have a detailed knowledge of the sociological, developmental, and psychodynamic factors that may contribute to adolescent vandalism. They will also be able clinically to evaluate the significance and meaning of vandalism in adolescents.

GANG BEHAVIOR

Research on gangs has revealed that a surprising number of adolescents who do not have major psychopathologies migrate to gangs during times of developmental stress. If these individuals are not harmed by the gang experience, they may go on to complete their psychological development in a relatively normal fashion.

Medical students should be aware of the contemporary significance of gang behavior and the positive and negative influence of gangs. Residents will, in addition, have knowledge of the sociological, developmental, and psychodynamic contributions to this behavior. This knowledge will include the different needs of early, middle, and late adolescence. Fellows will have a more detailed knowledge of the sociological, developmental, and psychodynamic factors which contribute to gang behavior and of what the variety of gangs offer the young person. They will also be aware of prognostic factors and clinical interventions that may help to interrupt the recurring cycle of gang behavior.

CULT INVOLVEMENT

The vulnerabilities and pressures of adolescence may render some adolescents especially susceptible to the enticement of cults. There is also a growing body of knowledge concerning the psychological effects of cult involvement and the rehabilitation process.

Medical students should be aware of the general phenomenon of cults and why an adolescent may be vulnerable. Residents will, in addition, be knowledgeable about the psychological sequelae of cult involvement. Fellows will have an extensive knowledge of the sociological, developmental, and psychodynamic factors that render adolescents vulnerable to cult involvement, and knowledge of the therapeutic interventions that may ameliorate the psychological problems assiciated with cult involvement.

RUNAWAY

Runaway behavior is surprisingly frequent and encompasses a large spectrum of severity. The behaviors subsumed under this heading range from adolescents who provocatively disappear only to stay with a friend overnight, to those who hitchhike cross country, and to those who sever all ties with family and friends.

Medical students should be aware of the extent of the problem and the heterogeneity of the population that engages in this behavior. They should also be aware of the health needs of this population and the importance of providing them with appropriate resources. Residents should in addition understand common family dynamics and have an expanded cognizance of the psychodynamic stressors which lead to and result from runaway behavior. Fellows will, in addition, have a knowledge of treatment and programmatic interventions that have proven successful in reuniting the runaway with their family or alternative safe and nurturing living environments.

PSYCHOPATHOLOGIC DISORDERS

Familiarity with child and adolescent psychopathology is essential to the training of medical students, general psychiatrists, and child and adolescent psychiatry fellows (see Table 4).

By the end of a psychiatry clerkship, a medical student should be able to speak the language of psychiatry. Medical students should know and understand the criteria of major diagnostic categories, how adolescent patients present differently from adults, the interviewing and therapy techniques for working with adolescents and their families, and have some exposure to psychiatric treatment as specifically applied to adolescents.

Usually the objectives just described are best taught through lectures, assigned reading, and working side by side with residents and faculty. Medical students usually should not be responsible solely for managing an adolescent patient but should serve a valuable function in data gathering and acting as a coworker or cotherapist.

A medical student should be able to develop a differential diagnosis that includes the most common Axes I and II diagnoses. Residents and

TABLE 4

Psychopathological Disorders	Medical Student	Resident	Fellow
Pervasive Developmental Disorders	1	1	3
Attention-Deficit Hyperactivity Disorder	1	2	3
Conduct Disorder	1	2	3
Oppositional Defiant Disorder	1	2	3
Tic Disorders	1	2	3
Substance Abuse Disorders	1	2	3+
Schizophrenic Disorders	1	2	3+
Other Psychoses (e.g., Delusional Disorders, Brief Psychotic Disorder	1	2	3
Mood Disorder	1	2	3+
Anxiety Disorder	1	2	3+
Obsessive-Compulsive Disorders	1	2	3
Posttraumatic Stress Disorder, including Neglect and Abuse	1	2	3+
Somatoform Disorder	1	1	3
Dissociative Disorder	1	1	2
Gender Identity Disorder	1	1	3
Eating disorder	1	2	3+
Impulse Control Disorders	1	2	3
Adjustment Disorders	1	2	3+
Personality Disorder	1	2	3

fellows should be able to develop and understand a DSM IV differential diagnoses that includes the major diagnostic categories on all five axes. Fellows in addition should recognize minor disorders.

PSYCHIATRIC EVALUATION

Techniques for effective interviewing of adolescent patients are essential for medical students, residents, and fellows. These include the ability to establish rapport with the adolescent and the family and thus to elicit the important information necessary to make both a differential diagnosis and a formulation of the important issues involving the adolescent and the family (see Table 5). Interviewing skills should be learned through the observation of and supervision by skilled interviewers.

TABLE 5

Psychiatric Evaluation	Medical Student	Resident	Fellow
Interviewing Techniques	2	3	3+
Collection of Relevant Information	2	3	3+
Differential Diagnosis	1	2	3
Formulation and Integration	1	2	3
Treatment Planning	1	2	3
Referral	1	2	3
Specialized Evaluations			
Crisis	2	3	3
Comprehensive (includes integration of medical, educational, psychological, psychiatric information	1	2	3
Forensic	1	2	3
Custody	1	2	3
Abuse/Neglect	2	2	3
Consultation	2	2	3

Adolescent patients frequently feel more comfortable talking to and identifying with medical students because the students tend to be closer to the patient's age and usually have more time to talk with the patient than do other members of the treatment team. Medical students should acquire the ability to interview patients and their families, to accurately diagnose the most common disorders of childhood and adolescence, and to know about treatments used for the most common clinical problems.

Psychiatry residents, in addition, should be expected to evaluate, diagnose, and formulate a treatment plan for a variety of the diagnostic entities seen in children and adolescents. Residents should be under close faculty supervision (including case supervision) and should be expected to follow cases as long as possible. Psychiatry residents should learn about the complexities of diagnosis, the frequency of comorbidity, and the unanswered questions about the treatment of child and adolescent psychopathology. Residents should also learn the limits of their expertise and should recognize when to refer a patient and his family to a specialist in adolescent psychiatry.

Optimally, fellows should evaluate, diagnose, and treat patients and families representing every diagnostic category of psychopathology. Obviously, some training programs may not have services for all

426

adolescent patients. Child and adolescent psychiatry resident training, however, can be supplemented by videotapes and electives with special populations.

Most important for medical students and residents is the ability to know when, where, and how to refer effectively an adolescent patient to the appropriate specialist or facility. Specialized adolescent evaluations should be familiar to all fellows. This includes evaluations of adolescents in a crisis, such as following a suicide attempt or when acutely psychotic. The medical student should be able to accurately assess the situation and know when and how to seek the help of an adolescent psychiatrist. Crisis evaluations should be a basic skill for both residents and fellows. Both should be capable of making a comprehensive evaluation of an adolescent. They should be able to integrate information from multiple sources including medical, educational, and psychological and psychiatric material into a thorough formulation, differential diagnosis, and treatment plan.

Forensic evaluations include such areas as competency to stand trial, court commitments to treatment facilities, and termination of parental rights. Also included are custody evaluations both for divorcing parents and for state custody related to abuse and neglect. Knowledge of the guidelines and requirements for the identification and reporting of abuse and neglect in adolescents is essential for all medical trainees. The ability to perform other specialized forensic evaluations are basic skills expected more for residents and fellows than for medical students.

PSYCHIATRIC TREATMENT

This section describes treatments about which trainees at different levels would be expected to attain differing degrees of experience, knowledge, and skill (see Table 6).

Trainees at all levels should be knowledgeable about the components of a psychiatric evaluation, with residents and fellows able to provide adequate assessments, treatment planning, and disposition in a crisis situation. When treatment is indicated, the establishment of a therapeutic alliance is crucial to the success of most approaches. All trainees should attempt this task, and indications of greater skill would be expected from trainees with more frequent direct clinical experience with adolescent patients. Knowledge of the elements of the pertinent therapies listed above would be expected of medical students. At a

TABLE 6

Psychiatric Treatment	Medical Student	Resident	Fellow
Establishing a Therapeutic Alliance	2	3	3
Integration of Treatments	1	3	3
Administration of Treatment Team	1	1	3
Individual Psychotherapies			
Psychodynamic (Transference & Countertransference	1	2	2
Cognitive Therapy	1	2	3
Behavioral Therapy	1	2	3
Supportive & Counseling Therapies	1	3	3
Work with Parent/Custodian	1	3	3
Family Psychotherapy	1	2	3
Pharmacotherapy	1	2	3
Group Psychotherapy	1	2	3
Adjunctive Therapies (Expressive Therapies, Social Skills)	1	2	3
Milieu Therapy	1	2	3

more advanced level, residents would be expected to attempt an integration of these treatments in compatible fashion during direct patient care, and fellows would be expected to develop sophistication in the administration of these combined therapies.

Psychiatric intervention is provided not only through direct patient responsibility but also by the coordination of patient care, particularly in more restrictive settings. Exposure of medical students to such settings can be beneficial and resident exposure under supervision, while functioning as part of a team, is a valuable and desired experience. Fellows must learn to incorporate the fundamentals of these administrative skills through exposure to such settings during training, and by assumption of some team leadership responsibilities.

Most treatment approaches with adolescents involve individual meetings with the patient. The most commonly utilized individual-focused treatments include psychodynamic, behavioral, and cognitive psychotherapeutic approaches. Supportive and counseling interventions, while individual-focused, are generally conducted with less intensity or for briefer periods of time. It is useful for medical students to have an elementary understanding of these approaches, while residents at a minimum should have the experience of providing supportive interventions. Moreover, resident experience with more intensive individual therapy should be encouraged. It is essential that fellows have clinical experience in applying these treatments with adolescents, possibly in their more pure or distinct forms, and definitely in an integrated fashion.

Inasmuch as adolescents are generally engaged in the process of autonomous development while not as yet having achieved adult capacities, issues surrounding developing independence may become prominent. The treatment of adolescents, therefore, often involves mutually shifting feelings between the patient and the psychiatrist. In other words, transference and countertransference phenomena frequently arise and need to be acknowledge and addressed. Medical students should have an awareness of these aspects of adolescent treatment, residents ideally should get a clinical taste of these interpersonal exchanges, and it is essential that fellows have the opportunity to experience these phenomena via comprehensive clinical experience and knowledgeable supervision.

A variety of acute and chronic psychopathological syndromes that manifest during adolescence will require or benefit from the provision of pharmacotherapeutics, as either the primary or an adjunctive treatment approach. Many psychological illnesses manifesting during this developmental period are treated with psychotropic medications that may include typical and atypical neuroleptics, selective serotonin reuptake inhibitors (SSRI's), tricyclic and heterocyclic compounds, mood stablizators, central nervous system stimulants, and alpha adrenergic agonists. In addition, various anxiolytic agents are utilized to a limited degree. Medical students should have knowledge of these medications, residents should have familiarity with their clinical use with adolescents, and fellows should develop confidence in utilizing these medications, with the objective of learning to integrate pharmacological treatment with other therapies. In addition, trainees at all levels should be aware that differing body maturities lead to considerable pharmacokinetic variations among patients in this age range.

Appreciation of the considerable importance of therapeutic work with parents, guardians and other family members should be expected of trainees at all levels. Residents should be expected to engage in such family contacts, while fellows should develop clinical competence in the skill of family interventions and therapies, techniques which are essential to the provision of adolescent treatment.

Group therapy is a potentially powerful and useful tool in treatment, especially in light of the common tendency of adolescents to form peer clusters. Clinical experiences can be obtained in both patient care and school settings. Medical students should have an awareness of this modality, whereas residents may get clinical exposure through observation of, or participation in, adolescent therapy groups. Fellows should have the experience of participating in, and leading new groups.

Psychiatric coordination of care in more restrictive settings usually implies a managerial approach for the handling of patients, who are treated both as individuals and as a group. The psychiatrist may be asked to provide direction for other professionals and staff involved in care of the adolescents, including nurses, social workers, psychologists, teachers, and leaders of adjunctive (e.g., recreational, art, and vocational) and social skills therapies. The composite of this care is often termed milieu treatment. Medical students should be aware of the existence of such facilities and of milieu therapy, while residents would benefit from clinical exposure to such programs. Fellows are required and expected to competently provide treatment in these milieus, and to assimilate administrative experience.

Athough the above discussion generically describes treatment interventions, specific treatment approaches are required for some distinct psychopathological syndromes. Thus, unique treatments have been devised for disturbances that most commonly emerge during adolescence, including eating disorders, substance abuse, and violent conduct disorders. Medical students and residents may have an awareness of these treatments, while fellows should have access to clinical experience with these populations.

EXPERIENCES IN SETTINGS
WHERE ADOLESCENTS ARE TREATED

Supervised experience in the programs and facilities where adolescents are treated is invaluable in developing skills in adolescent psychiatry (see Table 7). Most training programs have access to a variety of these settings but few have access to all the possibilities. Basic program experience for all levels of training include inpatient units, outpatient centers, and crisis evaluation programs. Experiences in specialized settings such as substance abuse and eating disorder programs, day hospitals, and schools and community based programs will depend on availability. Several of these settings should be

TABLE 7

Experiences in Setting Where Adolescents Are Treated	Medical Student	Resident	Fellow
Inpatient Treatment of Adolescents			
Short-Term Patients	1	3	3
Long-Term Patients	1	1	3
Substance Abuse	1	1	3
Eating Disorder	1	1	2
Day/Partial Hospital	1	1	2
Crisis	2	3	3
Outpatient Treatment			
Brief Term	1	3	3
Long Term	1	1	3
Hospital Consultation/Liaison	1	2	3
Pediatric Clinic	1	1	2
School Consultation	1	1	3
Agency Consultation	1	1	3
College Mental Health	1	2	2
Community Based Programs	1	2	3
Residential Treatment Centers	1	1	2
Group Homes	1	1	2
Detention Centers	1	1	2
Juvenile Court Clinic	1	1	2

available for resident and fellow training based on the special emphasis of the adolescent psychiatry program.

All trainees should have a general understanding of the continuum of care and the suitability of the different levels of structure and restrictiveness for the degree of disturbance exhibited by the adolescent. For the medical student this consists of a familiarity with the components of the continuum and a general understanding of the disturbances that can be treated in each setting. The resident should be able to evaluate an adolescent and make recommendations about treatment settings with the backup consultation of an adolescent psychiatrist if necessary. The fellow should be able to perform a complete evaluation of an adolescent, identify all of the important criteria necessary to make an appropriate referral to a suitable treatment setting, and be capable of performing the treatment at each level of care.

Experience on an inpatient unit where adolescents are treated should lead to a familiarity with evaluation of and criteria for admission, treatment and discharge planning, management of aggressive behavior, effective interdisciplinary team relationships and integration, appropriate involvement of families and social agencies, and principles of milieu treatment. The medical student should have an exposure to management and administrative issues, while the resident should be directly involved with these issues, and the child and adolescent psychiatry fellow should be involved in the leadership of the unit. Issues affecting length of stay such as the nature of the adolescent's psychiatric disorder, level of support in the environment, third party coverage, including Medicaid reimbursement and pressures from managed care and administration, should become part of the knowledge base of all medical trainees, with the fellow learning to effectively deal with these pressures and ethical dilemmas.

OTHER TOPICS

Certain adolescent training programs are likely to find a number of topics listed previously that they will emphasize. The topics listed on Table 8 include additional general topics important to all programs.

Administrative issues are gaining increasing importance in the success of every clinical psychiatric program for adolescents. Today, a successful program depends not only on a good clinical program but also on a sound administration. The successful clinical administrator must learn the essential principles of hospital administration both through training and experience. This includes a familiarity with and

TABLE 8

Other Topics	Medical Student	Resident	Fellow
Administrative Issues	1	3	3=
Ethical Issues	3	3	3+
Public Relations and Education	1	3	3+
Patient Advocacy	2	3	3
Court Testimony	1	2	3
Working with Other Professionals Who Work with Adolescents	2	2	3
Research Methodology	2	2	3
Medical Economics	2	2	3

understanding of current health care funding and economics including managed care, hospital policy and regulations, strategic planning, effective leadership styles, and the ability to work effectively with others in the administration of the hospital. This information is essential for residents and fellows.

Medical professionals at all levels of training must be familiar with the ethical issues and guidelines particular to adolescents. Some of the important issues include the doctor–patient relationship, confidentially, patient rights, and for whom the doctor is working (e.g., the adolescent, the parents, the insurance company, the state). Ethical guidelines such as those of the American Academy of Child and Adolescent Psychiatry should be familiar to all medical professionals working with adolescents in mental health settings. Educating adolescents, their families, and the general public about mental illness and the need for and availability of mental health services in an accurate, nonstigmatizing manner is an important skill for all health care professionals. The health care professional interested in adolescents should also possess skills in public relations including the effective use of the media. It is increasingly necessary for adolescent psychiatrists to convincingly advocate for adequate adolescent mental health care for all adolescents due to unequal funding, public misunderstanding, and the lack of preparedness of adolescents to advocate for themselves.

Adolescent psychiatrists are often called upon to testify in court regarding such issues as court commitment, competence to stand trial, the impact of mental illness on behavior, and custody. Competence as an expert witness requires developing skills seldom taught in medical training. Teaching and supervision are necessary to develop competence as an expert witness.

A variety of other professionals work with adolescents and often consult adolescent psychiatrists when they encounter mental health problems. These include pediatricians, adolescent medicine specialists, psychologists, social workers, teachers, clergy, juvenile probation officers, and state social workers. The frequency with which they seek consultation often depends on the skills of the adolescent psychiatrists to effectively collaborate with these professionals.

All medical trainees should be familiar with what constitutes good research. Medical students should know how to evaluate the validity of a study in adolescent psychiatry. The psychiatry resident should be able to evaluate the usefulness of a study in adolescent psychiatry, and the child and adolescent psychiatry fellow should be capable of identifying an issue relevant to the practice of adolescent psychiatry and of designing a research protocol to scientifically elucidate the issue. Trainees in adolescent psychiatry should be encouraged to pursue this research.

Conclusion

Evaluation of both the trainees and the educational program is essential. This includes didactics and seminars, clinical experiences, and faculty supervision. The evaluation should address the specific knowledge, skills, attitudes, and educational objectives of the program, and it should include receiving verbal and written feedback from examination and from supervision. An oral examination format similar to the board examinations is also a useful method of evaluation for medical students, residents, and fellows. Trainees should provide written feedback regarding their response to the effectiveness of the training program.

Adolescent psychiatry is an expanding field with rapid increases in knowledge and treatment modalities. Program directors must make continued efforts to keep educational programs current and relevant. Both trainees and educators are engaged in a lifelong learning process. What is most important is that trainees obtain a solid theoretical and experiential background that inspires them to continue learning.

REFERENCES

Blos, P. (1967), The second individualation process of adolescence. *The Psychoanalytic Study of the Child*, 22:162–186. New York: International Universities Press.

Bowlby, J. (1988), Developmental psychiatry comes of age. *Amer. J. Psychiat.*, 145:1–10.

Eisenberg, L. (1980), The relativity of adolescence: Effects of time, place, and person in adolescent psychiatry. *Developmental and Clinical Studies*, Vol. 7. Chicago: University of Chicago Press. pp. 25–40.

Erikson, E. (1968), Identity, *Youth and Crisis*. London: Faber.

Flaherty, L. T. (1989), A model curriculum for teaching adolescent psychiatry. *Adolescent Psychiatry*, 16:491–520.

Freud, A. (1958), Adolescence. *The Psychoanalytic Study of the Child*, 13:255–278. New York: International Universities Press.

Gilligan, C. & Murphy J. M. (1979), Development from adolescence to adulthood: The philospher and the dilemma of the fact. In: *Intellectual Beyond*, ed. D. Kuhn. San Francisco: Jossey-Bass.

Kohlberg, L. & Kramer, R. (1969), Continuities and discontinuities in childhood and adult moral development. *Human Develop.*, 12:93–120.

Looney, J. G., Ellis, W., Benedek, E. & Schowalter, J. (1985), Training in adolescent psychiatry for general psychiatry residents: Elements of a model curriculum. *Adolescent Psychiatry*, 12:94–103. Chicago: University of Chicago Press.

Masterson, J. F. (1968), The psychiatric significance of adolescent turmoil. *Amer. J. Psychiat.*, 124:1549–1554.

Offer, D. (1969), The psychological world of the teenager. New York: Basic Books.

Piaget, J. (1969), The intellectual development of the adolescent. In: *Adolescence*, ed. G. Caplan & S. Lebovici. New York: Basic Books, pp. 22–26.

Tanner, J. M. (1962), *Growth at Adolescence*. Oxford: Blackwell.

THE AUTHORS

MARIE ARMENTANO, M. D. is an Instructor in Psychiatry at Harvard Medical School.

MARY E. BAKER-SINCLAIR, PH. D. is a pediatric psychologist in practice in Chapel Hill, North Carolina.

JONATHAN COHEN, PH. D. is Adjunct Associate Professor in Psychology and Education, Doctoral Program in Clinical Psychology; and Director of The Program for Social and Emotional Learning, Teachers College, Columbia University.

DARIN DOUGHERTY, M. D. is Chief Resident in Psychopharmacology at Massachusetts General Hospital and Clinical Instructor in Psychiatry at Harvard Medical School.

LOIS T. FLAHERTY, M. D. (editor) is Clinical Associate Professor of Psychiatry, University of Pennsylvania, Philadelphia; and Adjunct Associate Professor at the University of Maryland, Baltimore.

BENJAMIN GARBER, M. D. is a Training and Supervising Analyst, Chicago Institute for Psychoanalysis, and Director, Barr-Harris Center for the Study of Separation and Loss in Childhood.

BARONESS GHISLAINE D. GODENNE, M. D. is Director Emerita, Counseling and Psychiatric Services; and Professor of Psychiatry, Pediatrics, and Mental Hygiene, Johns Hopkins University.

SIMEON GRATER, M. D. is Assistant Professor of Family Practice and Psychiatry, Southern Illinois University School of Medicine.

MARTIN HARROW, PH. D. is Professor and Director of Psychology in the Department of Psychiatry, University of Illinois College of Medicine. He is a widely cited expert on schizophrenia and has published more than 200 scientific papers in this and related areas.

ROBERT HENDREN, D. O. is Professor and Director, Division of Child and Adolescent Psychiatry, University of Medicine and Dentistry of New Jersey-Robert Wood Johnson Medical School, Piscataway.

HARVEY HOROWITZ, M. D. (editor) is Clinical Associate Professor of Psychiatry, University of Pennsylvania School of Medicine, Philadelphia; and is a Past President of the American Society for Adolescent Psychiatry.

CHARLES M. JAFFE, M. D. is Assistant Professor of Psychiatry, Rush Medical College, Chicago; and Faculty, Chicago Institute for Psychoanalysis.

THOMAS JOBE, M. D. is Associate Professor of Psychiatry and Associate Director of the Division of Neuropsychiatry in the Department of Psychiatry, University of Illinois at Chicago. He has published in the area of brain models of schizophrenia.

MICHAEL G. KALOGERAKIS, M. D. is Clinical Professor of Psychiatry, New York University School of Medicine; and President of the International Society for Adolescent Psychiatry.

PHILIP KATZ, M. D., F. R. C. C. is Professor of Psychiatry, University of Manitoba (Winnipeg) and is a Past President of the American Society for Adolescent Psychiatry.

GUSTAVO A. LAGE, M. D. is a Past President, American Society for Adolescent Psychiatry, and is a psychoanalyst in private practice in Paradise Valley, Arizona.

RICHARD C. MAROHN, M. D. (deceased), Editor in Chief of Volume 20 of Adolescent Psychiatry, was Professor of Clinical Psychiatry, Northwestern University Medical School, and Faculty, Institute for Psychoanalysis Chicago.

THE AUTHORS

EDWIN J. MIKKELSON, M. D. is Associate Professor of Psychiatry, Harvard Medical School.

ELIZABETH PERL, PH. D. is Assistant Professor, Department of Psychiatry and Behavioral Sciences, Northwestern University Medical School; and Director, Extended Partial Hospitalization Program, Northwestern Memorial Hospital, Chicago.

LINDA M. PEROSA, PH. D. is Assistant Professor, Department of Physical Activity and Educational Services, The Ohio State University, Columbus.

SANDRA L. PEROSA, PH. D. is Associate Professor, Department of Counseling and Special Education, University of Akron, Ohio.

LYNN E. PONTON, M. D. is Professor of Child and Adolescent Psychiatry, University of California, San Francisco, and author of *The Romance of Risk.*

JOHN PORT, PH. D., M. D. is involved in functional brain imaging in the Department of Radiology at Johns Hopkins University School of Medicine; and has published in the area of electrophysiology of the thalamus.

RICHARD ROSNER, M. D. is Clinical Professor, Department of Psychiatry, New York University School of Medicine; and Medical Director, Forensic Psychiatry Clinic, Bellevue Hospital Center, New York City.

RICHARD M. SARLES, M. D. is Professor and Director, Division of Child and Adolescent Psychiatry, University of Maryland School of Medicine, Baltimore; and is a Past President of the American Society for Adolescent Psychiatry.

ROBERT SIMONS, PH. D. is Professor, Department of Psychology, University of Delaware, Newark.

ADRIAN N. SONDHEIMER, M. D. is Associate Professor of Clinical Psychiatry, University of Medicine and Dentistry of New Jersey, New Jersey Medical Center, Piscataway.

MAX SUGAR, M. D. is Clinical Professor of Psychiatry, Louisiana State University Medical Center and Tulane University Medical Center, New Orleans; a Past President of the American Society for Adolescent Psychiatry, he is the Editor of *Monographs of the International Society for Adolescent Psychiatry.*

PAUL V. TRAD, M. D. (deceased) was Associate Professor of Clinical Psychiatry and Director, Child and Adolescent Outpatient Department, The New York Hospital-Cornell Medical Center. He was also Editor-in Chief, *The American Journal of Psychotherapy.*

CLAUDE VILLENEUVE, M. D. is Coordinator, Family Therapy Unit, Allen Memorial Institute, and Assistant Professor of Psychiatry, McGill University and Université de Montréal.

BETH S. WARNER, PH. D. is Assistant Professor and Associate Director of the School Mental Health Program (SMHP), Department of Psychiatry, University of Maryland.

STEVEN M. WEINE, M. D. is Assistant Professor of Psychiatry, College of Medicine, University of Illinois at Chicago.

MARK D. WEIST, PH. D. is an Assistant Professor and Director of the School Mental Health Program (SMHP), Department of Psychiatry, University of Maryland.

CONTENTS OF VOLUMES 1–20

INDEX